Exercise Physiology

Exercise Physiology

A Thematic Approach

Tudor Hale
University College Chichester, UK

WILEY

This publication is designed to provide accurate and authoritative information in regard to
the subject matter covered. It is sold on the understanding that the Publisher is not engaged
in rendering professional services. If professional advice or other expert assistance is
required, the services of a competent professional should be sought.

Other Wiley Editorial Offices

John Wiley & Sons Inc., 111 River Street, Hoboken, NJ 07030, USA

Jossey-Bass, 989 Market Street, San Francisco, CA 94103-1741, USA

Wiley-VCH Verlag GmbH, Boschstr. 12, D-69469 Weinheim, Germany

John Wiley & Sons Australia Ltd, 33 Park Road, Milton, Queensland 4064, Australia

John Wiley & Sons (Asia) Pte Ltd, 2 Clementi Loop #02-01, Jin Xing Distripark, Singapore
129809

John Wiley & Sons Canada Ltd, 22 Worcester Road, Etobicoke, Ontario, Canada
M9W 1L1

Wiley also publishes its books in a variety of electronic formats. Some content that appears
in print may not be available in electronic books.

British Library Cataloguing in Publication Data

A catalogue record for this book is available from the British Library

ISBN 0 470 84682 8 (cloth)
ISBN 0 470 84683 6 (paper)

To my wife, Nan, for her love and steadfastness, to Nicola, Tim and Gavin for their unconditional love, and to our beautiful grand-children, Kimberley, Eleanor, Tamsin, Lucy, Megan, Jonathan and Cameron, for the joy they bring every day –

and to my parents

Mary Ceridwen Hale (1914–1950)

Samuel Thomas Hale (1910–1977)

without whom none of this would have been possible.

Contents

Series Preface

One of the most astonishing cultural phenomena of the twentieth century has been the exponential growth in our knowledge and understanding of the importance of sport and exercise to humankind. At the beginning of that century, sport was principally a force for moral development, whilst strenuous exercise, though necessary to ensure military personnel were fit to engage in combat, was medically proscribed. The academic study of sport – what there was of it – was restricted largely to the history of the Olympic Games and philosophical arguments for the moral case for team games. A hundred years later, the picture is very different. Four hundred million people turn on their television sets to watch the Opening Ceremony of the Olympic Games and soccer's World Cup Final; millions of people jog, go to the gym, or work out in front of the television; and the academic study of sport embraces physics, chemistry, biology, biomechanics, physiology, psychology, politics, sociology, social anthropology and business studies, as well as history and philosophy. Over the last twenty years the number of degree courses in the academic study of sport and exercise has grown phenomenally, attracting students from a wide range of backgrounds. It is against this background that the new series *Wiley SportTexts* was conceived.

This new series provides a collection of textbooks in Sport and Exercise Science that is rooted in the student's practical experience of sport. Each book covers the theoretical foundations of the contributing disciplines from the natural, human, behavioural, and social sciences, and provides the theoretical, practical and conceptual tools needed for the rigorous academic study of sport. Individual texts focus on a specific learning stage from the various levels of undergraduate to postgraduate study.

The series adopts a student-centred, interactive, problem-solving approach to key issues, and encourages the student to develop autonomous learning strategies through self-assessment exercises. Each chapter begins with clear learning objectives and a concise summary of the key concepts covered. A glossary of important terms and symbols familiarizes students with the language and conventions of the various academic communities studying sport. Worked examples and solutions to exercises, together with a variety of formative and summative self-assessment tasks, are also included, supported by key references in book, journal and electronic forms. The series will also have a dedicated web site with specific information on individual titles, supplementary information for lecturers, important developments in the academic study of sport, and links to other sites of interest.

It is intended that the series will eventually provide a complete coverage of the mainstream elements of taught undergraduate and postgraduate degrees in the study of sport.

Tudor Hale, Jim Parry and **Roger Bartlett**
April 2003

Acknowledgements

It is not possible to write a book like this without the help of others. The major source of inspiration for my interest in exercise physiology is Professor Rainer Goldsmith, who not only taught me about maximal oxygen uptake but also how to write. The late Dr Ernest Hamley supervised my masters degree at Loughborough, and the late Professor Gordon Cumming made the facilities of the Midhurst Medical Research Institute available for my doctoral studies. The former gave me a sound grounding in human biology, the latter, with his colleague Dr Keith Horsfield, told me more about the lung than I knew existed. Two heads of departments, Henry Uren at Aberdeen and Dennis Drinkwater at Bishop Otter College, and three College Principals, Gordon McGregor, John Wyatt and Philip Robinson at Chichester, gave practical and psychological support and encouragement throughout my career in higher education. I enjoyed the benefits of very good colleagues and undergraduates over 30 years spent at Chichester. My postgraduate students almost certainly taught me more than I taught them.

During the gestation of the book, I re-learned much of what I thought I knew. Most of this occurred through existing published material in book or journal form, but some came out of the aether via the Internet; the main sources are listed under 'Further reading'. My thanks go to the librarians at University College Chichester who have continued to provide their customary speedy and efficient services. However, it is impossible to acknowledge the unconscious use of the material in the public domain that has been absorbed over 30 years of teaching.

Alan Rees (Portsmouth), John Sproule (Edinburgh), Rob James (Coventry), and Simon Northcott (Chichester) read every chapter and made very useful suggestions for improving the material. David Bishop (Western Australia) provided similar service, from reading Chapters 2 and 9, and my long-time colleague and good friend Craig Sharp tidied up my efforts at a glossary of terms. None of the above is responsible for the errors that remain.

Andy Slade of Wiley gave sage advice at the outset of the project and at intervals thereafter. Celia Carden, Wiley's Development Editor, led me calmly through the intricacies of the publishing world, always offered sound advice, and maintained a good sense of humour and determined cheerfulness at all times. Special thanks go to Robert Hambrook for his skill at turning my illustrations into intelligible material. Finally, I have had the renewed pleasure of the company and good sense of my friends and Series Co-editors Roger Bartlett and Jim Parry.

                                                          Tudor Hale

Prologue

Introduction

Molecular oxygen is a diatomic, colourless, odourless gas. Discovered independently in 1772 by an English cleric, Joseph Priestley, and a Swedish chemist, Karl Scheele, but given its name in 1777 by the French chemist, Antoine Lavoisier, it is vital for human life. We can survive for weeks on a diet of bread and water, and for several days without water, providing we keep still and in the shade. But, without oxygen, we can survive for minutes only before irreversible brain damage and then death occurs. Molecular oxygen is essential because it is necessary for the production of a high-energy compound – adenosine triphosphate (ATP) – that drives all of our cellular activity. However, our stores of oxygen and adenosine triphosphate are very limited, so we need physiological mechanisms to provide both continuously.

At rest, our oxygen demands are quite modest – depending on our size and body composition, we consume about a quarter of a litre of oxygen each minute. During exercise, the position changes dramatically, and the oxygen needed to maintain sufficient adenosine triphosphate increases as much as twentyfold. Our early ancestors evolved a three-stage energy-producing system that ensured their survival. It enabled them to gather fruits, hunt for meat, and escape from predators; it also enables us to engage in a range of sport and exercise activities.

The first stage provides an initial burst of maximum speed, allowing them a quick dash to the nearest tree or cave. The same process enables some of us – Carl Lewis, Linford Christie, Dwain Chambers and Tim Montgomery for example – to run a 100 metres in under 10 seconds. The second stage gives a

Exercise Physiology: A Thematic Approach   Tudor Hale
© John Wiley & Sons, Ltd   ISBN: 0 470 84682 8 (cloth), ISBN 0 470 84683 6 (pbk)

slightly better chance of survival by providing energy for a sustained burst of speed over about a quarter of a mile. This process allowed two of us – Butch Reynolds and Michael Johnston – to run the 400-metres in less than 43.3 seconds. The third stage was necessary for the hunt with bows and curare-tipped arrows. When hit, the prey runs off, but dies slowly and quietly through progressive muscle paralysis. The hunter jogs after the animal until it collapses, kills it and gathers its meat. The chase requires large amounts of oxygen. It enables some of us – Steve Ovett, Seb Coe and Steve Cram – to run a mile (1.609 km) in well under 4 minutes, and Paula Radcliffe to run more than 26 miles (42.195 km) faster then most men.

The most interesting feature of the first two stages is the fact that we can achieve such high speeds without using very much oxygen during the actual events. In the 100-m, we use another high-energy compound called creatine phosphate (CrP) to maintain the adenosine triphosphate (ATP) availability needed for muscle contraction. In the 400-m, the process requires the break-down – technically called catabolism – of glucose to deliver a limited supply of adenosine triphosphate and producing lactic acid. The process that allows these astonishing achievements without oxygen is *anaerobic* metabolism. The third, oxygen-dependent, stage of the system is *aerobic* metabolism. It underpins all of our everyday activities – working, sleeping, playing, eating, thinking and exercising, and breaks down carbohydrate (glycogen) and fat (lipids) into carbon dioxide and water.

Maximal oxygen uptake

Maximal oxygen uptake ($\dot{V}_{O_2max}$) describes our ability to transport and consume the greatest amount of oxygen breathing air at sea level. A laboratory-based maximal oxygen uptake test is a measure of our cardiovascular, respira-tory, and skeletal muscle biochemical capabilities and is a feature of almost all sport and exercise science courses. During maximal exercise the average sport and exercise science student consumes between three and four litres of oxygen a minute, or about 45 to 55 millilitres for each kilogram of body mass. An elite endurance athlete doubles this to around six litres of oxygen each minute, roughly 24 times resting oxygen consumption. The process allows some of us to run 1500 m in under 3.5 min, and a marathon in just over 2 hours at an average speed of nearly 21 km $\cdot$ hr^{-1} (12 mi $\cdot$ hr^{-1}). At the other end of the scale, patients with heart or lung disease struggle to reach symptom-limited oxygen uptake values of 1–1.5 litres of oxygen per minute. The need to understand the physiological processes that take oxygen from the atmosphere to the muscle cell is a key feature of all exercise physiology texts and provides the central theme for this book. There are innumerable ways of doing this, but in this book we shall be using a fairly simple equation – the Fick equation for oxygen – as the framework around which to introduce key physiological processes that underpin much of sport and exercise physiology.

The Fick equation

In 1870, a German physiologist, Adolf Fick, was interested in measuring cardiac output – the amount of blood pumped out of the heart in one minute. This is what he said to one of his contemporaries.

> *It is astonishing that no one has arrived at the following method by which it [the measurement of cardiac output] may be determined, at least in animals. One measures how much oxygen an animal absorbs from air in a given time, and how much carbon dioxide it gives off. During the experiment one obtains a sample of arterial and venous blood; in both the oxygen and carbon dioxide content are measured. The difference in oxygen content tells us how much oxygen each cubic centimetre of blood takes up in its passage through the lungs. As one knows the total quantity of oxygen absorbed in a given time one can calculate how many cubic centimetres of blood passed through the lungs in this time.*

Put more simply, Fick was saying: 'Cardiac output ($\dot{Q}_C$) is oxygen consumption ($\dot{V}_{O_2}$) divided by the difference in the oxygen content (C_{O_2}) of arterial and mixed venous blood (a-$\bar{v}$)' – i.e.

$$\dot{Q}_C = \frac{\dot{V}_{O_2}}{C_{a-\bar{v}O_2}}$$

However, Fick's idea was ahead of its time. The process he described in 1870 was not testable on humans because no one had invented the methods for sampling mixed venous and arterial blood. Consequently, it took another 60 years, when arterial catheters were developed and arterial blood sampling became possible, to confirm his prediction. In 1956 Verner Forssman, Andre Cournand and Dickson W. Richards received a Nobel Prize for developing the technique.

Now, it doesn't take much to rearrange the Fick principle to read: 'Oxygen uptake equals cardiac output multiplied by the difference in oxygen content of arterial and mixed venous blood' – i.e.

$$\dot{V}_{O_2} = \dot{Q}_C \cdot C_{a\text{-}\bar{v}O_2}$$

This simple equation, the Fick equation for oxygen, provides us with a framework for investigating the physiology that underpins maximal oxygen uptake. However, to understand the logical chain of events that governs oxygen uptake, we need to re-arrange the equation and consider the *sequential* order of the physiological mechanisms involved. The logic behind this rearrangement is quite straightforward. We breathe in oxygen molecules from the atmosphere which then combine with the blood passing through the lungs to give us oxygenated blood – so first we consider the oxygen content of arterial blood (C_{aO_2}). The heart then pumps this oxygenated blood around the body to the cells; this is our whole body flow ($\dot{Q}_C$) or cardiac output. The oxygen delivered to the muscle cells enables them to contract and us to exercise in a variety of ways and at different speeds. These cells extract oxygen from the blood as it passes through the capillaries of muscle groups. The aerobic breakdown of glycogen and fats consumes oxygen and produces carbon dioxide and water, and the oxygen content of the venous blood ($C_{\bar{v}O_2}$) falls. The oxygen content of this systemic venous blood tells us how effective the muscle cells are at oxygen extraction. The venous blood returns to the right side of the heart and then the lungs where the carbon dioxide produced from the breakdown of glucose and fats is excreted and oxygen picked up to start the whole process again. This sequential approach to understanding the physiology of maximal oxygen uptake provides the general structure of this book.

At this point it is important to say that what is set out in this book is a summary of what we *think* we know about the cascade of oxygen from atmosphere to muscle cell. However, all scientific knowledge is *provisional*, and what we now think of as facts may well turn out to be false in the future. This is how science has progressed from the fifteenth century. It was then that Nicolaus Copernicus, a Polish priest, astronomer and doctor, first showed that the earth travelled around the sun, thus refuting the second century geocentric universe theory of Egyptian astronomer and geographer, Ptolemy. So, do not be lulled into thinking that we are dealing with irrefutable facts; even Einstein thought that some of his findings could not be true.

Equally important are the findings from research into learning strategies. These indicate that if the sole strategy is simply *reading* the text, learners retain only about 10 per cent of the information. *Discussion* improves retention to about 50 per cent; but the greatest retention level occurs when *explaining* what you have learned to others. Experience shows that students learn a great deal by talking to tutors, even more from their postgraduate peers, and most by working in small friendship groups by talking through difficulties and discussing possible solutions.

General structure of the book

Each chapter begins with a list of things you should be able to do if you

(a) read the chapter carefully,

(b) attempt the exercises and questions, and

(c) clear away any uncertainties by discussion amongst your peers or with your tutors.

An objective test follows to assess your current level of knowledge. Attempt these tests before reading the subsequent chapter; photocopy the page and file the answers in your notes. After all, if you know most of the answers you may wish to skip that particular chapter. Thirty-three per cent or more 'Don't know' responses suggest that the chapter should form part of further private study.

The exercises and questions within the text have been designed to achieve two things. First, they reinforce the material; second, they provide a respite from the periods of intense concentration needed for careful reading. Research shows that learning is most effective in short bursts, interspersed with rest periods of a few minutes, or a change of activity. If you are not sure of the answer, read on a little further and come back to the question. The answers to the exercises and questions, with explanations, are at the end of the each chapter. Don't look at the answers until you have finished the chapter.

Before moving on to the next chapter, take the objective test again to monitor your progress. You can check your answers from the lists provided at the end of the book, but you will only get 'right' or 'wrong' responses here. You will find additional information on the *Wiley SportTexts series* website. A success rate of less than 40 per cent – i.e. a fail grade in most institutions – suggests that you have not understood the material sufficiently. This has two consequences: the first is failure in examinations, and the second is that you may find subsequent material difficult to grasp. The least you should do is seek tutorial advice. A success rate of 50–55 per cent is adequate, but only just; more than 65 per cent augurs well for the future. If you file your answers, they can act as a useful reminder of the areas where additional revision is necessary around examination time.

Each chapter also includes a list of the symbols and abbreviations in current use in journal articles and textbooks. Become comfortable with them, and use them whenever you can in your written work – it saves time and paper, and confirms to your tutors that you are becoming familiar with the everyday conventions of exercise physiology. It is important to recognize that the dots over volume data $(\dot{V})$ carry precise information – namely, that time, usually minutes, is involved; any symbol carrying a bar above it $(\bar{v})$ indicates that the figure is a mean (average) value.

Some material – abbreviations, symbols and units for example – appears in several places in the text. This is deliberate. Firstly, repetition in itself is a good learning strategy; secondly putting material into slightly different contexts can aid understanding; thirdly, repetition helps those who only read selected chapters rather than the whole book. At the end of each chapter, a short summary acts as a quick revision aid.

Chapter 1 introduces an important piece of practical work that underpins the rest of the book, namely the maximal oxygen uptake test. All sport and exercise science courses use this laboratory practical to introduce the concept of the oxygen cascade and to give students some experience of collecting and analysing raw data. Chapters 2 to 9 cover sequentially the specific physiological systems involved in oxygen delivery and consumption. The chapters are built around the concept of levels. Each one contains typical data that might be recorded during one of your practical sessions; this is an attempt to link practice and theory, a link too often ignored by many students. Try not to treat lectures and practical laboratory exercises as separate entities. Study the data carefully, and see how they fit in with the lectures. After the practical examples, there is a basic outline of the physiological mechanisms at work during a particular part of the oxygen uptake chain; this aims to provide a foundational account of the information needed to pass the course. A fuller account follows giving more detailed information on the theoretical underpinning of the mechanisms at work; if the theories are understood and applied appropriately to examination questions, laboratory reports and assessed coursework assignments, higher grades should result.

The final two chapters (10 and 11) are slightly different and take the form of coursework essays that try to critically evaluate current theories on particular topics. They deal with two important issues that are likely to confront sport and exercise science students during their study of exercise physiology. The first examines the factors likely to limit maximal oxygen uptake, a topic that has been the subject of debate, sometimes heated, since the 1920s. Understanding of such physiological limitations is important in grasping the fundamentals of exercise physiology.

The second deals with the complex relationships between exercise, fitness and health. This topic has become the concern in many of the rich, industrialized countries worried about the cost of diseases of affluent societies, where the physical labour that once fuelled the industrial revolution of the nineteenth century has all but disappeared. No sport and exercise science student can ignore these issues and claim to be adequately educated.

The four appendices contain supplementary material that may help knowledge and understanding. The first offers suggestions for additional reading material that can be found in encyclopaedias, key textbooks, journal articles and websites. Two words of caution are necessary here. The first relates to the referencing of material, and the second to the use of websites.

The Editors of the *Wiley SportTexts series* made a conscious decision to place all reference material at the end of the book rather than within the text or at the end of each chapter. The decision was taken to facilitate ease of reading and to maintain the continuity of the text and flow of ideas. *However, this is not conventional academic practice and students should not follow this example in their written work. Each sport and exercise department will have specific guidelines for referencing written work. Students would be foolish to ignore these guidelines.*

Web sites can provide some very interesting and useful material, not only in the form of text but with diagrams and animations. However, the quality is very variable ranging from the very basic to PhD level and users should be selective in what they choose to use. *Whatever that is, be sure you acknowledge the source of the material.*

The second appendix provides a glossary that may help clarify some of the technical terms used. The third gives the roots of some of the words we use, and demonstrates how much we owe to the Greeks and Romans for our present-day language. These roots may help in understanding and memory. Finally, there is the appendix containing the answers to the objective tests.

1 The Maximal Oxygen Uptake Test

Learning Objectives

By the end of this chapter, you should be able to

- distinguish between aerobic and anaerobic metabolism

- define maximal oxygen uptake

- give the Fick equation for maximal oxygen uptake

- outline the procedures entailed in the indirect calculation of oxygen uptake

- list the physiological characteristics indicating the achievement of maximal oxygen uptake

- describe the safety procedures to be undertaken before a maximal oxygen uptake test

- explain the differences between discontinuous and continuous exercise test protocols

- describe three commonly used ergometers along with their strengths and weaknesses

- outline the calibration procedures for gas analysers and gas meters

- calculate values for oxygen uptake, carbon dioxide excretion and the respiratory exchange ratio

Exercise Physiology: A Thematic Approach   Tudor Hale
© John Wiley & Sons, Ltd   ISBN: 0 470 84682 8 (cloth), ISBN 0 470 84683 6 (pbk)

Objective test

Say whether the following answers are true (T) or false (F). If you do not know, say so (D) – not knowing is not an academic crime, but not finding out is. Try not to look at the answers until you have worked your way through the chapter and completed the test a second time. In this way, you can monitor your progress.

	Pre-test			Post-test		
	T	F	D	T	F	D
1. A. V. Hill first reported the O_2 plateau during maximal exercise						
2. $\dot{V}_{O_2max}$ is defined as a plateau in an O_2 uptake–power graph						
3. $\dot{V}_{O_2max}$ is the greatest $\dot{V}_{O_2}$ consumed breathing air at altitude						
4. Aerobic exercise requires increased oxygen consumption						
5. The $\dot{V}_{O_2max}$ test is the best measure of anaerobic performance						
6. Large quantities of oxygen are consumed during the 100-m						
7. At rest about 0.25 L of oxygen is consumed each minute						
8. Elite endurance athletes have reached $\dot{V}_{O_2max}$ of $6\ L \cdot min^{-1}$						
9. The Fick equation for oxygen is $\dot{V}_{O_2} = \dot{Q} \cdot C_{a-\bar{v}_{O_2}}$						
10. The indirect calculation of $\dot{V}_{O_2}$ requires $\dot{V}_I$ measurement						
11. Pure inspired air contains 3% CO_2						
12. Expired air contains 20.93% O_2						
13. Calculation of $\dot{V}_{O_2}$ assumes that nitrogen is metabolically inert						

	Pre-test			Post-test		
	T	F	D	T	F	D
14. Various forms of ergometer can regulate exercise intensity						
15. A set of steps, and a treadmill can be used to measure power output						
16. An infrared gas analyser measures the O_2 fraction in expired air						
17. A paramagnetic analyser measures the CO_2 fraction in expired air						
18. 'White spot' N_2 sets the baselines of both O_2 and CO_2 analysers						
19. Fresh air is used to set the upper limits of the CO_2 analyser						
20. 15% O_2–5% CO_2 in N_2 is used to check analyser accuracy						
21. Expired air is measured by a dry gas meter						
22. Inspired and expired air volumes are always the same						
23. The volume of O_2 consumed $= \dot{V}_{O_2}$ inspired $+ \dot{V}_{O_2}$ expired						
24. $\dot{V}_{O_2} = \dot{V}_E \cdot \{[(1 - F_{EO_2} - F_{ECO_2}) \cdot 0.265] - F_{EO_2}\}$						
25. $\dot{V}_{CO_2} = \dot{V}_E \cdot (F_{ECO_2} - 0.0003)$						
26. $\dot{V}_{CO_2}/\dot{V}_{O_2}$ is called the respiratory exchange ratio (RER)						
27. RER is affected by the energy source – fat or carbohydrate – used						
28. RER is always <1						
29. Maximum heart rates can be estimated from 220 + subject's age						
30. A 20–50 mL blood sample is needed for lactate analysis						

Symbols, abbreviations and units of measurement

ambient pressure	P_{amb}	Pa; kPa; mmHg
arterio-venous	a-v	
barometer, barometric	B	
barometric pressure	P_B	Pa; kPa; mmHg
breathing rate, respiratory frequency	f_R	$br \cdot min^{-1}$
carbon dioxide fraction	F_{CO_2}	
cardiac output/whole body blood flow	$\dot{Q}_C$	$L \cdot min^{-1}$
expiratory	E; exp	
frequency	f	min^{-1}; s^{-1}
gas fraction	F_{GAS}	
gas fraction expired	F_{EGAS}	
gas fraction inspired	F_{IGAS}	
heart rate, cardiac frequency	f_C	$bt \cdot min^{-1}$
inspiratory	I; insp	
kilogram	kg	
lactate concentration of blood	$[La_{bl}]$	mM; $mmol \cdot L^{-1}$
litre	L	
mass	m	kg
maximum	max	
maximum oxygen uptake	$\dot{V}_{O_2max}$	$L \cdot min^{-1}$
oxygen fraction	F_{O_2}	
pascal; kilopascal	Pa; kPa	
pressure	P	Pa; kPa; mmHg
standard temperature and pressure dry	STPD	0°C; 101.1 kPa; 760 mmHg
volume	V	L
volume of gas flow in unit time	$\dot{V}$	$L \cdot min^{-1}$
volume expired in unit time	$\dot{V}_E$	$L \cdot min^{-1}$
volume inspired in unit time	$\dot{V}_I$	$L \cdot min^{-1}$
venous	v	
venous (mixed)	$\overline{v}$	

Introduction

With modern equipment and techniques, it is quite possible to calculate oxygen consumption in the way Fick described, i.e.

$$\dot{V}_{O_2max} = \dot{Q}_{Cmax} \cdot C_{a\text{-}\bar{v}O_2max}$$

It occurs routinely in certain medical investigations requiring cardio-respiratory information. However, it is an invasive process and entirely unsuitable for the everyday testing of athletes and sport and exercise science students. This is especially so when we can obtain a perfectly good estimate from analysing the gases in the breath we exhale. If we do this whilst undertaking progressive exercise, we get a relationship that looks like that shown in Figure 1.1. This indirect calculation of oxygen consumption merely requires a note of

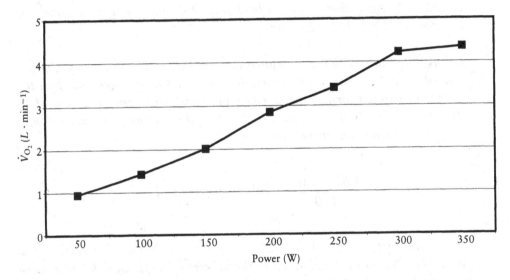

Figure 1.1 A schematic representation of the systematic increase in oxygen uptake as exercise intensity increases until the point at which no further increase in oxygen uptake occurs in spite of an increase in exercise demand

(a) the prevailing barometric pressure (P_B), and ambient temperature;

(b) a collection of expired gas and a record of the fractions of oxygen and carbon dioxide in it;

(c) a note of its volume and temperature.

It is not clear who first discovered the method, but it appears that someone measured oxygen consumption in some form even earlier than 1888.

Question 1.1   *How do we know this?*

An English physiologist, John Scott Haldane, is widely credited with devising the method for calculating oxygen consumption from expired air only, and it has carried his name – the Haldane Transformation – ever since. This is how he described the process in 1912 in his book, *Methods of Air Analysis.*

Let us suppose, for instance, that the volume of air expired in exactly ten minutes was 70.4 litres, and that the temperature of the gas meter was 18.5°, and the barometric pressure 748 millimetres. From the table the factor for correction [given earlier] is evidently about 0.902, and the reduced volume is therefore 70.4 × 0.902 = 63.5 litres.

Let us now suppose that the inspired air was pure, and contained 20.93 per cent of oxygen, 0.03 of carbon dioxide, and 79.04 of nitrogen; and that the sample of expired air contained 16.41 per cent of oxygen, 3.62 of carbon dioxide, and 79.97 of nitrogen. It is clear that the volume (at 0° and 760 mm dry) of carbon dioxide given off was

$$\frac{3.62 - 0.03}{100} \times 63.5 = 2.280 \ litres.$$

The volume of oxygen absorbed is less easy to calculate, however, as the volume of dry air has diminished in the process of respiration, because more oxygen has been taken up than carbon dioxide has been given off. Since nitrogen is neither taken up nor given off in respiration it is evident that for every 100 volumes of air there corresponded in the air not 20.93 volumes of oxygen but

$$20.93 - \frac{79.97}{79.04} = 21.18 \ volumes.$$

Hence the oxygen which disappeared was

$$\frac{21.18 - 16.41}{100} \times 63.5 = 3.029 \; litres;$$

and the respiratory quotient was 2.280/3.029 = 0.753.

However, it is uncertain whether Haldane thought of this method independently in 1912, or whether he knew of it from the work of two German physiologists, J. Geppert and N. Zuntz, who, 24 years earlier, had reported it as follows.

The content of oxygen in expired air does not say how much oxygen has disappeared from inspired air, because the quantity of expired air is not the same as inspired air when both gases are thought to be free of water. Normally the volume of expired air will be smaller because more oxygen is used than carbon dioxide acid is given off. Only the amount of nitrogen remains unchanged. We can, under the assumption of a constant relation between oxygen and nitrogen in atmospheric air, calculate the amount of inspired oxygen from the nitrogen of the expired air. We just have to multiply the latter by the constant 20.93/79.07.

Although Haldane's description is easier to follow, scientific convention indicates that the least we must do is to describe the method as the Geppert–Zuntz–Haldane (GZH) Transformation. However, Haldane invented a very precise chemical method of analysing the oxygen and carbon dioxide fractions in expired air, and his work has been a critical factor in developing our understanding of oxygen consumption at rest and during exercise.

Using the Haldane gas analyser and the GZH Transformation, an English physiologist, Archibald Hill, examined the effects of exercise on oxygen consumption. In a series of experiments on himself and other colleagues in the 1920s, he measured the amount of oxygen consumed during running around a grass track at different speeds. The concept that underpinned the experiments was very imaginative, but by today's standards the process was rather crude. The subjects ran with a wooden, A-shaped frame tied to their back. Attached to this frame was a tube connecting a one-way mouthpiece to a large rubberized canvas bag – called the Douglas bag after one of Hill's colleagues – that was used to collect the runners' expired air. The subjects ran at a constant speed for about five minutes and the expired air collection occurred during the last minute. Hill analysed the contents of the bag for oxygen and carbon dioxide concentrations, and measured the total volume of the expired gas in the bag. He repeated the process on separate occasions at higher speeds until the subjects were unable to run any faster.

On the basis of these data, Hill and his colleagues claimed that oxygen uptake increased with increasing speed up to a point at which, no matter how much faster the subject was able to run, oxygen uptake did not increase any further. He showed this phenomenon quite clearly in one of his subjects (Subject J), a particularly skilled runner who was able to run faster than any other subject. This gave rise to the term 'the oxygen plateau', which is still regarded as the main criterion for determining an individual's maximal oxygen uptake ($\dot{V}_{O_2max}$) by most practising exercise physiologists. However, there are also other physiological indicators including maximum heart rates, the respiratory exchange ratio, and the level of lactic acid in the blood. Often, in the absence of the plateau, we use these second-level indicators to determine the maximal level. Some people would argue that this is an unjustified step and that the term 'peak oxygen uptake' is the more appropriate term to use.

If we repeat Hill's intermittent exercise experiment and plot oxygen uptake against running speed the outcome is the classical graph as shown in Figure 1.2. Oxygen uptake rises linearly with growing oxygen demand until the final increase in speed results in a levelling off in oxygen consumption. An immediate question that arises is 'What is the energy source for completing that final increment in exercise intensity?' The obvious answer is that subjects complete the final stage with the aid of supplementary anaerobic breakdown of glucose

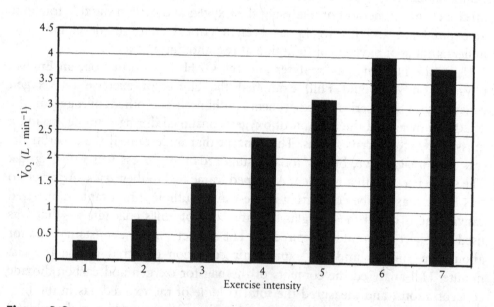

Figure 1.2 A typical A. V. Hill graph obtained from a discontinuous progressive exercise test

to lactic acid. High levels of blood lactate recorded after a maximal test support this view.

Intuitively, that explanation seems to make some kind of sense. Several chemical reactions follow a similar pattern. Our own experience of running at maximum effort shows speed increasing up to our maximum rate, being maintained for a time before the effects of fatigue become too great and we stop. So for now, the notion of a plateau in oxygen uptake at maximal levels is a useful starting point for trying to understand the processes involved in oxygen consumption when we exercise. However, not everyone believes that this classical graph gives an entirely satisfactory picture of what really happens, and that is an issue we will return to in which Chapter 10 deals with factors limiting oxygen uptake.

Collecting data

The most effective way of starting to understand the physiology underpinning maximal oxygen uptake is to take part in a laboratory test to measure it in two roles – as a subject, and then as a data recorder. The procedures are now routine and relatively easy to perform, but if the test is to be useful, it must be done very carefully and with as much precision as possible.

Informed consent

There is an ethical, and perhaps even legal, obligation to take every precaution to ensure the safety and well-being of every subject. Thus, the most important pieces of preliminary information required of subjects are their willingness to undertake the test, and their state of health. The test procedures need to be explained carefully and fully so that the subjects are in no doubt about what is going to happen to them and can give their informed consent. This means that they fully understand the kinds of discomforts they are likely to experience in a test to exhaustion, and that they can withdraw from the test at any time. After signing an informed consent form, subjects complete a health questionnaire. This attempts to identify three main things: the likelihood of exercise-induced asthma; the familial risks of cardiovascular insufficiency, particularly important in older subjects prone to erratic heart rhythms; and that subjects are not suffering from the presence, or after-effects, of musculo-skeletal problems, colds, influenza or viral infections which may affect their ability to perform the test safely.

Preliminary measures

In a reasonably equipped laboratory, there are devices for assessing the blood profile of the subjects, and monitoring their lung function. The former measures the ratio of the solids to fluids, and counts of the number of white cells present in the sample. High white cell counts may indicate infection. The number of red blood cells is recorded and the amount of haemoglobin present; low levels may indicate anaemia. The latter focuses particularly on the subject's ability to move large quantities of air into and out of the lungs quickly. If any of these measures are abnormal, the test should not proceed. We routinely measure the subject's height and body mass; a stadiometer and a set of calibrated scales are standard pieces of equipment. We attach a heart rate monitor to the subject's chest.

It is important to maintain constant laboratory conditions. A laboratory lacking air-conditioning needs industrial fans to help prevent the subjects becoming over-heated during the test. It is necessary to record temperature, pressure and relative humidity regularly. A room thermometer, a barometer with a vernier scale, and a whirling hygrometer to record wet and dry-bulb temperatures are required.

Question 1.2   *Why do we need to record room temperature and pressure?*

Test protocols

Maximal tests must be progressive in terms of the physical demands made on the subject and can be either continuous or discontinuous (Figure 1.3). The original work undertaken by A. V. Hill took the discontinuous form, and consisted of subjects running at increasing speeds around a grass track with a Douglas bag strapped to their back, interspersed with recovery periods. The favoured procedure for teaching purposes is a 5-min warm-up followed by continuous, incremental exercise consisting of 5-min stages. Research studies also employ 3-min increments, and a continuous ramp test. We record all data in the final minute of each increment, except for the ramp test where data collection is continuous. The starting intensity varies and depends on the

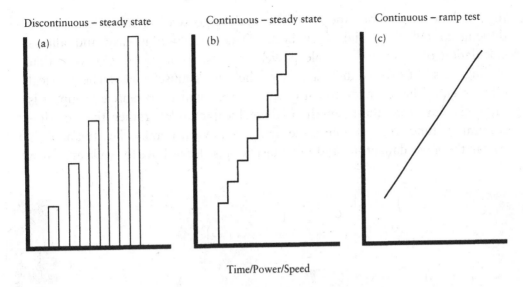

Discontinuous – steady state Continuous – steady state Continuous – ramp test

(a) (b) (c)

Time/Power/Speed

Figure 1.3 Graphical representations of various $\dot{V}_{O_2max}$ protocols. (a) Discontinuous. (b) Continuous – steady-state. (c) Continuous – ramp test

subject's perceived fitness level. The finishing point is the volitional exhaustion of the subject. It is worth pointing out here that different protocols do influence the final maximal oxygen uptake figure. In general, treadmill running gives higher values than cycle ergometry, and short, continuous ramp tests give higher values than longer tests.

Ergometers

The next requirement is some kind of ergometer – from the Greek for work 'erg', and measure 'metron'; it is simply a means of measuring the intensity of exercise undertaken. The simplest device consists of a set of steps of varying heights and a metronome; probably the most helpful is a cycle ergometer because it allows the measurement of power output and is generally safer; increasingly popular is a treadmill that allows increases in the speed and incline of the belt.

Each ergometer has strengths and weaknesses. Steps require the subject to maintain a constant rhythm; this is not easy as fatigue approaches. Theoretically, power output can be measured; multiply the subject's mass the height of the step and the number of steps, and divide by time. Again, this requires the subjects to straighten their legs every step-up; it is difficult to be certain that this is done throughout the test. The cycle ergometer is the safest – it is difficult to fall off a stationary cycle. Data collection is easy and allows calculation of valid and reliable power outputs. Its major weakness is that cycling does not involve the majority of the body's muscle mass. The physical effort requires heavy involvement of mainly the quadriceps muscle group. It is often the case that the strength of these local muscles, rather than cardio-respiratory function, determines the maximal oxygen uptake. The treadmill is by far the most dangerous and all subjects must learn how to walk and then

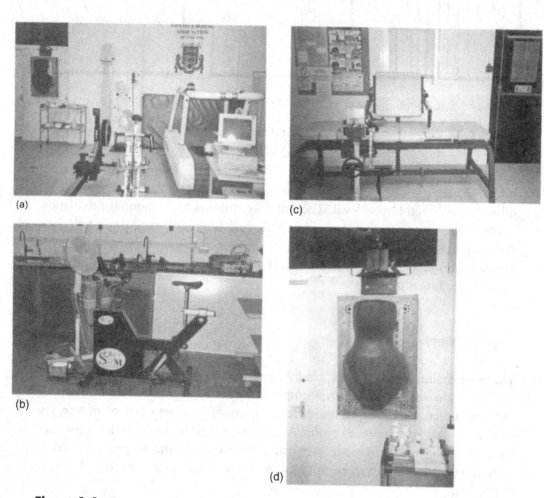

Figure 1.4 Ergometers. (a) A range of ergometers – starting from the right with a treadmill, a cycle ergometer, a rowing ergometer, and on the wall a purpose-built punching ergometer. (b) An isokinetic cycle ergometer. (c) An isokinetic bench for arm, leg and back exercise. (d) Close-up of a sport-specific ergometer for boxing. It consists of a boxing manikin attached to a force platform suspended on a wall. (Reproduced with permission of University College Chichester)

run on it before the start of any tests. This is a process called 'habituation'. Data collection is more difficult because the subject is on the move. It has major strengths, however; running is a natural action, and is a whole body movement. Sport-specific ergometery is becoming more important for assessing the training status of elite athletes, and so electrically braked cycles and rowing machines are now available commercially; but purpose-built dinghy-sailing, sail-board and boxing ergometers have been reported at Sports Science Conferences and in journals.

> **Question 1.3** *Why is sport-specific ergometry necessary?*

Gas collection

The calculation of the volumes of oxygen consumed ($\dot{V}_{O_2}$) and carbon dioxide excreted ($\dot{V}_{CO_2}$) depend on the volume of expired gases, and rely on the assumption that nitrogen is neither produced nor consumed. A method is required for separating the inspirate and the expirate and collecting the latter. A one-way valve system together with a mouthpiece and a nose-clip ensures the separation. Lightweight, leak-proof tubing connects the expiratory port of the valve-box to the T-shaped tap of a large plastic Douglas bag. A stopwatch times the collection of expired air. All of the connections must be airtight to prevent leakage to and contamination from the atmosphere, and the subject must be encouraged to concentrate on keeping the mouthpiece in place to prevent the air leaking around its edges.

We now need to measure the fraction (F_{GAS}) or percentages of the gases in the expirate. The most accurate method for measuring oxygen and carbon dioxide concentrations is a chemical one using the Lloyd–Haldane apparatus. However, this requires training and a degree of technical aptitude. It is also rather slow and has fallen out of favour, and has been replaced by paramagnetic and infrared analysers for the oxygen and carbon dioxide and respectively. Precise calibration of these analysers is vital before use; they must be checked regularly during extended testing sessions.

> **Question 1.4** *Why is this calibration necessary?*

(a)

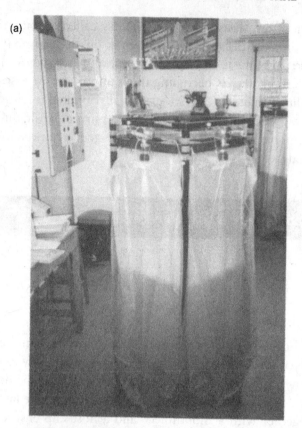

(b)

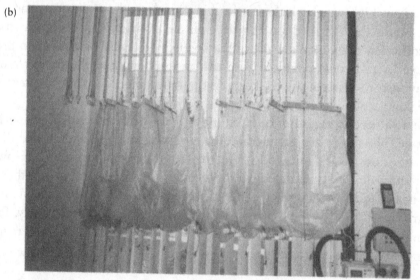

Figure 1.5   Expired gas collection. (a) A movable set of Douglas bags suitable for simple class experiments. (b) An arrangement of Douglas bags for multiple collections required for research projects. (Reproduced with permission of University College Chichester)

Calibration

The process normally requires three cylinders of gas. One contains pure nitrogen (N_2), called white-spot nitrogen; the second holds 0.08 to 0.10 (8 to 10 per cent) CO_2 in nitrogen; and the third a mixture of about 0.15 (15 per cent) O_2 and 0.05 (5 per cent) CO_2 and 0.8 (80 per cent) N_2. In addition, we need a pump that draws in fresh air from outside the laboratory. We pass the white-spot nitrogen through the two analysers to give the zero baseline for the measurements, and the fresh air and the 0.10 CO_2 through the oxygen and carbon dioxide analysers respectively to set the upper ranges. We use the gas mixture of 0.15 O_2 and 0.05 CO_2 to check the accuracy of the analysers. A small pump draws a sample of expired gases, known as an aliquot, from the Douglas bag through the analysers. We take readings when the digital display has remained steady for 10 to 15 s. Plenty of practice ensures that the entire process should take no longer than a minute.

Finally, expired volume is measured accurately. The most popular arrangement is a Havard gas meter, similar in principle to the one in your house belonging to your local gas company. A graduated calibration syringe of precise volume is also required to check the meter's accuracy at regular intervals. The inlet port of the gas meter is connected to a Douglas bag containing the expired air. Leak-proof tubing links the exit port of the gas meter to a vacuum pump, which is usually a small household vacuum cleaner. A variable transformer controls the suction rate, and is determined by trial and error. The meter is set to zero, the Douglas bag tap opened and the vacuum switched on; when the bag is empty the reading is recorded. Because pressure and temperature affect gas volume, a fast-response thermometer inserted close to the exit port of the meter, and a barometer with a vernier scale, are needed to record the temperature and pressure of the expired air as it passes through the meter. Remember to add the volume of the *sample* removed from the Douglas bag during the analysis of gas fractions to the *volume* measured by the gas meter to avoid errors.

The importance of calibration is not restricted to gas analysers. For example, the weights used to exert force on the flywheel of the cycle ergometer and the belt speed of the treadmill need verification. An example of the lengths taken for research activity appears in Figure 1.7.

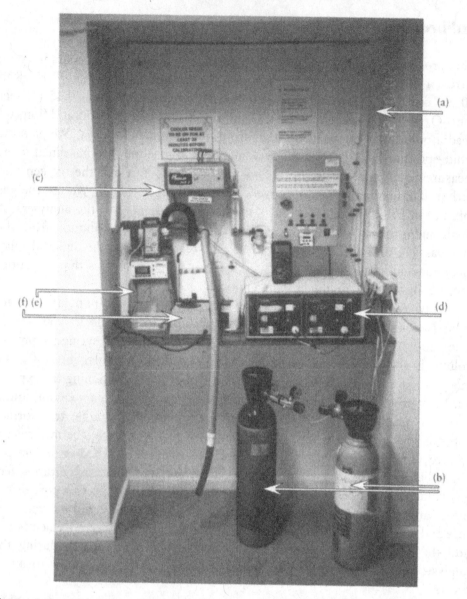

Figure 1.6 A typical arrangement of equipment for analysing gases and recording gas volume. (a) Inlet from atmosphere with drying tube. (b) Calibration gases. (c) Sample flow-meter and condenser which draws expired gas from the Douglas bag and dries it. (d) Oxygen and carbon dioxide analysers. (e) Vacuum pump. (f) Havard dry gas meter with thermometer to measure gas temperature. (Reproduced with permission of University College Chichester)

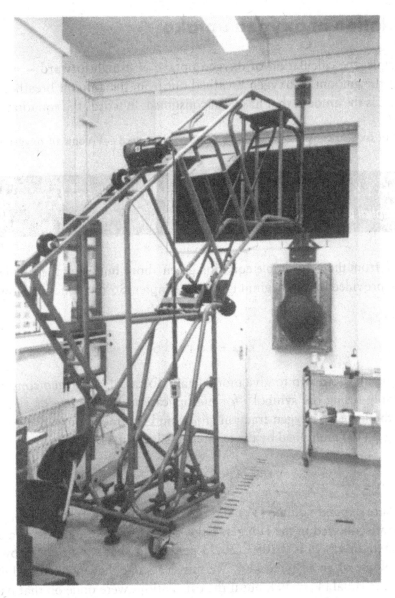

Figure 1.7 A purpose-built device for calibrating the punching ergometer. Weights of varying mass can be attached to a pendulum to generate different forces. The cradle can be moved into different positions to simulate punches of different kinds – straight, uppercut and hook – arising from various positions. (With permission of Dr R. Dyson, University College Chichester, and Mr L. Janaway, Brunel University)

Calculation of oxygen uptake

In principle, the calculation of oxygen uptake is straightforward – we simply subtract the amount of oxygen breathed out from the amount breathed in; the difference is the amount that has been consumed. In words the equation is

Volume of oxygen consumed = Volume of oxygen inspired − Volume of oxygen expired

> **Question 1.5** *From the information you have at your disposal, can you spot the potential problem in solving that equation?*

We begin from the very simple equation given above but using the conventional symbols provided at the beginning of the chapter. So the equation now looks like this

$$\dot{V}_{O_2} = \dot{V}_{O_2I} - \dot{V}_{O_2E}$$

We can break this down to give more detail. To calculate oxygen consumption we multiply (using the symbol · for multiplication) the volume of air inspired ($\dot{V}_I$) by the inspired oxygen fraction (F_{IO_2}) and subtract from it the volume of expired gas ($\dot{V}_E$) multiplied by the expired gas fraction (F_{EO_2}), i.e.

$$\dot{V}_{O_2} = \dot{V}_I \cdot F_{IO_2} - \dot{V}_E \cdot F_{EO_2}$$

We measure expired volume ($\dot{V}_E$) and the expired oxygen fraction (F_{EO_2}) from the expirate collected in the Douglas bags, and we know the oxygen fraction in the inspired air (F_{IO_2}) is 0.2093 (20.93 per cent); what we do *not* know is the actual volume of air inspired ($\dot{V}_I$). We might assume that inspired and expired volumes are equal ($\dot{V}_I = \dot{V}_E$), but if the calculations were done on that basis the answer would give only a rough estimate of actual oxygen uptake ($\dot{V}_{O_2}$). However, inspired and expired volumes are not always equal ($\dot{V}_I \neq \dot{V}_E$). This is because energy sources change as exercise intensity increases. At low levels of exercise the energy source is largely fat, whereas the source for severe exercise is carbohydrate. Fat requires more oxygen to break it down into a usable substrate, and carbon dioxide excretion increases during severe exercise. As a result, the ratio of carbon dioxide excreted to oxygen consumed ($\dot{V}_{CO_2}/\dot{V}_{O_2}$) known as the respiratory exchange ratio (RER), is not always 1. If the ratio is less than one (<1), the number of oxygen molecules taken from inspired air is not replaced with the same number of molecules of carbon dioxide in expired air and thus expired volume is less than inspired volume ($\dot{V}_E < \dot{V}_I$).

Thus far, nitrogen, the most plentiful of the respiratory gases, has not entered our thinking.

Question 1.6 *Can you see another problem in solving the equation? Can you also see the solution to it?*

We know from standard tables that the inspired nitrogen fraction (F_{IN_2}) is 0.7904. So in a litre of inspired air 79.04 per cent of the molecules will be nitrogen molecules. However, nitrogen is an inert gas and does not take any part in metabolic activity (unless a high intake of protein has preceded the test), so the *number* of nitrogen molecules will be the same in both inspired and expired air. If the volume expired is less than a litre the same number of nitrogen molecules will be taking up more space and so the relative nitrogen *concentration* is increased. This is where Geppert and Zuntz, and Haldane, were clever enough to see that the difference between expired and inspired volumes ($\dot{V}_E$ and $\dot{V}_I$) would be directly proportional to the difference between expired and inspired nitrogen fractions (F_{EN_2} and F_{IN_2}). In other words

$$\dot{V}_I \cdot F_{IN_2} = \dot{V}_E \cdot F_{EN_2} \quad \text{or} \quad \dot{V}_I = \dot{V}_E \cdot \frac{F_{EN_2}}{F_{IN_2}}$$

There is only one final problem – we do not record the nitrogen fraction of expired air. It is possible to do this through the Lloyd–Haldane analyser or an electronic N_2 analyser. However, the first is technically demanding and time-consuming, the other expensive. However, the solution is simple, quick, and inexpensive.

Question 1.7 *Have you spotted it yet*

Simple subtraction gives the nitrogen fraction in the expired air, i.e.

$$F_{EN_2} = 1 - F_{EO_2} - F_{ECO_2}$$

We are now in a position to calculate $\dot{V}_{O_2}I$

$$\dot{V}_{O_2I} = \dot{V}_E \cdot \left[\frac{(1 - F_{EO_2} - F_{ECO_2})}{F_{IN_2}} \cdot F_{IO_2} \right]$$

Expired volume of oxygen ($\dot{V}_{O_2E}$) is easily obtained by multiplying the volume of expired air ($\dot{V}_E$) collected in the Douglas bag by the difference in the oxygen fractions of the inspirate, 0.2093, and the expirate (F_{EO_2})

$$\dot{V}_{O_2E} = \dot{V}_E \cdot (0.2093 - F_{EO_2})$$

We are now in a position to calculate oxygen consumption:

$$\dot{V}_{O_2} = \left\{ \left[\dot{V}_E \cdot \left(\frac{1 - F_{EO_2} - F_{ECO_2}}{0.7904} \right) \right] \cdot 0.2093 \right\} - \{ \dot{V}_E \cdot F_{EO_2} \}$$

Simplifying, we get the following, which is easier to use

$$\dot{V}_{O_2} = \dot{V}_E \cdot \{ [(1 - F_{EO_2} - F_{ECO_2}) \cdot 0.265] - F_{EO_2} \}$$

Question 1.8   *Can you see how we derive the figure 0.265? Think about the two gas fractions that are constant.*

The calculation of carbon dioxide excreted ($\dot{V}_{CO_2}$) follows a similar path. The volume excreted is the difference between the expired and inspired volumes

$$\dot{V}_{CO_2} = \dot{V}_{CO_2E} - \dot{V}_{CO_2I}$$

The volume expired ($\dot{V}_{CO_2E}$) is the volume of the expirate ($\dot{V}_E$) multiplied by the fraction of carbon dioxide in the expirate (F_{ECO_2})

$$\dot{V}_{CO_2E} = \dot{V}_E \cdot F_{ECO_2}$$

The volume inspired ($\dot{V}_{CO_2I}$) is the volume of air inspired ($\dot{V}_I$) multiplied by the fraction of carbon dioxide in the atmosphere (F_{ICO_2})

$$\dot{V}_{CO_2I} = \dot{V}_I \cdot F_{ICO_2}$$

Since the carbon dioxide fraction in the atmosphere is very small, 0.0003, the equation can be simplified to

$$\dot{V}_{CO_2} = \dot{V}_E \cdot (F_{ECO_2} - 0.0003)$$

Atypical inspired gas fractions

The Geppert–Zuntz–Haldane Transformation for calculating oxygen consumption and carbon dioxide excretion assumes standard laboratory conditions where inspired fractions of oxygen and carbon dioxide are 0.2093 and 0.0003 respectively. However, it has been shown that in poorly ventilated laboratories with an inspired oxygen fraction just lower than normal, e.g. 0.2083, the calculated oxygen uptake values would be ~4 per cent lower than the actual value assuming normality. Similar problems arise with higher than normal carbon dioxide levels. Air-conditioning, or open windows, usually solve this particular problem.

It is important to realize that the calculation you have just completed will only be an approximate answer because we have not taken the effects of temperature or pressure into account. We will deal with those issues in more detail when we discuss the ventilation of the lungs.

Exercise 1.1

Using the following information recorded during a typical exercise test calculate $\dot{V}_{O_2}$, $\dot{V}_{CO_2}$ and RER:

$$\dot{V}_E = 50_{STPD}\ L \cdot min^{-1};\ F_{EO_2} = 17.00\%;\ F_{ECO_2}\ 3.50\%$$

Use the long and the short methods.

N.B. Remember to convert the gas *percentages* into *fractions*.

Other variables recorded

Important though the measurement of maximal oxygen uptake is, it does not cover the whole range of measurements taken during a maximal oxygen uptake test. Heart rates (f_C), before, during and after the test, provide important information. These data are now routinely monitored from two electrodes attached to the chest which are linked to a miniaturized transmitter; this sends the signals to a recorder which updates the heart rate every five beats or so.

Maximum heart rates are taken as supporting evidence that maximal oxygen uptake has been achieved. Individual maximum rates vary, but a useful guide is given by the equation

$$f_{Cmax} = 220 - age \ (\pm 10\%)$$

Respiratory rate (f_R) is recorded from the time taken for 10 movements of the valves in the one-way valve box, or by inserting a fast-response thermistor near to the subjects' lips. The thermistor reacts to the changes in temperature between inspired air ($\sim 20°C$) and expired ($35°C$) gases, and produces a signal that can be recorded on computer or chart recorder and counted. Most laboratories also record the presence of lactate (La) and the rate at which it accumulates in the blood. This requires a small drop ($20-50 \ \mu L$) of blood obtained from fingertip or ear-lobe punctures by a short, fine, sterile needle during and after the test. High post-exercise blood lactate concentrations [La_{bl}] of more than 8 mmol $\cdot L^{-1}$ are also taken as an indicator that maximal oxygen uptake has been reached.

A laboratory notebook is essential. The data, and any unusual events that may affect the results, should be recorded accurately. Although it is easy to calculate oxygen uptake and carbon dioxide excretion with a hand-held calculator the operations are somewhat tedious and time-consuming. All laboratories have their own bit of software on a computer that does all of the necessary calculations and prints out the results in a standardized format. It is advisable that you become proficient in doing the calculations the long way for two reasons. First, you demonstrate your understanding of the process; second, a computer may not always be at hand, particularly in fieldwork.

A typical record of a discontinuous, progressive test of 5-minute increments found in a laboratory notebook resembles that shown in Table 1.1.

Key points

- The indirect method of calculating oxygen requires collection of expired air in a Douglas bag.

- The process depends on the discovery, by the French chemist Antoine Lavoisier, that nitrogen does not take part in the aerobic breakdown of fats and carbohydrates.

Table 1.1 A typical data sheet obtained from a continuous steady-state cycle ergometer test

Project no: .. Date of test: ...... Subject: .... Gender: M/F

Date of birth: ...... Height: .....m Mass: ....kg

Consent form: Y/N Health questionnaire: Y/N

Blood profile: Y/N Lung function: Y/N

Ambient pressure (P_B): .... Ambient temperature (T_{amb}): ......

Relative humidity: ...... Ambient (P_{H_2O}): ....

POWER (W)	f_C (bt·min⁻¹)	f_R (br·min⁻¹)	$\dot{V}_{E\,STPD}$ (L·min⁻¹)	$\bar{V}_T$ (L·br⁻¹)	F_{EO_2} (%)	F_{ECO_2} (%)	$\dot{V}_{O_2}$ (L·min⁻¹)	$\dot{V}_{CO_2}$ (L·min⁻¹)	RER	La_{bl} (mmol·L⁻¹)
50	116	13	20.110	1.547	16.45	3.75	0.945	0.748	0.79	1.05
100	132	15	27.001	1.800	15.85	4.35	1.430	1.166	0.81	1.26
150	149	17	37.023	2.176	15.69	4.55	2.015	1.672	0.83	1.79
200	165	19	50.007	2.632	15.41	4.89	2.855	2.430	0.85	2.56
250	181	25	64.998	2.601	15.75	4.99	3.224	3.405	0.94	4.01
300	196	38	95.011	2.498	16.49	4.51	4.256	4.256	1.01	7.76
350	201	55	131.071	2.383	17.55	3.72	4.343	4.836	1.11	11.58

- The English physiologist Archibald Hill discovered a linear relationship between sub-maximal exercise and oxygen consumption.

- He also described the plateau in oxygen consumption that indicates an individual's maximal oxygen uptake.

- Each subject must undergo a health check before the test takes place.

- Laboratory environments should be temperature-controlled ventilated.

- Pre-test routines must include records of ambient temperature and pressure, calibration of the gas analysers and gas meter, and records of the test date and time and the subject's height and body mass.

- Record heart rates, respiratory frequency, and blood lactates.

- A classical test protocol involves 5-min bouts of progressive exercise with recovery between each bout.

- Collect expired air during the last minute, analyse it for oxygen and carbon dioxide fractions, and measure its volume.

- Most laboratories now employ continuous tests of various descriptions.

- Treadmills and cycle ergometers are the favoured devices for delivering controlled bouts of exercise.

- Oxygen uptake is calculated by subtracting the volume of oxygen expired from the volume inspired ($\dot{V}_{O_2I} - \dot{V}_{O_2E}$).

- The gas volume multiplied by the oxygen fraction gives the volume of oxygen expired ($\dot{V}_{O_2E} = \dot{V}_E \times F_{EO_2}$).

- Calculate the inspired volume ($\dot{V}_I$) by multiplying the expired volume ($\dot{V}_E$) by the ratio of expired and inspired nitrogen fractions (F_{EN_2}/F_{IN_2}).

- Obtain this ratio by subtracting the expired oxygen and carbon dioxide fractions from 1 and dividing the result by a constant 0.7904.

- Multiply this by the fraction of oxygen in pure air (F_{IO_2}), a constant 0.2093, to give the volume of oxygen inspired ($\dot{V}_{IO_2} = \dot{V}_I \times 0.2093$).

- The volume of carbon dioxide excreted is the expired volume ($\dot{V}_E$) multiplied by the expired gas fraction (F_{ECO_2}) minus the inspired gas fraction (F_{IO_2}), which is a constant 0.0003 ($\dot{V}_{CO_2} = \dot{V}_E \times (F_{ECO_2} \times 0.0003)$).

- The ratio of carbon dioxide excreted and oxygen consumed ($\dot{V}_{CO_2}/\dot{V}_{O_2}$) is the respiratory exchange ratio (RER).

Answers to questions in the text

Question 1.1
Adolf Fick seemed to be measuring oxygen uptake in 1870 according to the material quoted in the Prologue on the measurement of cardiac output.

Question 1.2
Temperature and pressure fluctuate within and between days; both will affect the measurement of expired gas volumes, and therefore the volumes of oxygen consumed and carbon dioxide excreted.

Question 1.3
Treadmills and ergometers measure general cardio-respiratory fitness adequately. However, elite sportsmen and women need to know how fit they are for their sport. Testing swimmers and rowers on a treadmill, for example, will give some idea of their general fitness but not their fitness for the actual sports at which they excel.

Question 1.4
Equipment calibration is an essential feature of the preparation for a maximal oxygen uptake test for two reasons. First, the machines themselves are prone to change over time; second, the environmental conditions are changing constantly and may affect the responses of the equipment.

Question 1.5
The problem is that the Douglas bag method only collects *expired* gas; we can calculate the volume of oxygen *expired* easily enough, but there is still the problem of recording the volume of oxygen inspired.

Question 1.6

Although we know the *inspired* nitrogen fraction – it is 0.7904 (79.04 per cent) – we do not *measure* the nitrogen fraction of the *expired* air. However, we can calculate the expired nitrogen fraction by simple subtraction of the expired oxygen and carbon dioxide fractions from 1.

Question 1.7

Given expired oxygen and carbon dioxide fractions of 0.15 (15 per cent) and 0.05 (5 per cent) respectively, the nitrogen fraction in that mixture is $1 - 0.15 - 0.05 = 0.80$ (80 per cent)

Question 1.8

There are only two constants in the oxygen uptake equation. These are the fractions of oxygen and nitrogen of inspired air, 0.2093 and 0.7904, respectively, highlighted below.

$$\dot{V}_{O_2} = \left\{ \dot{V}_E \cdot \frac{(1 - F_{EO_2} - F_{ECO_2})}{0.7904} \cdot 0.2093 \right\} - \left\{ \dot{V}_E \cdot (0.2093 - F_{EO_2}) \right\}$$

Dividing 0.2093 by 0.7904 gives us the 0.265 seen in the simplified equation below.

$$\dot{V}_{O_2} = \dot{V}_E \cdot \left\{ [(1 - F_{EO_2} - F_{ECO_2}) \cdot 0.265] - F_{EO_2} \right\}$$

Answer to exercise in the text

Exercise 1.1

$$\dot{V}_E = 50 \ L \cdot min^{-1}{}_{STPD}; \ F_{EO_2} = 0.17 \ (17.00\%); \ F_{ECO_2} = 0.035 \ (3.50\%)$$

Method 1

$$\dot{V}_{O_2} = \left\{ \left[\dot{V}_E \cdot \frac{(1 - F_{EO_2} - F_{ECO_2})}{F_{IN_2}} \right] \cdot F_{IO_2} \right\} - \left\{ \dot{V}_E \cdot F_{EO_2} \right\} L \cdot min^{-1}$$

$$= \left\{ \left[50 \cdot \frac{(1 - 0.17 - 0.035)}{0.7904} \right] \cdot 0.2093 \right\} - \left\{ 50 \cdot 0.17 \right\}$$

$$= \left\{ 50 \cdot \left[\frac{(0.7950)}{0.7904} \right] \cdot 0.2093 \right\} - 8.500$$

$$= \{[50 \cdot 1.0058] \cdot 0.2093\} - 8.500$$

$$= \{[50.2910] \cdot 0.2093\} - 8.500$$

$$= 10.526 - 8.500$$

$$\dot{V}_{O_2} = \underline{2.03 L \cdot min^{-1}}$$

Method 2

$$\dot{V}_{O_2} = \dot{V}_E \cdot \{[(1 - F_{EO_2} - F_{ECO_2}) \cdot 0.265] - F_{EO_2}\}$$

$$= 50 \cdot \{[(1 - 0.17 - 0.035) \cdot 0.265] - 0.17\}$$

$$= 50 \cdot \{[0.7950) \cdot 0.265] - 0.17\}$$

$$= 50 \cdot \{0.2107 - 0.17\}$$

$$= 50 \cdot 0.0407$$

$$\dot{V}_{O_2} = \underline{2.03 L \cdot min^{-1}}$$

$\dot{V}_{CO_2}$

$$\dot{V}_{CO_2} = \dot{V}_E \cdot (F_{ECO_2} - F_{ICO_2})$$

$$= 50 \cdot 0.035 - 0.0003$$

$$= 50 \cdot 0.0347$$

$$\dot{V}_{CO_2} = \underline{1.735 L \cdot min^{-1}}$$

$$RER = \dot{V}_{CO_2} / \dot{V}_{O_2}$$

$$= 1.735 / 2.03$$

$$RER = 0.85$$

2

Oxygen from Atmosphere to Blood

Learning Objectives

By the end of this chapter, you should be able to

♦ identify the static and dynamic volumes and capacities of the lungs

♦ describe the effects of exercise on various volumes and capacities

♦ explain the effects of temperature and pressure on gas volumes

♦ convert volumes from ATPS to BTPS and STPD and explain the need for such conversions

♦ calculate partial pressures of gases

♦ explain the development of the oxygen pressure gradients between the atmosphere and the blood

♦ describe the factors that affect diffusion of gases from the alveoli to the blood and from the blood to the alveoli

♦ identify the main features of the lungs' airways and their structures

♦ outline the main features of the pulmonary circulation

♦ describe the effects of exercise on the airways

♦ indicate the major muscles involved in inspiration and expiration at rest and during exercise

♦ outline the major elements of the control of ventilation at rest and during exercise

Exercise Physiology: A Thematic Approach   Tudor Hale
© John Wiley & Sons, Ltd   ISBN: 0 470 84682 8 (cloth), ISBN 0 470 84683 6 (pbk)

Objective test

Say whether the following answers are true (T) or false (F). If you do not know, say so (D) – not knowing is not an academic crime, but not finding out is. Try not to look at the answers until you have worked your way through the chapter and completed the test a second time. In this way, you can monitor your progress.

	Pre-test			Post-test		
	T	F	D	T	F	D
1. Each lung is covered with a membrane called the pleural sac						
2. The upper respiratory tract warms and moistens inspired air						
3. The diameter of the trachea is between 15 and 20 cm						
4. The trachea consists mainly of smooth muscle						
5. Alveoli begin to appear on the bronchioles						
6. The conductive zone is often called the anatomical dead space						
7. The functional unit of respiration is called the acinus						
8. The alveoli are lined with a single layer of epithelial cells						
9. There are about 3 million alveoli in an adult male lung						
10. At rest the main active inspiratory muscle is the abdominal group						
11. At rest the main active expiratory muscle is the diaphragm						
12. Resting tidal volume in male adults is about 500–700 mL						
13. A typical value for adult residual volume is about 4.5 L						
14. $V_{TLC} = V_{VC} + V_{RV}$						

	Pre-test			Post-test		
	T	F	D	T	F	D
15. $V_{FRC} = V_{ERV} + V_{RV}$						
16. The FRC prevents large swings in alveolar P_{O_2} and P_{CO_2}						
17. Exercise increases the FRC						
18. $V_T \times f_R = VC$						
19. The symbol for volume expired in 1 minute is $\dot{V}_E$ $L \cdot min^{-1}$						
20. As barometric pressure increases gas volume increases						
21. Ambient temperature and pressure $= 0°C$ and 101.1 kPa/760 mmHg						
22. The partial pressure of water vapour varies with temperature						
23. The partial pressure of water vapour at BTPS is 6.3 kPa/47 mmHg						
24. O_2 diffuses faster than CO_2 in the gas phase						
25. CO_2 diffuses faster than O_2 in the liquid phase						
26. O_2 partial pressure in the trachea is 20.7 kPa/159 mmHg						
27. Resting alveolar O_2 partial pressure $\sim$13.7 kPa/103 mmHg						
28. O_2 partial pressure in mixed venous blood is 13.3 kPa/100 mmHg						
29. Arterial partial pressure of CO_2 is 6.1 kPa/46 mmHg						
30. Mixed venous partial pressure of CO_2 is 5.3 kPa/40 mmHg						

Symbols, abbreviations and units of measurement

alveolus, alveolar	A	
alveolar pressure	P_A	kPa; mmHg
ambient	amb	
ambient pressure	P_{amb}	kPa; mmHg
ambient temperature and pressure saturated	ATPS	
arterial	a	
arterial pressure	P_a	kPa; mmHg
atmosphere, atmospheric	atm	
barometric pressure	P_B	kPa; mmHg
blood	bl	
body temperature and pressure saturated	BTPS	
capillary	c	
cerebrospinal fluid	CSF	
diffusing capacity of the lung	D_L	
gas	g	
hydrogen ion	H^+	
length	l	metre; m
litre	L	
pascal; kilopascal	Pa; kPa	
pulmonary	P	
pressure	P	kPa; mmHg
standard temperature and pressure dry	STPD	
tracheal pressure	P_{trach}	kPa; mmHg
ventilation/perfusion ratio	V_A/Q	
volume	V	L; mL
volume of alveolar dead space	V_{DA}	L; mL
volume of series dead space	V_{DS}	L; mL
volume of alveolar ventilation	V_A	L; mL
volume expired	V_E	L; mL
volume inspired	V_I	L; mL
volume of single breath, tidal volume	V_T	L; mL
volume of gas flow in unit time	$\dot{V}$	$L \cdot min^{-1}$
volume expired in unit time	$\dot{V}_E$	$L \cdot min^{-1}$
volume inspired in unit time	$\dot{V}_I$	$L \cdot min^{-1}$
venous	v	

| venous pressure | P_v | kPa; mmHg |
| mixed venous | $\bar{v}$ | |

Lung volumes and capacities

expiratory reserve volume	ERV; V_{ER}	L; mL
forced expiratory volume in 1 second	$FEV_{1.0}$	L; mL
functional residual capacity	FRC	L; mL
inspiratory capacity	IC	L; mL
inspiratory reserve volume	IRV; V_{IR}	L; mL
residual volume	RV; V_{res}	L; mL
tidal volume	TV; V_T	L; mL
total lung capacity	TLC	L; mL
vital capacity	VC	L; mL

Introduction

The primary function of the lung is the exchange of oxygen and carbon dioxide between the atmosphere and the blood. The amount of air moved in and out of the lungs to ensure this exchange is the product of the rate of breathing – respiratory frequency (f_R br $\cdot$ min^{-1}) – and mean volume per breath – tidal volume ($\bar{V}_T$ mL $\cdot$ br^{-1})

$$\dot{V} = \bar{V}_T \cdot f_R$$

At rest, breathing is largely subconscious as we move about 8–10 litres of air in and out of the lungs every minute. By the end of the maximal oxygen uptake test ($\dot{V}_{O_2 max}$) this volume may well have risen to between 100 and 200 $L \cdot$ min^{-1}, as the body's physiological mechanisms respond to the need to excrete carbon dioxide and increase oxygen availability. A typical expired volume response to progressive exercise appears in Figure 2.1. Note that the relationship is curvilinear, and quite different to the power–oxygen uptake relationship we saw in Chapter 1.

In this chapter, we concentrate mainly on the oxygen transfer from the atmosphere to the blood via lung ventilation; in Chapter 9 we explain more fully the movement of carbon dioxide in the opposite direction. We begin with an examination of the static and dynamic volumes and capacities of the lung.

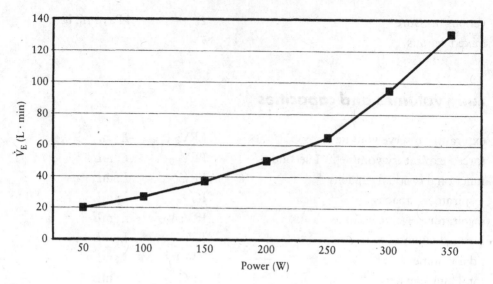

Figure 2.1 A typical relationship between power (*W*) and ventilation ($\dot{V}_E$) resulting from a maximal oxygen uptake test

Lung volumes and capacities

At rest only a small proportion of the lungs' capacities is used, but like most physiological systems, there are considerable reserves that are called upon during exercise. A simple experiment using a wet spirometer (see Figure 2.2) is a good way of looking at resting lung volumes and capacities and the changes that occur during exercise. We get similar data using the more up-to-date, but more expensive, device called a pneumotachograph.

We fit the subject with a nose-clip and mouthpiece and then allow her or him time to become familiar with this equipment. We call this familiarization period 'habituation'; it is an important feature of all physiological experiments and is essential for valid and reliable data. When the subject is relaxed, we open the tap into the spirometer, and switch on a device to record the output from the spirometer or pneumotachograph. After a few normal breaths, the subject takes the maximum inspiration possible, holds it for a splitsecond, and then exhales maximally.

The trace produced (Figure 2.3) allows us to measure a range of respiratory variables. The major ones are total lung capacity (TLC), vital capacity (VC), inspiratory capacity (IC), tidal volume (V_T), and the inspiratory and expiratory

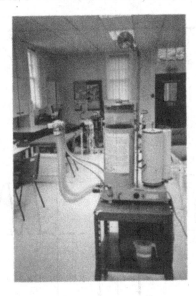

Pneumotachograph

$\dot{V}$

P_x P_y

P_{x-y}

Screen (Lilly)

Recording drum

Gas sample tube

Tap

One-way
valve box

Motor

$\dot{V}$

P_x P_y

P_{x-y}

Soda-lime container

Capillary (Fleisch)

Wet spirometer

Figure 2.2 Photograph and cross-sectional diagram of a Warren–Collins wet spirometer. The more sophisticated devices are typical screen and capillary pneumotachographs. These devices record gas flow over time. The screen and capillary mesh provide a resistance which is proportional to flow. The pressure difference across the resistance is converted into flow which is integrated to give volume. (Pneumotachographs based on Tammeling (1980))

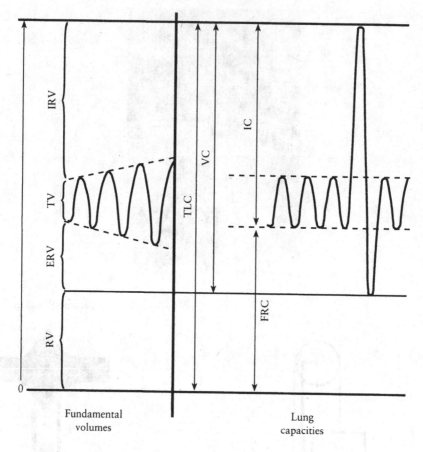

Figure 2.3   Static and dynamic lung volumes and capacities

reserve volumes (V_{IR}, and V_{ER}). Respiratory frequency (f_R) and expired volume in one minute ($\dot{V}_E$) can also be calculated.

Question 2.1   *How can the volume of air expired in one minute (V_E) be calculated? Note: there are two ways.*

We measure vital capacity from peak to trough of the maximum inspiration and expiration manoeuvre. We measure inspiratory capacity from the end of a normal exhalation to the peak of maximal inspiration; inspiratory reserve volume is the maximum volume that can be inspired following a normal inspiration. The expiratory reserve volume is the maximum volume that can be expired following a normal exhalation.

However, no matter how forcefully we exhale, some gas will always remain trapped deep within the lung. This arises because of the increased pressure within the chest (intra-thoracic pressure) causing the small airways to close; the trapped air is the residual volume (V_{res}). We seldom measure this volume directly; instead, we measure functional residual capacity (FRC) by indicator dilution, nitrogen clearance or whole-body plethysmography, and subtract the expiratory reserve volume. Most sport and exercise laboratories do not have the equipment to perform any of these procedures.

We can now complete the final measurements. The functional residual capacity is the expiratory reserve volume added to the residual volume. The total lung capacity is vital capacity added to residual volume, or inspiratory capacity added to functional residual capacity. The boundaries of all of the volumes and capacities are summarized in Figure 2.3.

Although we have introduced functional residual capacity, we have not yet defined it. It is the volume of gas remaining in the lung after expiration. This capacity is important. The gas left in the lung after expiration contains a mixture of gases – about 80 per cent (0.80) is nitrogen, 15 per cent (0.15) is oxygen, and 5 per cent (0.05) is carbon dioxide. Fresh air contains 79.04 per cent (0.7904) nitrogen (together with traces of other gases), 20.93 per cent (0.2093) oxygen, and 0.03 per cent (0.0003) carbon dioxide. When this fresh air is inhaled it mixes with the gases already present in the lungs, and the functional residual capacity acts as a buffer which prevent large swings in alveolar partial pressure of oxygen within the gas exchange units of the lung. If there were no functional residual capacity, the alveolar partial pressures would change from almost 20 kPa (150 mmHg) at the end of inspiration to 5.3 kPa (40 mmHg) at the end of expiration, and would affect oxygen content of arterial blood. At rest, the swings are negligible, less than 0.5 kPa (3–4 mmHg), but can rise to about 4 kPa (30 mmHg) at maximal exercise because of the increased inspired tidal volumes. We deal with concept of partial pressures in some detail later in the chapter.

After obtaining resting values, we now ask the subject to perform two bouts of progressive exercise.

Exercise 2.1

Before studying Figure 2.4 jot down the changes in lung volumes and capacities you would expect to see in this little experiment.

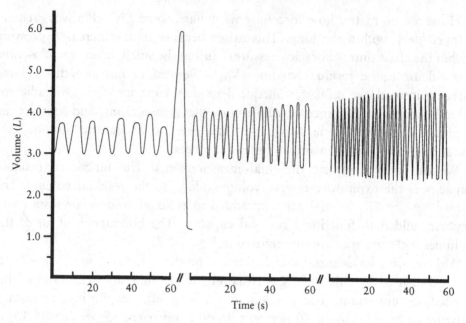

Figure 2.4 A diagrammatic representation of resting and exercising lung volumes and capacities

During the last minute of each bout, we record the spirometer output. Figure 2.4 above is a schematic representation of a typical record of the exercise from a wet spirometer to which we have added a typical residual volume.

Question 2.2 *What happens to the ratio of V_T to VC as exercise increases? Do you think V_T will increase to such an extent that at maximal exercise it becomes equal to VC?*

Exercise 2.2

Using the data from Figure 2.4 complete the volumes, capacities, frequencies, symbols and units shown in blank Table 2.1. Compare the actual data with your guesses from Exercise 2.1

Table 2.1 Lung volumes and capacities at rest and during exercise

Variable	Units	Symbol	Resting values	Exercise 1	Exercise 2
Vital capacity					
Residual volume					
Total lung capacity					
Inspiratory capacity					
Mean tidal volume					
Functional residual capacity					
Inspiratory reserve volume					
Expiratory reserve volume					
Minute volume					
Respiratory frequency					

The Vitalograph lung function test

Before the maximal oxygen uptake test, we usually ask the subject to take a lung function test using a more modern device called a Vitalograph (Figure 2.5). It is a quick, easily performed test designed to examine a subject's ability to move air out of the lungs quickly, but unlike the spirometer only gives limited information.

The subject takes a maximal inspiration and then exhales as fast, and for as long, as possible. We record three useful measures affected by age, height and gender, and compare them against normal values. The first is forced vital capacity (FVC), which is maximum volume of air that can be expired forcefully in a single breath. The second is the volume of air expired in the first second of a forced manoeuvre; it is the forced expiratory volume in one second ($FEV_{1.0}$), and is measured in litres. Finally, there is the peak expiratory flow (PEF); this is the greatest flow sustained for 10 milliseconds (ms) during a forced expiration measured in litres per minute. The normal value for $FEV_{1.0}$ in young adults (20–25 years) is 80–85 per cent of the forced vital capacity. Values less than this suggest narrowing of the airways as in acute bronchitis or asthma. Elite endurance athletes invariably have above average population values in all three measures but also often show reduced peak flow after exercise test indicating short-lived airway constriction. The three lung function traces shown in Figure 2.6 allow you to estimate FVC and $FEV_{1.0}$.

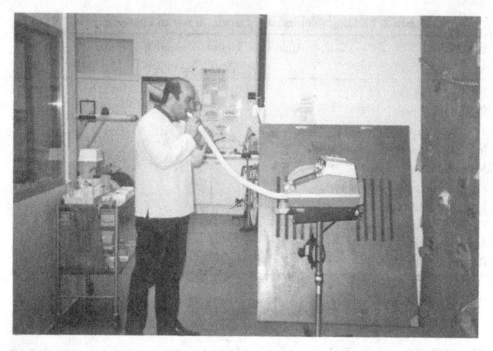

Figure 2.5 The Vitalograph used to record forced expiratory manoeuvres. (Reproduced with permission of University College Chichester)

Exercise 2.3

What are your estimates? Assuming the subjects are the same gender, age, height and ethnic group, say which of the three traces is 'normal', which one might belong to an 'athlete', and which one is an asthmatic. Why might athletes produce above average values?

The effects of pressure and temperature on gas volumes

The fact that pressure and temperature affect gas volume is now well known. The Italian physicist Evangelista Torricelli invented the barometer in 1643, making the measurement of barometric pressure possible.

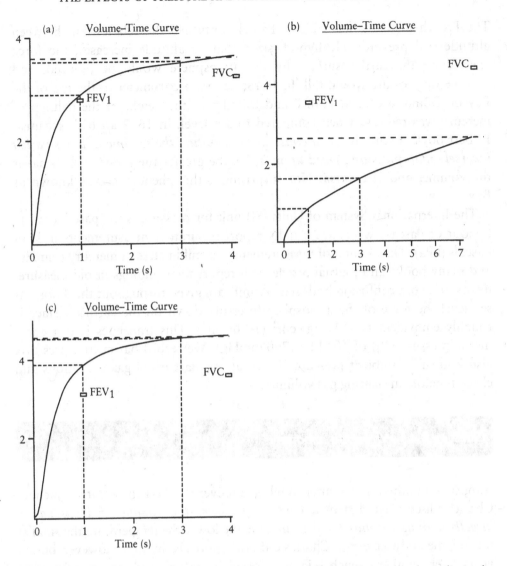

Figure 2.6 Typical graphs from lung function tests. (The labelled rectangles indicate the predicted value for a person of similar age, height and gender.) (With permission of Dr M. Buckman, King Edward VII Hospital, Midhurst)

Question 2.3   *Would the volume of gas collected during an exercise test at sea level be the same as the volume collected performing the same exercise test at altitude?*

The French mathematician Blaise Pascal confirmed the relationship between altitude and pressure. He hypothesized that as altitude increases, the force exerted on the earth's surface by the atmosphere would be reduced, and barometric pressure would fall. In 1648, he sent a barometer to the top of the Puy de Dôme in central France and found that the height of the column of mercury was reduced when compared to sea level. In 1662 an Irish scientist, Robert Boyle, found that *at a constant temperature the volume of a gas varied inversely with pressure placed upon it*, i.e. the greater the pressure the smaller the volume, and vice versa. Not surprisingly, this phenomenon is known as Boyle's law.

The International System of Units (SI) unit for pressure is the pascal (Pa), in honour of Pascal's work; we usually report respiratory measurements in kilopascals (kPa). The old unit of measurement was millimetres of mercury (mmHg) and many books and journal articles still report their findings in old measurements; to avoid confusion both sets of units are given throughout this book. At sea level the force of the atmosphere pressing down on the earth's surface is roughly equivalent to $6.41 \, \text{kg} \cdot \text{cm}^2$ ($14 \, \text{lb} \cdot \text{in}^2$). This translates into a barometric pressure (P_B) of 101 kPa (760 mmHg). We record barometric pressure, also known as ambient pressure (P_{amb}), at the start of all gas collections and check it before measuring gas volumes.

Question 2.4   *Why is this important?*

Almost a hundred years after Boyle's discovery a French scientist, Jacques Charles, discovered that *at a constant pressure the volume of a gas varied directly with its absolute temperature*, i.e. the lower the temperature the smaller the volume and vice versa. Charles did not report his findings, however, but 25 years later another French scientist, Joseph Gay-Lussac discovered the same effect and did report it. The law, known as the Charles–Gay-Lussac law, recognizes the work of both men. During the maximal oxygen uptake test the expired air is collected in Douglas bags at close to body temperature, i.e. 37°C. These bags then stand around in the laboratory in an ambient temperature of $\sim 20°C$ until we have time to analyse their contents.

Question 2.5   *What happens to the volume of expired gas in the bags as they stand around in the laboratory? Why?*

Temperature not only influences the volume of gas collected, but also the amount of water vapour held by that volume, and we need to be aware of this. When reporting gas volumes, we have to take account of three key measures of temperature. These are body temperature (normally 37°C, but this can change as a result of exercise), ambient temperature (the temperature existing at the time of the experiment), which varies widely, and standard temperature (0°C) which is a constant.

The lung volumes and capacities are measured at body temperature and ambient pressure saturated with water vapour (BTPS). However, air expired into a Douglas bag is collected at ambient temperature and pressure saturated (ATPS). Temperature and pressure vary widely, not only daily and seasonally in any one location, but also from place to place. Physiological data collected in different places and at different times need to be standardized for temperature (0°C) and pressure (101 kPa, 760 mmHg), and without the influence of water vapour, before valid and reliable comparisons can be made. Thus oxygen uptake values are always reported at standard temperature and pressure dry (STPD).

We can change gas volumes from ATPS to BTPS and STPD; the equations required are as follows:

ATPS to BTPS

$$\dot{V}_{E\,BTPS} = \dot{V}_{E\,ATPS} \times \frac{273 + \text{body temp}}{273 + \text{ambient temp}} \times \frac{P_B - \text{ambient } P_{H_2O}}{P_B - P_{H_2O} \text{ at body temp}}$$

ATPS to STPD

$$\dot{V}_{E\,STPD} = \dot{V}_{E\,ATPS} \times \frac{273}{273 + \text{ambient temp}} \times \frac{P_B - \text{ambient } P_{H_2O}}{\text{standard pressure}}$$

To grasp the full effect of different ambient conditions on gas volumes it is always useful to work through an example.

Exercise 2.4

Given the following information convert the ATPS gas volumes to BTPS and STPD. Older texts and journal articles may not use the SI units so do the calculations using both SI units and the older unit of mmHg so that you become familiar with both sets of figures.

$V_{E\,ATPS} = 100$ litres; body temp $= 37°C$; ambient temp $= 23°C$; ambient $P_{H_2O} = 2.79$ kPa (21 mmHg); P_{H_2O} at body temp $= 6.25$ kPa (47 mmHg); $P_B = 97.09$ kPa (730 mmHg)

Lung structure and function

The two lungs consist of a system of 25 generations of asymmetrical branching airways embedded in soft, spongy tissue covered by a continuous membrane. They are cone-like in shape with their concave base in contact with the major respiratory muscle, the diaphragm. Inspired air is cleaned, warmed and moistened as it passes through nose, mouth, pharynx and larynx into the major airway known as the trachea. Imagine an inverted tree with the trachea as the trunk, the two bronchi as the two main branches, the smaller airways as the branches and twigs, and the leaves as the alveoli and you get a reasonable picture of the structure of the airways. The membrane that covers the lungs is the visceral pleura and the part that sticks to the wall of the rib cage is the parietal pleura. The space in between is lubricated by a small amount of pleural fluid. The combined system forms an airtight covering that is open to the atmosphere via the pharynx and the nasal cavities.

The bronchial tree

In the lungs, the trachea divides into two main branches called stem bronchi. These two stem bronchi each produce two further branches; each of these four branches produce two further offspring – and so on for about 25 generations, ending in blind sacs called the alveoli. The photograph in Figure 2.7 of the cast of the bronchial tree with the alveoli and respiratory bronchioles removed shows the branching nature of the airways. This process – asymmetrical dichotomous branching – does not lead to symmetry of the airways; we can see

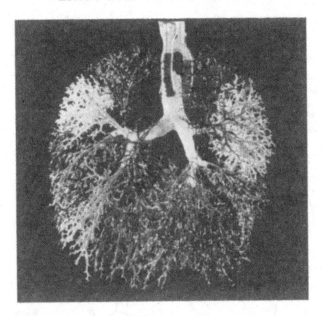

Figure 2.7 Photograph of the cast of the bronchial tree down to the terminal bronchioles. (With permission of Dr K. Horsfield Midhurst Medical Research Institute)

the differences in Figure 2.8. This airway asymmetry becomes important when we talk about gas transfer from the lungs to the blood.

The trachea consists of incomplete rings of cartilage supported by a layer of smooth muscle on its dorsal side. It is the largest airway in the lung with a diameter of 15–20 mm. About 10–15 cm from the larynx, at a point called the carina, the trachea divides into two stem bronchi that feed the right and left lungs. The right stem is the more upright, wider and shorter of the two. The right lung is the larger and consists of three lobes, whereas the left lung consists of only two due to the asymmetrical position of the heart. These airways feed the subdivisions of the lungs – the lobes, segments, sub-segments, lobules, bronchioles, terminal bronchioles and, the ultimate unit of respiration, the acinus. The acinus (Latin for a cluster of grapes) is made up of the respiratory bronchioles, the alveolar ducts and the alveolar sacs. In the typical adult human lung there are about 200 000 respiratory bronchioles and 300 million alveoli, but this latter figure depends on body size and can vary from 200 to 600 million.

As the asymmetrical dichotomous branching progresses deeper into the lungs the diameter of the individual airways become progressively narrower with each generation, and they vary in length and diameter. Typical diameters of the trachea range from 15 to 20 mm whilst the diameter of an alveolus is about 0.2 mm. The cross-sectional area of the trachea is about 3 cm^2. By the time the

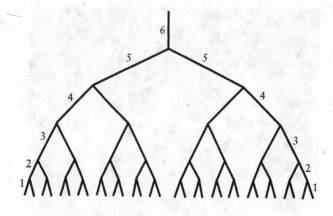

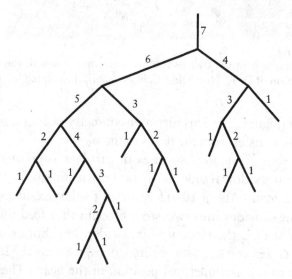

Figure 2.8 Symmetrical and asymmetrical branching patterns. (With permission of the American Physiological Society from the originals by Dr K. Horsfield (1968) and (1990))

respiratory bronchiole is reached the total cross-sectional area of all of the airways has increased to about 400 cm². If all of the alveoli could be laid out one layer thick they would cover an area the size of a tennis court, or about 80 m². To get a picture of the way that the cross-sectional area of the airways develops as we go deeper into the lung, imagine an inverted drawing pin – very narrow at the trachea and very extensive at the alveolar level.

The structure of the airways also changes as we go deeper into the lung. The walls of the first nine generations of airways, stretching from the trachea down to the bronchioles, consist mainly of cartilage with some smooth muscle. But the walls of the next five generations, made up of bronchioles, contain mainly smooth muscle.

Smooth muscle

We need to digress for a moment here to talk briefly about smooth muscle. There are three types of tissue: involuntary smooth muscle, involuntary striated cardiac muscle, and voluntary striated skeletal muscle. All three have one thing in common: in each type the contractile mechanism depends on the chemical interaction of two protein filaments called actin and myosin. However, their overall structure differs, along with the way each muscle functions. In cardiac and skeletal muscle, which are discussed in the chapters dealing with blood transport by the heart, and oxygen uptake by skeletal muscle, the actin and myosin filaments are arranged in such a way that under a microscope they appear as distinct light and dark bands. In smooth muscle the internal organization of the filaments is much less distinct so the dark and light bands do not appear (Figure 2.9).

Smooth muscle cells are usually short (about 0.5 cm), containing a single nucleus, and are a common feature of hollow tubes throughout the body. They are controlled by the autonomic nervous system that is designed to keep the internal environment of the body relatively stable.

The action of the smooth muscle of the airways consists of dilatation or constriction of the particular vessel. In the lung the airways are dilated during exercise because of the action of a hormone called adrenaline (also known as epinephrine). This widening of the airways allows more air into the lungs to assist in ventilating the blood. Conversely, an asthma attack – sometimes induced by exercise – leads to broncho-constriction (narrowing of the bronchial airways) and results in difficulty in moving air into and out of the lungs, and results in the typical wheezing of asthmatics. An aerosol inhaler containing adrenaline or one of its derivatives often relieves the problem and allows sufferers to take part in exercise.

Conductive and diffusive zones

The airways just described make up the *conductive* zone of the lungs, because the walls of the airways are too dense and thick for gas exchange to take place. Although the next four generations of respiratory bronchioles also contain some smooth muscle, alveoli begin to appear indicating the start of the *diffusive*

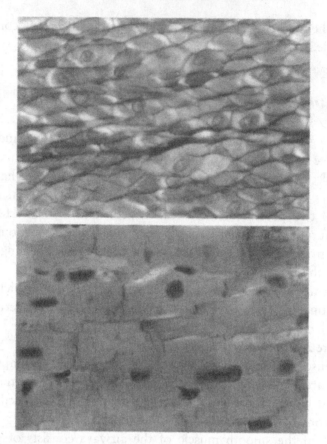

Figure 2.9 Micrographs of involuntary smooth muscle and striated cardiac muscle. (Reproduced with permission of Philip Harris Education Ashby-de-la-Zouch.)

zone. The walls of the last four generations of the airways – respiratory bronchioles and alveolar ducts – consist only of one layer of epithelial cells so that maximum exchange of gases from the lungs into the pulmonary blood supply can take place. Together with the alveoli they make up the acinus (see Figure 2.10).

Exercise 2.5

Using the information given above identify the major features indicated in the diagrammatic representation of the lungs and the acinus shown in Figure 2.11.

As we have seen, the structure of the lung gives rise to two zones – the

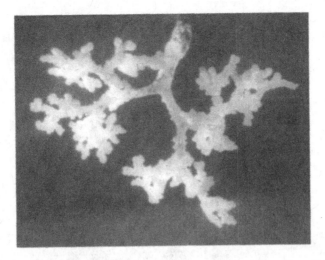

Figure 2.10 Photograph of the cast of an acinus. (With permission of Dr K Horsfield, Midhurst Medical Research Institute)

conductive and diffusive zones – and gas exchange only takes place from the alveoli of the respiratory bronchioles and the acinus. On inspiration, the larger airways from the mouth down to the respiratory bronchioles contain air with an oxygen concentration that is very little different from atmospheric air.

Question 2.6 *What are the two differences that will be apparent?*

This volume of air in these airways is generally described as the 'anatomical dead space' ($V_{D_{anat}}$). This is because no gas exchange takes place, and so it represents wasted ventilation. The real situation is a little more complicated and is dealt with in Chapter 10 – 'The factors limiting maximal oxygen uptake'.

The pulmonary circulation

The oxygen molecule has now reached the point where gas exchange can take place between alveolar air and pulmonary blood. It is sensible at this point to introduce information regarding the pulmonary circulation (the systemic circulation will be discussed in detail in Chapter 5). The pulmonary circulation holds about 12 per cent of total blood volume. The four main blood vessels feeding the lungs are the left and right pulmonary arteries, carrying deoxygenated blood

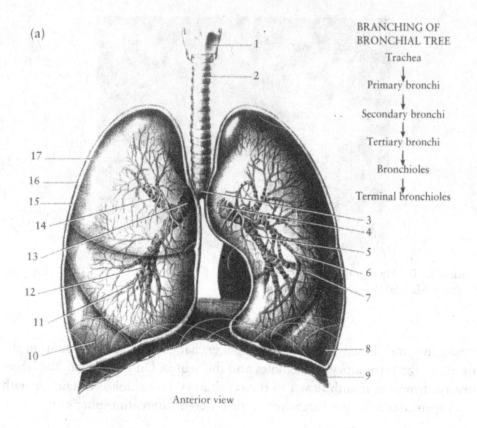

(a)

BRANCHING OF
BRONCHIAL TREE

Trachea
↓
Primary bronchi
↓
Secondary bronchi
↓
Tertiary bronchi
↓
Bronchioles
↓
Terminal bronchioles

Anterior view

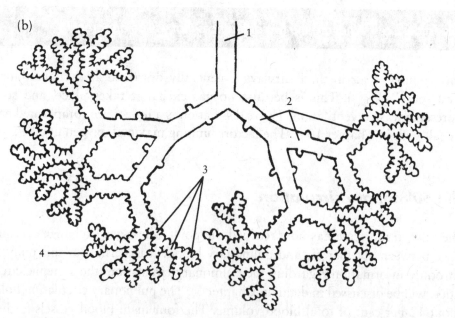

(b)

Figure 2.11 (a) General features of the lungs. (b) Diagrammatic representation of an acinus. (With permission (a) John Wiley & Sons, Ltd from the original in Tortura and Grabowski (2003); and (b) Dunsel, Paris. From the original in Cumming G, (1980))

from the right atrium, and the left and right pulmonary veins, returning the oxygen-enriched blood to the left side of the heart.

Question 2.7 *At this point it is appropriate to ask you to define arteries and veins.*

These major blood vessels branch into smaller arteries and veins leading eventually to the pulmonary capillary bed. The walls of the arteries and veins contain smooth muscle that regulates blood flow to the various regions of the lungs. The capillaries invade the lung tissue and wrap themselves around alveoli rather like a fine-meshed net; the walls consist of single endothelial cells that permit exchange of gases.

The position of the heart in relation to the lungs means that the force needed to propel blood through the pulmonary vascular bed is low; the mean pulmonary arterial pressure is about 12–15 mmHg (blood pressure measurements are invariably given in mmHg, not kPa). In the upright position at rest, cardiac output (Q_C), assisted by gravity, is distributed preferentially to the lower lobes of the lungs. This leads to a mismatch between ventilation and blood flow – and is described by the ventilation/perfusion ratio (V_A/Q). The upper regions of the lung are relatively well ventilated (hyperventilated) but poorly perfused (hypoperfused), and so the ratio is high ($V_A/Q > 3$), whereas the lower regions are well perfused, but relatively hypoventilated, so the ratio is low ($V_A/Q < 1$). During exercise, when blood flow through the pulmonary circulation increases, the increased pressure results in dilatation of the small arterioles. Adrenaline, released during exercise, also acts as a vasodilator and increases blood supply to the lung. Both of these responses mean that more blood is distributed to the upper regions of the lung, and there is a better match between ventilation and perfusion of the lung; however, it is important to realize that gas and blood are never perfectly matched across the entire lung.

Lung ventilation and gas transfer

Convection and diffusion

The physical process involved here is mass transport. Mass transport, can be subdivided into two differing physical processes. The first is convection, whereby air is moved from the atmosphere into and out of the branching airways of the lung via the action of the respiratory muscles; the second is diffusion, a process whereby atoms and molecules move from an area of high to an area of low concentration by thermal agitation. As inspired air approaches the respiratory bronchioles where gas exchange takes place, the number of airways, and more importantly their cumulative cross-sectional area, have increased substantially. This increase results in a progressively slower forward convective movement of the air, rather like the slowing flow rate of a river as it enters its delta. By the time the inspirate reaches the respiratory bronchioles the convective process has come to a halt. However, the oxygen concentration in the airways is higher than in the alveoli and the blood; thus, oxygen moves by diffusion from the respiratory bronchioles into the alveoli, and from the alveoli into the blood.

Before diffusion can occur there must be a difference in the concentration of a substance between two adjacent areas. Imagine a small water tank divided into two compartments by an impermeable but removable screen. One half contains pure water; in the other water has been coloured by a vivid red dye; a red dye concentration gradient exists between the two compartments. If the screen is removed the molecules of the red dye will diffuse down this concentration gradient until the entire tank contains an even distribution of the dye. A similar situation occurs if gases are used rather than water.

Five factors determine the rate of diffusion in the lung. They are

(a) the length of the diffusion pathway;

(b) the partial pressure gradient;

(c) the density of the gas;

(d) the solubility of the gas; and

(e) the thickness of the alveolar capillary membrane.

We know that the airways differ in length and diameter because of the process of asymmetric dichotomous branching. Indeed, one terminal bronchiole may appear after twelve branchings whilst another may occur after twice that number. So the time taken for a molecule of oxygen to reach the acinus will depend on the airway route taken.

Partial pressure

To understand the next part of the process we have to tackle the concept of the partial pressure of gases in a mixture. The actual calculation of the partial pressure of a gas is very simple. In a sample of fresh air at standard pressure of 101 kPa (760 mmHg), there are two main components: nitrogen and oxygen. Their respective fractions are 0.7904 and 0.2093. John Dalton, an English chemist, published his law of partial pressures in 1803; it says that *the pressure of a gas in a mixture is equal to the pressure it would exert if it occupied the same volume alone at the same temperature.*

The equation used to calculate the partial pressure of a gas (P_{GAS}) is the barometric pressure (P_B) multiplied by the gas fraction (F_{GAS}).

$$P_{GAS} = P_B \cdot F_{I\,GAS}$$

Take as an example a gas fraction of 0.1 (10 per cent) with a total pressure of 66.5 kPa (500 mmHg); the partial pressure of that gas is

$$P_{GAS} = 66.5 \cdot 0.1 = 6.65 \text{ kPa (50 mmHg)}$$

If the fraction was 0.9 (90 per cent)

$$P_{GAS} = 66.5 \cdot 0.9 = 59.85 \text{ kPa (450 mmHg)}$$

It is also important to become familiar with the symbols used in respiratory physiology; they represent a useful shorthand way of presenting information in reports and essays. When the gases are passing through the *lung*, upper-case symbols indicate alveolar (A) partial pressures i.e. P_{AO_2} and P_{ACO_2}. When the gases are carried in the *blood*, lower-case symbols indicate whether the partial pressures are those found in arterial (a) blood, i.e. P_{aO_2} and P_{aCO_2}, or venous (v) blood, i.e. P_{vO_2} and P_{vCO_2}.

Exercise 2.6

Given standard pressure of 101 kPa (760 mmHg) and oxygen, nitrogen and carbon dioxide concentrations of 0.2093, 0.7904 and 0.0003 respectively, calculate the partial pressures of each gas – P_{O_2}, P_{N_2}, P_{CO_2} – in the atmosphere. Calculate both kPa and mmHg units of measurement.

Now look at what happens to ambient partial pressures at the top of Everest. The P_B is 30.59 kPa (230 mmHg) but the gas concentrations remain unchanged.
What are the partial pressures now? Does the change in P_{O_2} suggest why exercising at altitude becomes more difficult?

Given the standard pressure of 101 kPa (760 mmHg) and an oxygen fraction of 0.2093, the partial pressure of oxygen in the atmosphere (P_{O_2amb}) is

$$P_B \times F_{IO_2} = 101 \text{ kPa} \times 0.2093 = 21.3 \text{ kPa}$$

$$P_B \times F_{IO_2} = 760 \text{ mmHg} \times 0.2093 = 159 \text{ mmHg}$$

The partial pressure of oxygen changes as the gas moves from the mouth to the alveoli. During its passage through the upper airways the air is warmed and moistened; this adds the additional factor of water vapour into the calculations. Normal body temperature is 37°C. At this temperature the water vapour content of the air exerts a pressure of 6.25 kPa (47 mmHg). As a result the partial pressure of oxygen in the trachea $P_{O_2\,trach}$ is reduced as follows:

$$(P_B - P_{H_2O}) \times F_{IO_2} = (101 - 6.25 \text{ kPa}) \times 0.2093 = 19.83 \text{ kPa}$$

$$(P_B - P_{H_2O}) \times F_{IO_2} = (760 - 47 \text{ mmHg}) \times 0.2093 = 149 \text{ mmHg}$$

This is the partial pressure of oxygen (P_{IO_2}) delivered to the respiratory bronchioles each inspiration.

As oxygen and carbon dioxide are in a state of continual exchange, the partial pressures of the two gases fluctuate over the course of a single breath. Within the alveoli, oxygen is diffusing into the blood and its concentration is constantly changing, so a precise alveolar partial pressure (P_{AO_2}) will depend on the point of the respiratory cycle at which we take the measurement. For example, if a sample is taken from the first 100 mL of the expirate, the oxygen concentration is found to be little different from atmospheric oxygen.

Question 2.8 *Explain this.*

On the other hand, if we take the sample from the last 100 mL of a deep exhalation – called the 'end-tidal' sample – the oxygen fraction lies somewhere between 0.14 (14 per cent) and 0.15 (15 per cent). This figure is representative of the oxygen in the alveoli and gives us a better idea of conditions deep within the lung.

Using 0.145 as an approximate end-tidal oxygen fraction, we calculate the alveolar partial pressure (P_{AO2}) in the usual way:

$$P_{AO_2} = (101-6.25 \text{ kPa}) \times 0.145 = 13.7 \text{ kPa}$$

$$= (760-47 \text{ mmHg}) \times 0.145 = 103 \text{ mmHg}$$

The difference in oxygen partial pressure (P_{O_2}) between the terminal bronchioles (19.8 kPa or 149 mmHg) and alveolar air (13.7 kPa or 103/104 mmHg) reveals a *pressure gradient* that leads to oxygen molecules diffusing from the alveolar duct into the alveoli.

The alveoli come into very close contact with the small blood vessels called capillaries. The wall of each structure is only one cell thick and this allows gases to diffuse through them easily. The blood returning to the lungs, called mixed venous blood ($\bar{v}$), has had some of its oxygen removed by the working cells of the body. The partial pressure of oxygen in resting venous blood, P_{VO_2}, reflects this and is usually about 5.3 kPa (40 mmHg). This means that the pressure gradient between the alveoli (13.7 kPa; 103/104 mmHg) and this oxygen-reduced blood (5.3 kPa; 40 mmHg) is very large (8.4 kPa, 63 mmHg). Oxygen diffusion down this pressure gradient results in a typical resting partial pressure of oxygen in arterial blood (P_{aO_2}) of 13.3 kPa (100 mmHg).

Question 2.9 *The difference between alveolar and arterial P_{O_2} is only 0.4 kPa (3 to 4 mmHg). What does this tell us about the membrane that separates the alveoli from the blood?*

Thus far the partial pressure of carbon dioxide has not been mentioned. The fraction of this gas in the atmosphere is very low, 0.0003, so its partial pressure in the terminal bronchioles is effectively zero. However, when considering partial pressure of the carbon dioxide in the alveoli (P_{ACO_2}) the picture changes. Carbon dioxide is a waste product of the breakdown of glucose and fats in the presence of oxygen at the muscle cell. It is carried in the blood to the lungs where it is continually diffusing into the alveoli and is excreted into the atmosphere during exhalation. Its fraction in the alveolar spaces is about 0.055 (5.5 per cent), so the P_{ACO_2} is calculated as

$$P_{ACO_2} = (101 - 6.25 \text{ kPa}) \times 0.055 = 5.3 \text{ kPa}$$

$$= (760 - 47 \text{ mmHg}) \times 0.055 = 40 \text{ mmHg}$$

The amount of carbon dioxide carried in the blood varies according to the level of activity being undertaken. At rest, its fraction in mixed venous blood ($P_{\bar{v}CO_2}$) is about 0.065 (6.5 per cent); the partial pressure therefore is

$$P_{\bar{v}CO_2} = (101-6.25 \text{ kPa}) \times 0.065 = 6.12 \text{ kPa}$$

$$= (760-47 \text{ mmHg}) \times 0.065 = 46 \text{ mmHg}$$

Here the pressure gradient from blood to the alveoli is less than 1 kPa (6 mmHg), but although much smaller than the gradient for oxygen, it is still sufficient for the carbon dioxide to diffuse into the alveoli and be excreted into the atmosphere. The explanation for the differences in pressure gradients between the atmosphere and the blood for the two gases is given below.

The importance of differences in partial pressure between the atmosphere and the blood for effective gas transfer to take place is evident from these calculations of partial pressures. However, *density* and *solubility* of gases also affect diffusion. In the lung, there are two phases; there is a gaseous phase in the acinus, and a liquid phase across the alveolar–capillary membrane. Oxygen and carbon dioxide behave differently in gaseous and liquid conditions. Thomas Graham, a Scottish physical chemist, reported in 1829 that *diffusion rates between two gases are inversely proportional to the square root of their densities*. Molecular oxygen is lighter than carbon dioxide; its molecular weight is 32 compared to 44 for carbon dioxide. The square roots of 32 and 44 are 5.6 and 6.6 respectively, so during the *gaseous* phase in the acinus oxygen diffuses slightly faster than carbon dioxide. However, the situation is reversed in the *liquid* phase. William Henry, an English chemist, published a law in 1803 dealing with the solubility of gases in liquids. The law says *the volume of gas carried by a given volume of a liquid is directly proportional to its partial pressure.*

Carbon dioxide is much more soluble in water than oxygen; its solubility is 0.59, whereas that of oxygen is 0.024. Thus, carbon dioxide diffuses faster than oxygen in the liquid that bathes the alveolar–capillary membrane. If the two laws are combined we see that relative rates for diffusion of the two gases are

$$\frac{\text{Diffusion rate for } CO_2}{\text{Diffusion rate for } O_2} = \frac{5.6}{6.6} \times \frac{0.59}{0.024} = \frac{20.9}{1}$$

Because carbon dioxide diffuses 21 times faster than oxygen, carbon dioxide excretion is never a problem for healthy lungs. However, during very heavy exercise the ability of the lungs to transfer oxygen to pulmonary blood does seem compromised for some athletes. This issue is discussed under the factors that limit maximal oxygen uptake in Chapter 10.

The mechanics of breathing

A healthy adult breathes somewhere between 14 000 and 15 000 times a day without conscious thought or effort. It is time to look at the mechanisms that drive this life-giving process. We deal first with the mechanics, then with the control of ventilation.

The lungs lie in the thoracic cavity. Each lung is covered with a continuous membrane, which also lines the chest wall, and is called the pleural sac. Air is drawn into the lung by a fall in pressure within the thorax, brought about by the action of the respiratory muscles. Two muscles are mainly involved. The first, the diaphragm, is a dome-shaped sheet of muscle separating the contents of the abdomen from the lungs and heart. This muscle flattens on contraction. The second, the external intercostal muscles, lift the ribs forwards and upwards. The combined action of these two muscle groups increases the volume of the thorax, producing a drop in intra-thoracic pressure that, providing the nose and mouth are not artificially blocked, draws in air from the atmosphere. Inspiration ends when stretch receptors in the lung send a signal to the respiratory centre to stop the two muscle groups from contracting further. The muscles relax and the thorax falls under its own weight, reducing its volume and pushing the air back into the atmosphere. At rest expiration is largely the result of passive recoil of the chest wall and diaphragm. This phenomenon is called the Breuer–Hering reflex. In some books, we find the names reversed, but Breuer was Hering's student, and it seems that it was the student rather than the supervisor who discovered the reflex; but as is sometimes the case even today, the supervisor seems to claim seniority! During heavy exercise, when the demands for oxygen intake and carbon dioxide excretion are increased, accessory muscles of respiration – mainly the scalene, pectoral and sterno-cleido-mastoid in inspiration, and the abdominal muscles and internal inter-costals during expiration – become increasingly active.

It is worth looking at the relationships between ventilation, respiratory frequency and mean tidal volume during the maximal oxygen uptake test (see Figure 2.12). None of them is rectilinear. There is a disproportionate increase in ventilation as exercise becomes more severe; this is the result of increasing frequency and an inverted-U-shaped tidal volume response.

In the drive to increase total ventilation, we sacrifice tidal volume for breath-

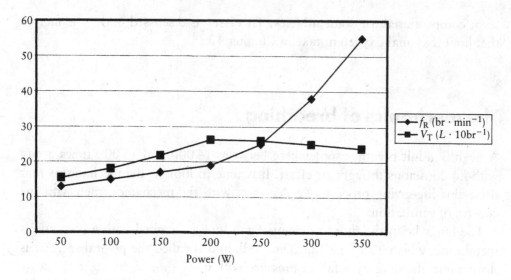

Figure 2.12 The relationships between power and tidal volume and respiratory frequency during progressive exercise

ing rate. This has a knock-on effect in terms of expired gas fractions. We might reasonably expect the respective gas fractions to mimic similar existing linear relationships between progressive exercise, oxygen uptake and carbon dioxide excretion. This is not the case, as Figure 2.13 shows.

There is a logical explanation to this apparent anomaly. Expired gas in the Douglas bags is a mixture consisting of air that does not take part in gas exchange – the dead space air (F_{IO_2} = 0.2093 (20.93 per cent) and negligible carbon dioxide) – and gas from the alveoli (e.g. F_{EO_2} = 0.15 (15 per cent), F_{ECO_2} = 0.06 (6 per cent)) where gas exchange has taken place. During exhalation, the dead space air dilutes the alveolar gas so that the Douglas bag gas fractions are roughly 0.17 (17 per cent) for oxygen and 0.035 (3.5 per cent) for carbon dioxide. In moderate exercise, the volumes of oxygen consumed and carbon dioxide excreted rise, and ventilation increases because of greater *tidal volumes* rather than faster breathing; the gas fractions change in line with our expectations – oxygen *falls* carbon dioxide *increases*. In severe exercise, there is a disproportionate increase in ventilation because of increased *breathing frequency* and falling tidal volumes. This leads not only to larger expired dead space volumes but also to more of them per unit time. The increased total dead space volume is sufficient to dilute the alveolar gas, resulting in *rising* oxygen and *falling* carbon dioxide fractions.

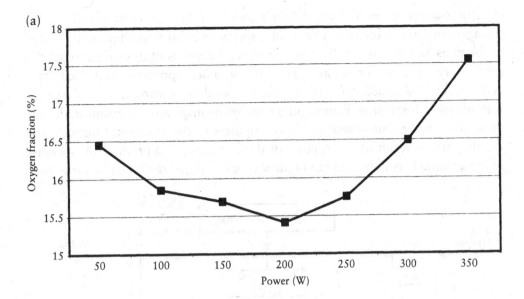

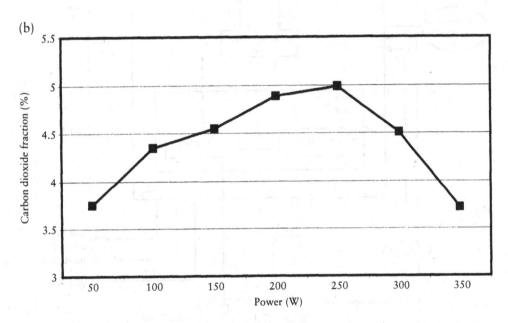

Figure 2.13 The response of gas fractions to progressive exercise. (a) Oxygen fraction. (b) Carbon dioxide fraction

Control of ventilation

The nervous control of breathing is still not entirely understood. It is clear that the primary function of the lungs is the maintenance of adequate levels of oxygen to support metabolism and the removal of the waste product of aerobic metabolism, carbon dioxide. The main respiratory control mechanism is located in the pons and medulla of the lower brain and consists of three interconnected respiratory centres. These are the pneumotaxic, apneustic and medullary centres; the last-named consists of separate bundles of inspiratory and expiratory neurons. Inspiration is brought about by the inspiratory neurons under the control of the apneustic centre. Nerve impulses to the intercostal muscles and the diaphragm result in contraction of these muscles and produce the increase in intra-thoracic volume and fall in intra-thoracic pressure that cause air to rush

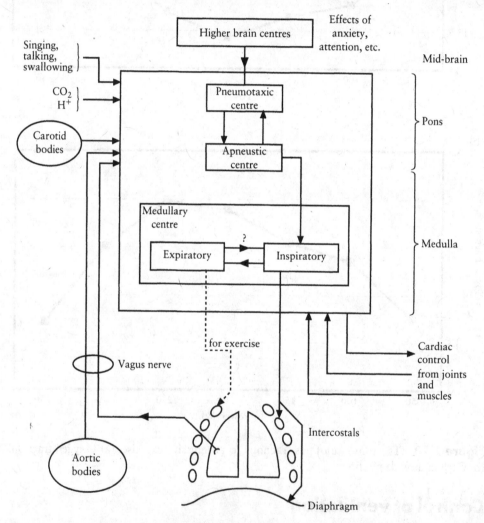

Figure 2.14 Schematic representation of the neural mechanisms controlling lung function. (With permission of the Open University – The Human Respiratory System (T241 13/14) Systems Behaviour Module 7 (1973))

into the lungs. Impulses from the inspiratory neurons are also transmitted to the pneumotaxic centre; as the lungs inflate, signals from stretch receptors embedded in the lung tissue are sent via the vagus nerve to this centre. At the peak of the inspiratory movement signals from the pneumotaxic centre to the apneustic centre bring about a cessation of activity from the inspiratory neurons. Inspiration stops and expiration occurs passively. The expiratory neurons only come into play during exercise when forced expiration is necessary to maintain lung ventilation (see Figure 2.14).

The respiratory centres are continually bombarded with information from several regions of the body. Ventilation increases immediately at, and often even before, the start of exercise. In the latter case, the anticipatory increase is almost certainly produced under impulses from higher-brain activity as breathing is under a degree of voluntary control. The increase at the commencement of exercise is too sudden to be the result of changes in blood gases, and is thought to originate from impulses from stretch receptors in the exercising joints and muscles.

Two other important sensors are located in two major blood vessels, namely the aorta and the carotid artery. These aortic and carotid bodies detect changes in the partial pressure of oxygen and are stimulated at altitude. Other receptors located in the lower brain are sensitive to two things; first the hydrogen ion concentration $[H^+]$ – that is changes in the level of acid – in the blood and cerebrospinal fluid; and second the partial pressure of carbon dioxide in the blood. These chemoreceptors are especially stimulated during strenuous exercise.

Exercise 2.7

Consider the following data arising from a set of experiments using a spirometer.

Experiment 1
The spirometer is filled with fresh air. The subject is asked to breathe into and out of it for several minutes. The gas concentrations are continually monitored. At the start of the experiment, V_T is 600 mL per breath and f_R is 12 min^{-1}. Over 10–15 minutes, both volume and frequency increase until breathing becomes laboured and V_T and f_R are doubled. The O_2 and CO_2 fractions are now 0.12 (12 per cent) and 0.08 (8 per cent) respectively. What explanations can you give for the increase in ventilation?

Experiment 2

The spirometer now is filled with medical grade oxygen and the experiment repeated. The results are very similar to those recorded in Experiment 1, except that oxygen fraction is now 0.60 (60 per cent). How do you explain these increases in V_{VT} and f_R?

Suppose you wanted to test your explanations knowing that a substance that removed carbon dioxide from the expired air was available. What experiment would you conduct? What would the gas concentrations be at the end of your experiment? What have these experiments shown?

Key points

- The primary function of the lung is the exchange of oxygen and carbon dioxide.

- Contraction of the diaphragm and internal intercostal muscles produces a fall in intra-thoracic pressure resulting in inspiration.

- Expiration is passive, except during exercise when accessory muscles of respiration (abdominal and external intercostals) are used.

- The upper airways consist mainly of cartilage with some smooth muscle.

- The smaller airways contain mainly smooth muscle that can change the diameter of the airways.

- The functional unit of the lung is the acinus, consisting of alveolar ducts, alveolar sacs and alveoli.

- Gas *transport* is by convection and diffusion (mass transport) via the system of branching airways; gas *exchange* takes place via diffusion.

- Diffusion rate is affected by (a) the diffusion pathway length; (b) the concentration gradient; (c) the density and solubility of a gas; and (d) the thickness of the alveolar capillary membrane.

- During exercise, the respiratory centres in the lower pons and medulla of the brain receive stimuli from joints and muscles, the blood, and the cerebrospinal fluid.

- These stimuli lead to increases in respiratory rate and tidal volume.

- Even at maximal exercise, tidal volume never reaches the level of an individual's vital capacity.

Answers to questions in the text

Question 2.1
Remember that

$$\dot{V}_E L \cdot \text{min}^{-1} = \overline{V}_T L \cdot f_R \text{br} \cdot \text{min}^{-1}$$

Multiply the mean tidal volume by respiratory frequency over 60 s, or simply sum the peaks of individual tidal volumes over 60 s.

Question 2.2
As tidal volumes increase, the inspiratory and expiratory reserve volumes fall along with functional residual capacity. Given a vital capacity of $4\,L$ and a resting tidal volume of $600\,mL$, the ratio of tidal volume to vital capacity (V_T/VC) is $0.6/4.0 = 0.15$. During strenuous exercise, the vital capacity remains unchanged, but tidal volumes can reach $3\,L$; thus, the ratio now is $3/4 = 0.75$. Because of the drive to increase respiratory frequency, it is difficult for tidal volume to ever take up all of the vital capacity of the lung.

Question 2.3
The short answer is that volumes will increase.

Mexico City lies some 2300 m (7500 ft) above sea level where the barometric pressure is about 73 kPa (550 mmHg). If the original $\dot{V}_{E\,\text{BTPS}} = 10\,L \cdot \text{min}^{-1}$, body temperature is 37°C and sea level pressure is 101 kPa (760 mmHg) we can use the gas laws of Boyle and Charles–Gay-Lussac to see how altitude affects volume as follows. The combined gas laws look like this

$$\frac{P_1 \cdot V_1}{T_1} = \frac{P_2 \cdot V_2}{T_2}$$

The left-hand side of the equation holds the sea level data; the right-hand side the data at Mexico City

$$\frac{101.1 \cdot 10}{37} = \frac{73 \cdot V_2}{37}$$

Rearranging to give V_2 we get

$$\frac{101.1 \cdot 10 \cdot 37}{37 \cdot 73} = 13.9 \ L \cdot min^{-1}$$

The volume has increased from 10 to almost 14 $L \cdot min^{-1}$. The pressure at the top of Everest is 30 kPa (230 mmHg). You can do your own calculations to see the change in volume.

Question 2.4

Pressure fluctuates, sometimes on an hourly basis. The pressure recorded at the start of an experiment will not necessarily remain constant throughout it.

Question 2.5

As the temperature of the expirate cools, its volume falls.

Core body temperature is 37°C, but the temperature of the outer shell is about 35°C. In air-conditioned laboratories, ambient temperature is usually set at about 20°C. Thus, expired air in the Douglas bag begins to lose heat to the atmosphere as soon as it is expired. If you want to know the volume of air in the lungs then you have to use the equation that adjusts volumes at ambient temperature and pressure saturated with water vapour (ATPS) to body temperature and pressure saturated (BTPS). Ultimately, all volumes will be reduced to standard temperature and pressure, dry (STPD).

Question 2.6

Inspired air is warmed and moistened as it passes through the upper airways. In the trachea, the temperature will equal core body temperature, i.e. 37°C. At that temperature, water vapour is added to the nitrogen, oxygen, and carbon dioxide inhaled and so has to be included in the calculation of partial pressures of the various gases. The partial pressure of water vapour at body temperature is equivalent to 6.3 kPa (47 mmHg), and this figure must be subtracted from the ambient pressure to give the partial pressures of the remaining gases. Thus, the partial pressure of atmospheric oxygen at standard temperature (0°C) and pressure (101.1 kPa (760 mmHg)) dry is its fraction multiplied by its pressure, i.e.

$$P_{O_2amb} = 0.2093 \cdot 101.1 \text{ kPa (760 mmHg)} = 21.2 \text{ kPa (159.1 mmHg)}$$

In the trachea at body temperature and 101.1 kPa (760 mmHg) the partial pressure of oxygen is

$$P_{O_2 \text{trach}} = 0.2093 \cdot (101.1 - 6.3 \text{ kPa})(760 - 47 \text{ mmHg}) = 19.84 \text{ kPa} (149.2 \text{ mmHg})$$

So the effective oxygen partial pressure has fallen without any uptake of oxygen by the blood.

Question 2.7

Arteries are vessels that carry blood away from the heart, whereas veins carry blood to the heart. Confusion sometimes occurs when we talk about oxygenated blood carried by arteries and de-oxygenated blood carried by veins. This is true of the systemic circulation, but not of the pulmonary circulation. In the latter case the pulmonary artery carries deoxygenated blood from the right side of the heart, and the pulmonary veins carry oxygenated blood to the left side.

Question 2.8

In normal breathing, the oxygen fraction of the air in the dead space is identical with that of the atmosphere. Because the dead space air is contained within the convective zone, no gas exchange takes place because there are no alveoli on the walls of the airways. However, the volume of the dead space diminishes during breath-holding. This occurs because at the boundary of the convective and diffusive zones time is available for diffusion to take place between the fresh air inhaled and the gas in the alveoli that is low in oxygen.

Question 2.9

The small difference between alveolar gas and oxygenated blood flowing into the pulmonary veins indicates a very efficient gas exchange mechanism. Given the thickness of the alveolar–capillary membrane, this efficiency is remarkable. During severe exercise the arterial partial pressure of oxygen falls, possibly because the transit time of the red blood cell through the lung is too quick for equilibration between alveolar and pulmonary blood to take place. In conditions like fibrosing alveolitis and pulmonary oedema where the thickness of the alveolar–capillary barrier is increased, gas exchange is compromised, sometimes fatally so.

Answers to exercises in the text

Exercise 2.1

(a) Tidal volume (V_T) increases.

(b) Respiratory frequency (f_R) increases.

(c) Inspiratory reserve volume (V_{IR}) decreases.

(d) Expiratory reserve volume (V_{ER}) decreases.

(e) Functional residual capacity (FRC) decreases.

(f) Residual volume (V_{Res}) remains unchanged.

(g) Vital capacity (VC) remains unchanged.

(h) Total lung capacity (TLC) remains unchanged.

At rest, the FRC acts as a buffer between the air in the lungs and inhaled air. Increased tidal volumes result in a reduced FRC, with higher oxygen partial pressure in the alveoli.

Exercise 2.2

Check these results with the predictions you made in Exercise 2.1. Look at the tidal volume/vital capacity ratios. Now look at Figure 2.12 and see how tidal volume actually declines as we approach volitional exhaustion.

Variable	Units	Symbol	Resting values	Exercise 1	Exercise 2
Vital capacity	L	VC	4.800	4.800	4.800
Residual volume	L	RV	1.200	1.200	1.200
Total lung capacity	L	TLC	6.000	6.000	6.000
Inspiratory capacity	L	IC	3.600	3.600	3.600
Mean tidal volume	L	$\bar{V}_T$	0.750	1.250	1.925
Functional residual capacity	L	FRC	3.000	2.765	2.660
Inspiratory reserve volume	L	IRV	2.250	1.985	1.415
Expiratory reserve volume	L	ERV	1.800	1.565	1.460
Minute volume	$L \cdot min^{-1}$	$\dot{V}_E$	6.25	18.750	51.975
Respiratory frequency	$br \cdot min^{-1}$	f_R	8	15	27

Exercise 2.3

The normal subject is trace is (a). The lung function of the asthma sufferer is trace (b); the key indicators here are FVC, $FEV_{1.0}$ and Peak Expiratory Flow values which represent 24, 60 and 35 per cent of the population average. The lung function of the athlete is trace (c); here, the $FEV_{1.0}$ and FVC values are 127 and 124 per cent respectively of the population average. Training that involves sustained, strenuous exercise results in increased ventilation over substantial periods. This, in turn, leads to an improved respiratory muscle function that is lacking in untrained populations from which the predicted values are usually derived.

The actual data are given in the following table.

		Normal	Population norm (%)	Asthmatic	Population norm (%)	Athlete	Population norm (%)
FVC	L	3.62	101	2.67	60	4.59	127
$FEV_{1.0}$	L	2.91	102	0.87	24	3.89	124
$FEV_{1.0}/FVC$	%	80	100	33	42	85	103
PEF	$L \cdot min^{-1}$	454	105	183	35	489	115

Exercise 2.4

ATPS to BTPS

Converting volumes from ATPS to BTPS means that volumes will *increase* because in this example *temperature* and *water vapour tension* have increased; the volume increase is 8.72 litres.

$$\dot{V}_{E\,BTPS} = \dot{V}_{E\,ATPS} \cdot \frac{273 + \text{body temp}}{273 + \text{ambient temp}} \cdot \frac{P_B - \text{ambient } P_{H_2O}}{P_B - P_{H_2O} \text{ at body temp}}$$

$$= 100 \cdot \frac{273 + 37}{273 + 23} \cdot \frac{97.1 - 2.79}{97.1 - 6.25} \text{ kPa}$$

$$= 100 \cdot \frac{273 + 37}{273 + 23} \cdot \frac{730 - 21 \text{ mmHg}}{730 - 47} \text{ mmHg}$$

$$= \underline{108.72\ L \cdot min^{-1}}$$

ATPS to STPD

Converting volumes from ATPS to STPD means that volumes will *decrease* because in this example *temperature* and *water vapour tension* have decreased, and *pressure* has increased; the volume decrease is 13.96 litres

$$\dot{V}_{E\,STPD} = \dot{V}_{E\,ATPS} \cdot \frac{273}{273 + T_{amb}} \cdot \frac{P_B - \text{ambient } P_{H_2O}}{P_{Standard}}$$

$$= 100 \cdot \frac{273}{273 + 23} \cdot \frac{97.1 - 2.79 \text{ kPa}}{101.1} \text{ or } 100 \cdot \frac{273}{273 + 23} \cdot \frac{730 - 21}{760} \text{ mmHg}$$

$$= \underline{86.04\ L \cdot min^{-1}}$$

Exercise 2.5

(a)

1 = larynx; 2 = trachea; 3 = carina; 4 = left primary bronchus; 5 = left secondary bronchus; 6 = left tertiary bronchus; 7 = bronchiole; 8 = terminal bronchiole; 9 = diaphragm; 10 = terminal bronchiole; 11 = bronchiole; 12 = right tertiary bronchus;

13 = right primary bronchus; 14 = right secondary bronchus; 15 = pleural cavity; 16 = parietal pleura; 17 = visceral pleura.

(b)
1 = terminal bronchiole; 2 = respiratory bronchiole; 3 = alveolar ducts; 4 = alveoli.

Exercise 2.6

The partial pressure of any gas is the gas fraction multiplied by the ambient pressure

$$P_{GAS} = P_{B\,amb} \cdot F_{GAS}$$

Thus, at sea level

$$P_{O_2} = 101.1 \cdot 0.2093 = 21.2 \text{ kPa} \quad \text{or} \quad 760 \cdot 0.2093 = 159.1 \text{ mmHg}$$

$$P_{N_2} = 101.1 \cdot 0.7904 = 79.9 \text{ kPa} \quad \text{or} \quad 760 \cdot 0.7904 = 600.7 \text{ mmHg}$$

$$P_{CO_2} = 101.1 \cdot 0.0003 = 0.03 \text{ kPa} \quad \text{or} \quad 760 \cdot 0.0003 = 0.228 \text{ mmHg}$$

At the top of Everest, however

$$P_{O_2} = 30.59 \cdot 0.2093 = 6.4 \text{ kPa} \quad \text{or} \quad 230 \cdot 0.2093 = 48.1 \text{ mmHg}$$

$$P_{N_2} = 30.59 \cdot 0.7904 = 24.2 \text{ kPa} \quad \text{or} \quad 230 \cdot 0.7904 = 181.8 \text{ mmHg}$$

$$P_{CO_2} = 30.59 \cdot 0.0003 = 0.01 \text{ kPa} \quad \text{or} \quad 230 \cdot 0.0003 = 0.07 \text{ mmHg}$$

The very low ambient partial pressure of oxygen means that oxygen saturation (S_{aO_2}) and oxygen content (C_{aO_2}) are very low. Unacclimatized individuals would not survive without supplemental oxygen. The first successful ascent of Everest in 1953 was oxygen-assisted. Subsequent successful ascents have been made without oxygen.

Exercise 2.7

Experiment 1
It looks as if the increases in tidal volume and respiratory frequency are due either to a shortage of oxygen, or an excess of carbon dioxide, or a combination of the two. However, given the data provided we cannot be sure where the responsibility lies. Let us remind ourselves what has happened during the experiment.

The subject inspires from and expires into the spirometer; in other words, this is a closed system. Over time, the subject consumes oxygen at the rate of about $0.25 \ L \cdot min^{-1}$, and produces carbon dioxide at the rate of about $0.2 \ L \cdot min^{-1}$. The result is inhaling of gradually falling oxygen and gradually increasing carbon dioxide fractions. The final partial pressures of the two gases in the spirometer, assuming standard pressure, are

$P_{O_2} = (101.1 - 6.25) \cdot 0.12 = \underline{11.4 \text{ kPa}}$ or $(760 - 47) \cdot 0.12 = \underline{85.6 \text{ mmHg}}$

$P_{CO_2} = (101.1 - 6.25) \cdot 0.12 = \underline{7.6 \text{ kPa}}$ or $(760 - 47) \cdot 0.08 = \underline{57.0 \text{ mmHg}}$

compared to the normal values of 21.2 kPa (159.1) for oxygen and 0.03 kPa (0.23 mmHg) for carbon dioxide. The lower oxygen partial pressure, raised partial pressure of carbon dioxide, and increased acidity of the blood will be detected by the aortic and carotid bodies. The sensors in the respiratory centres in the medulla oblongata will also detect changes in the acidity of the cerebrospinal fluid. Tidal volume and respiratory frequency will be affected, but we cannot say which stimulus has the greater effect.

Experiment 2

The situation is now changed because during the entire experiment the subject is never short of oxygen. Indeed, when the experiment ends because of subject distress, the oxygen concentration in the spirometer is over three times the normal inspired oxygen concentration.

$P_{O_2} = P_{O_2} = (101.1 - 6.25) \cdot 0.60 = \underline{56.9 \text{ kPa}}$ or $(760 - 47) \cdot 0.60 = \underline{427.8 \text{ mmHg}}$

The carbon dioxide concentration however is similar to that of Experiment 1. This suggests that carbon dioxide is the major stimulus of ventilatory control. This suggestion is reinforced by research that has shown that, at rest, the partial pressure of oxygen in the atmosphere needs to fall to about 8 kPa (60 mmHg) before oxygen lack stimulates increased tidal volume and respiratory frequency.

3 Oxygen Content of the Blood

Learning Objectives

By the end of this chapter, you should be able to

♦ evaluate a blood profile in relation to normal values of RBC count, Hb content, WBC count and Hct

♦ describe the main functions of blood and its principal constituents

♦ outline the production and destruction of erythrocytes, and the structure of haemoglobin

♦ apply Henry's law to oxygen carriage in the plasma

♦ explain the differences between haemoglobin and myoglobin

♦ distinguish between oxygen capacity, content and saturation

♦ explain the benefits of the sigmoid nature of the oxyhaemoglobin dissociation curve for oxygen carriage by the blood

♦ describe the effects of changes in body temperature, P_{CO_2}, pH, and 2,3-diphosphoglycerate content on oxygen carriage by the blood

Exercise Physiology: A Thematic Approach   Tudor Hale
© John Wiley & Sons, Ltd   ISBN: 0 470 84682 8 (cloth), ISBN 0 470 84683 6 (pbk)

Objective test

Say whether the following answers are true (T) or false (F). If you do not know, say so (D) – not knowing is not an academic crime, but not finding out is. Try not to look at the answers until you have worked your way through the chapter and completed the test a second time. In this way you can monitor your progress.

	Pre-test			Post-test		
	T	F	D	T	F	D
1. Average blood volume is roughly equal to 20% of body mass						
2. On average men have a slightly greater blood volume than women						
3. The main component of blood is water						
4. Plasma makes up 75% of the blood						
5. Blood is a slightly acid fluid						
6. The pH of blood is 7.0						
7. Red blood cells (erythrocytes) are produced in the bone marrow						
8. Red blood cells contain nuclei						
9. Erythropoietin stimulates red blood cell production						
10. The average life span of a red blood cell is about 120 days						
11. Haemoglobin (Hb) is the main constituent of white blood cells						
12. Normal Hb values for men lie between 120 and 150 $g \cdot L_{bl}^{-1}$						
13. Normal Hb values for women lie between 140 and 170 $g \cdot L_{bl}^{-1}$						
14. The haematocrit (Hct) is the ratio between the RBC and plasma						

	Pre-test			Post-test		
	T	F	D	T	F	D
15. High white blood cell (WBC) may indicate some kind of infection						
16. Oxygen dissolves easily in the plasma						
17. 2.7 mLO_2 are dissolved per litre of blood at P_{O_2} 13.3 kPa (100 mmHg)						
18. Haemoglobin (Hb) is the main oxygen carrier in the blood						
19. Myoglobin (Mgb) is the main oxygen reserve in muscles						
20. Adult Hb consists of amino acids, a haem group and an iron atom						
21. The O_2 molecule attaches itself to the protein globin						
22. The relationship between Hb and O_2 is a rectilinear curve						
23. This curve, called the oxyhaemoglobin dissociation curve, is fixed						
24. When fully saturated a gram of Hb can combine with 1.34 mLO_2						
25. At rest Hb is about 97% saturated with O_2 when it leaves the lungs						
26. At rest Hb is about 75% saturated when it returns to the lungs						
27. The Hb–O_2 curve is affected by CO_2, temperature and blood acidity						
28. If the curve shifts to the right the Hb affinity for O_2 is increased						
29. Rises in P_{CO_2}, and body temperature result in less O_2 being released						
30. As blood pH falls less O_2 is being released						

Symbols, abbreviations and units of measurement

acidity/alkalinity	pH	
blood	bl	
diffusing capacity of the lung	D_L	
erythropoietin	EPO	
haematocrit	Hct	%
haemoglobin	Hb	$g \cdot L_{bl}^{-1}; g \cdot dL_{bl}^{-1}$
inspired oxygen fraction	F_{IO_2}	
maximal oxygen uptake	$\dot{V}_{O_2max}$	$mL \cdot min^{-1}; L \cdot min^{-1}$
myoglobin	Mgb	
oxygen content of blood	C_{O_2}	$mLO_2 \cdot L_{bl}^{-1}$
oxygen content of arterial blood	C_{aO_2}	$mLO_2 \cdot L_{bl}^{-1}$
oxygen content of venous blood	C_{VO_2}	$mLO_2 \cdot L_{bl}^{-1}$
partial pressure of oxygen	P_{O_2}	kPa; mmHg
partial pressure of carbon dioxide	P_{CO_2}	kPa; mmHg
red blood cell, erythrocyte	RBC	mm^3
saturation	S	%
saturation of arterial blood with oxygen	S_{aO_2}	%
saturation of blood with oxygen	S_{O_2}	%
saturation of venous blood with oxygen	S_{VO_2}	%
white blood cell	WBC	mm^3
2,3-diphosphoglycerate	2,3-DPG	

Introduction

We have now reached the final point of the gas *transfer* process. The oxygen molecule has been drawn into the lungs by an increase in thoracic volume and a fall in intra-thoracic pressure brought about by the actions of the respiratory muscles. It has diffused down the acinus and across the alveolar–capillary membrane and has entered the capillary blood of the pulmonary circulation. The rest of this chapter is concerned with factors that affect the oxygen content of the blood.

Oxygen is carried in the blood in two ways. The first is dissolved in the water of the plasma. The second, and much more important, is in chemical combination with haemoglobin in the red cells. But before we consider these two processes, we need to know something about blood and its constituents and discuss the information contained in the results of the blood profile test given before the maximal oxygen uptake ($\dot{V}_{O_2 max}$) test.

The blood profile

The main functions of blood are as follows: transporting oxygen, nutrients and hormones to working tissues; removing waste products to the lungs and the kidneys; assisting in regulating body temperature over a fairly narrow range; providing protection, in combination with the body's immune system, against infectious diseases; and assisting in maintaining fluid and salt balance.

Blood

Blood consists of two components – liquids and solids – and is slightly alkaline.

Question 3.1   *What is the measure of acidity/alkalinity?*

The liquid compartment contains dissolved proteins, glucose, lipids, vitamins, enzymes, hormones, immune bodies and inorganic materials such as sodium, potassium, calcium and phosphate. The dissolved materials and water – the dominant material (about 92 per cent) – make up the plasma, a pale straw-coloured fluid. Suspended in the plasma are the solids – red cells, white cells and platelets. Average blood volume is roughly 8 per cent of body mass, so the standard adult male of 70 kg has an average blood volume of about 5.5 litres; women being generally smaller have slightly smaller blood volumes. The typical resting pH of the blood is about 7.4.

The blood profile (Figure 3.1), obtained during the screening process for a maximal test, provides information on four main components of the individual's blood. The first is the number of red blood cells (RBC).

Erythrocytes (red blood cells)

Red blood cells are not true cells because in humans they do not contain a nucleus; it is more accurate to call them erythrocytes. They develop in the bone

HAEMATOLOGY — COULTER PART No. 9920060F — COULTER ELECTRONICS LTD., LUTON, BEDS., ENGLAND

TEST: ☐ CBC   PROFILE: ☐ WBC ☐ RBC

REQ'D BY: DATE:
PERFORMED BY: DATE:

TEST NO:

		NORMAL RANGE
6.0	WBC × 10⁹/L	M/F 3·6-9·6
5.5	RBC × 10¹²/L	M 4·5-6·3 / F 4-2·5·4
15.0	Hb g/dL	M 14-18 / F 12-16
45.	Hct Ratio	M 38-52 / F 36-46
.	MCV fL	M/F 82-97
.	MCH pg	M/F 27-33
.	MCHC g/dL	M/F 32-36

WHITE CELLS: Segs, Bands, Eos, Basos, Lymphs, Monos, Atyp. Lym., Imm. Gran. / % Blasts, Other
RBC SIZE: Norm, Micro, Macro
RBC COLOUR: Norm, Hypo, Poly
RBC SHAPE: Norm, Poik
PLATELETS Inc. Nml. Dec / Appear
NRBC/100 WBC   Plt.Est. x10⁹/L
WBC Est. x 10⁹/L   TEST NO.
Review Code
COMMENTS:
COULTER COUNTER® MODEL M₊30. S₊60, S:70. DEC 86 (NOT FOR USE IN THE U.S.A. OR POSSESSIONS)

HAEMATOLOGY — COULTER PART No. 9920060F — COULTER ELECTRONICS LTD., LUTON, BEDS., ENGLAND

TEST: ☐ CBC   PROFILE: ☐ WBC ☐ RBC

REQ'D BY: DATE:
PERFORMED BY: DATE:

TEST NO:

		NORMAL RANGE
10.3	WBC × 10⁹/L	M/F 3·6-9·6
6.5	RBC × 10¹²/L	M 4·5-6·3 / F 4-2·5·4
18.0	Hb g/dL	M 14-18 / F 12-16
53.	Hct Ratio	M 38-52 / F 36-46
.	MCV fL	M/F 82-97
.	MCH pg	M/F 27-33
.	MCHC g/dL	M/F 32-36

(Same cell fields as above)
COULTER COUNTER® MODEL M₊30. S₊60, S:70. DEC 86 (NOT FOR USE IN THE U.S.A. OR POSSESSIONS)

HAEMATOLOGY — COULTER PART No. 9920060F — COULTER ELECTRONICS LTD., LUTON, BEDS., ENGLAND

TEST: ☐ CBC   PROFILE: ☐ WBC ☐ RBC

REQ'D BY: DATE:
PERFORMED BY: DATE:

TEST NO:

		NORMAL RANGE
9.0	WBC × 10⁹/L	M/F 3·6-9·6
4.5	RBC × 10¹²/L	M 4·5-6·3 / F 4-2·5·4
12.	Hb g/dL	M 14-18 / F 12-16
37.	Hct Ratio	M 38-52 / F 36-46
.	MCV fL	M/F
.	MCH pg	M/F 27-33
.	MCHC g/dL	M/F 32-36

(Same cell fields as above)
COULTER COUNTER® MODEL M₊30. S₊60, S:70. DEC 86 (NOT FOR USE IN THE U.S.A. OR POSSESSIONS)

Figure 3.1 Typical outputs from standard blood profile tests using a Coulter counter. (The data, in descending order, are WBC, RBC, Hb and Hct)

marrow of large flat bones like the skull and pelvis, and in the ends of long bones like the femur. There are four stages in erythrocyte production; it begins with a large immature cell, called an erythroblast, containing a nucleus but no haemoglobin. During the next two stages the erythroblast changes to a normoblast and then a reticulocyte; the cell becomes progressively smaller, its nucleus degenerates, and haemoglobin begins to appear. The final stage is the erythrocyte packed with haemoglobin and lacking a nucleus. The process is stimulated by the hormone erythropoietin (EPO), produced mainly by the kidneys in response to low partial pressures of oxygen.

Erythrocytes take the form of discs with concave surfaces. As they are only about 7 micrometres (μm) in diameter – 1 μm is a thousandth of a millimetre – and flexible they are able to pass through the capillaries of the circulatory system. Men have between 5.0 and 5.5 million and women between 4.5 and 5.0 million erythrocytes in 1 microlitre (μL) of blood. Subjects with a low red blood cell count may be anaemic and haemoglobin levels should be checked to confirm this. A lack of vitamins B_{12} and folic acid in the diet, or their inadequate take-up in the digestive tract leads to immature erythrocyte production. This results in fragile membranes that break up readily, leading to poor oxygen-carrying capacity.

> **Question 3.2** *Can you work out the total number of circulating erythrocytes in the average man and woman? Remember, there are 1000 μL in 1 mL, and 1000 mL in a litre.*

Erythrocytes age, have an average life span of about 120 days, and production is a continuous process at a rate of something approaching 140 million every minute. In the mature state the erythrocytes have no nucleus and so repair processes necessary for survival and optimal functioning cannot take place. Over time the wear and tear of being driven down arteries and veins, sometimes at high speeds, and of being squeezed through the capillaries of the circulatory system lead to protein loss and failing biochemical activity. The erythrocytes absorb water, become spherical in shape, are captured and digested by phagocytes, and finally destroyed in the liver and spleen. However, the important material is not lost as the proteins are re-synthesized, and iron is stored in bone marrow for future use in erythrocyte production. It is thought that in endurance athletes in particular the erythrocyte life cycle may be shortened in response to the punishing training programmes undertaken by these athletes.

Haemoglobin

The second element concerns the measurement of haemoglobin (Hb), the main constituent of the erythrocyte. The normal value for men ranges between 140 and 170 g $\cdot$ L_{bl}^{-1}, and for women between 120 and 150 g $\cdot$ L_{bl}^{-1}. Haemoglobin consists of the protein globin, bonded to which are four chains of amino acids each leading to a haem group and an atom of iron. In normal adult haemoglobin the four amino acid chains are made up of two identical alpha (α) chains of

141 amino acids, and two identical beta (β) chains of 146 amino acids. The four iron atoms serve as the oxygen-binding sites. Haemoglobin deficiency results in anaemia and may be particularly problematic for endurance athletes. Indeed the anaemic endurance athlete seems to be a contradiction in terms, because decreased levels of haemoglobin result in reduced oxygen-carrying capacity of the blood. However, there is evidence from a study of elite Swedish endurance athletes of fairly low (143 gHb $\cdot$ L_{bl}^{-1}) haemoglobin levels. The most common source of low haemoglobin levels is an iron deficiency in the diet, but inadequate intake of the vitamin B complex is also a factor.

The haematocrit

Thirdly, we obtain the ratio of erythrocytes to plasma, known as the haematocrit (Hct), by centrifuging a blood sample. During this process the heavier erythrocytes are forced to the bottom of the tube whilst the plasma floats on top. Between the two is a small layer, known as the buffy coat, consisting of white cells and platelets (Figure 3.2).

Haematocrit values for men lie between 42 and 52 per cent, and for women between 36 and 46 per cent. A high value may indicate a transient shift of fluid from the blood following exercise, some level of dehydration, a very recent blood transfusion as in blood doping (i.e. within 24 hours), or high levels of erythropoietin, a precursor for erythrocyte production.

Question 3.3　*What condition would result in a low Hct? Can you think of three conditions that are likely to stimulate production of red blood cells?*

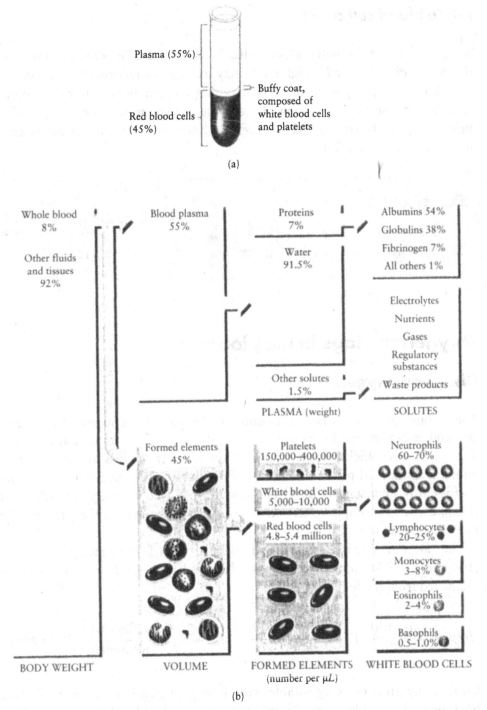

Figure 3.2 The major blood components (a) after separation by a centrifuge; (b) erythrocytes (red blood cells) and leukocytes (white blood cells). (With permission of John Wiley & Sons, Ltd from the original in Tortura and Grabowski (2003))

White blood cell count

Finally, we count the white blood cells. Typical values lie between 5000 and 10 000 per microlitre (μL); high levels may indicate some form of infection and should lead to postponement of a maximal oxygen uptake test. Strenuous exercise can result in a doubling of the white cell count, hence blood profiling must take place before the maximal test and preferably at least 24 hours after any preceding exercise bouts.

Exercise 3.1

You are now in a position to evaluate the blood profiles shown in Figure 3.1. Are they normal? What might be an explanation for any abnormalities?

Oxygen carriage in the blood

Dissolved oxygen

The amount of a gas carried in solution in the plasma is governed by Henry's law and is determined by its solubility coefficient (α) and its partial pressure. The solubility coefficient is the volume of the gas that will dissolve in 1 mL of a liquid at a standard pressure (101 kPa; 760 mmHg). For oxygen in plasma the coefficient is a constant 0.0209. The amount dissolved is dependent on partial pressure and is a simple rectilinear relationship – the greater the pressure the more oxygen dissolved.

The arterial partial pressure of oxygen (P_{aO_2}) is typically 13.3 kPa (100 mmHg). The amount of oxygen dissolved in 100 mL of blood can be calculated from the following equation.

$$\text{Volume} = \frac{\alpha \cdot 100}{P_B} \cdot P_{O_2} = \frac{0.0209 \cdot 100}{101.1 \text{ kPa}} \cdot 13.3 \text{ kPa} = \frac{0.0209 \cdot 100}{760 \text{ mmHg}} \cdot 100 \text{ mmHg}$$

Clearly, oxygen is not very soluble. Very little is carried in solution in humans breathing air at sea level; at a partial pressure of 13.3 kPa (100 mmHg) a litre of blood holds only 2.7 mL of oxygen. If this were the only form of oxygen carriage by the blood, human life as we know it would be impossible.

Exercise 3.2

What is the total amount of dissolved oxygen carried in the plasma of an adult with a blood volume of 5 litres breathing air at sea level?

What is the amount if pure oxygen is being inspired? What is the amount if pure oxygen at 3 atmospheres (303.3 kPa; 2280 mmHg) is being inspired?

(N.B. Remember to take account of P_{H_2O} in your calculations.)

Oxygen carried in chemical combination

There are two sources of chemically bound oxygen. These are myoglobin (Mgb), an important oxygen *store* found in muscle tissue, and haemoglobin (Hb), an important oxygen *carrier* in the blood. We shall deal with myoglobin in more detail when we consider oxygen uptake by the muscle cell; it is sufficient to say here that its structure is very different to that of haemoglobin, and its very strong affinity for oxygen would make it a very poor oxygen carrier. Haemoglobin also has an affinity for oxygen, that is they combine very quickly to form oxyhaemoglobin. It was discovered by the English biochemist Robert Hill in 1937, with each haemoglobin molecule carrying four molecules of oxygen, i.e.

$$Hb_4 + 4O_2 = Hb_4(O_2)_4$$

However, the chemical bond is easily reversible by changes in the partial pressure of oxygen, and oxygen is released by haemoglobin as readily as it is captured.

Oxygen content, saturation and capacity

We need to recognize three measures of blood oxygen levels. The first is the oxygen *content* (C_{O_2}); this is defined as the amount of oxygen carried in combination with haemoglobin. When $P_{O_2} = 20$ kPa (150 mmHg), $P_{CO_2} = 5.3$ kPa (40 mmHg) and temperature $= 38°C$, each gram of haemoglobin attracts 1.34 mLO_2. For a level of 150 gHb $\cdot L_{bl}^{-1}$ the oxygen *content* is

$$150 \text{ gHb} \cdot L_{bl}^{-1} \cdot 1.34 \text{ m}LO_2 = 210 \text{ m}LO_2 \cdot L_{bl}^{-1}$$

This represents a haemoglobin saturation of 100 per cent and is the maximum amount that can be carried in this way. However, the partial pressure of oxygen in the alveoli (P_{AO_2}) is not 20 kPa (150 mmHg) – it is about 13.7 kPa (103 mmHg) and at this partial pressure haemoglobin is only 97.5 per cent saturated. Thus, arterial blood carries 205 $mLO_2 \cdot L_{bl}^{-1}$ (210 · 0.975) chemically bound to the molecule.

The next measure is the oxygen *capacity*; this is the maximum amount of oxygen that can combine with haemoglobin plus the amount of oxygen dissolved in the plasma. Unlike haemoglobin, which has a fixed saturation ceiling, dissolved oxygen is entirely dependent on the prevailing partial pressure of oxygen. As we saw earlier, at an alveolar partial pressure of oxygen of 13.7 kPa (103 mmHg), the amount dissolved is 2.7 $mLO_2 \cdot L_{bl}^{-1}$, making the oxygen *capacity* of arterial blood 207.7 $mLO_2 \cdot L_{bl}^{-1}$.

The third measure is oxygen saturation (S_{O_2}). This is the oxygen capacity expressed as a fraction of 100 per cent saturation of haemoglobin. For example, at a P_{O_2} of about 2.66 kPa (20 mmHg), the oxygen capacity is 70.6 $mLO_2 \cdot L_{bl}^{-1}$; the amount dissolved is 0.6 $mLO_2 \cdot L_{bl}^{-1}$. Thus, the oxygen content at this partial pressure is ~ 70.6 $mLO_2 \cdot L_{bl}^{-1}$ and the percentage saturation is

$$\frac{70.6 \ mLO_2 \cdot L_{bl}^{-1}}{210 \ mLO_2 \cdot L_{bl}^{-1}} = \sim 34 \text{ per cent}$$

Oxyhaemoglobin

However, the relationship between oxygen and haemoglobin is not simply rectilinear but S-shaped or sigmoid (Figure 3.3). The Danish physiologist, Christian Bohr, discovered the relationship in 1903, and it has very interesting and important consequences for anyone interested in understanding oxygen delivery to the working muscle. The shape of the curve is the result of the behaviour of the haemoglobin molecule in the presence of oxygen. The attachment of an oxygen molecule to the first iron-binding site affects the way in which the remaining three oxygen molecules bind to the other three haem sites. The technical term for this behaviour is 'cooperativity'. As soon as the first site is occupied – at an oxygen partial pressure (P_{O_2}) of less than 1 kPa (5 mmHg) – the amino acids that make up the molecule alter their position. This allows rapid binding to the second and third sites as the partial pressure rises to 8 kPa (60 mmHg). At this point a plateau is reached and the haemoglobin molecule is almost saturated. Very little more oxygen can bind to the fourth site as the

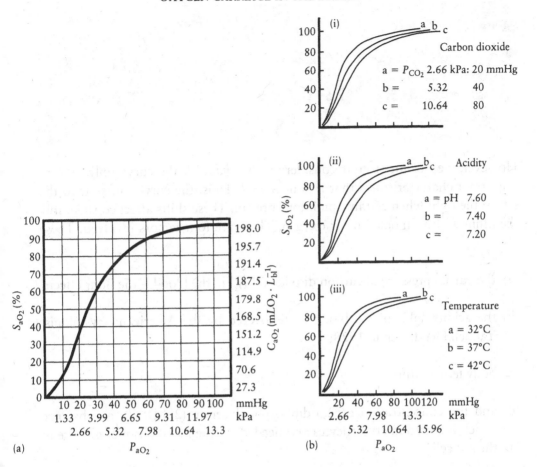

Figure 3.3 The oxyhaemoglobin dissociation curve, showing (a) the relationships between partial pressure, and oxygen saturation and oxygen content of arterial blood; and the effects of (b) (i) carbon dioxide; (ii) pH; and (iii) temperature on the shape and position of the curve

partial pressure rises from 8 kPa (60 mmHg) to the 13.3 kPa (100 mmHg) found in arterial blood.

Question 3.4   *The presence of the plateau in the oxyhaemoglobin curve is useful for those living at altitude. Can you say why?*

Exercise 3.3

Using the graph of Figure 3.3(a) construct a table estimating oxygen content, oxygen in solution, oxygen capacity, and oxygen saturation, for oxygen partial pressures ranging through 2.66 (20), 5.32 (40), 7.98 (60), 10.64 (80) and 13.30 (100) kPa (mmHg).

However, we do not stop at considering the *shape* of the curve only. A very important characteristic is that it is not *fixed*. Thus, the curve can shift to the left or the right when certain conditions prevail. These shifts affect considerably the affinity of haemoglobin for oxygen. There are four factors involved. These are

(a) the partial pressure of carbon dioxide (P_{CO_2}) in the blood – the Bohr effect;

(b) the acidity (pH) of the blood – discovered by the American physiologist Yandell Hendersen in 1928;

(c) body temperature;

(d) and the concentration of 2,3-diphosphoglycerate (2,3-DPG), a substance which is stored in erythrocytes and needed for the metabolism of glucose in the red cell.

Question 3.5   Use Figure 3.3 to calculate the amount of oxygen still combined with Hb at a partial pressure of 5.3 kPa (40 mmHg). Say in a couple of sentences what are the general effects of the curve moving (a) to the right, and (b) to the left?

We shall return to the oxyhaemoglobin dissociation curve in Chapter 7 on oxygen consumption in the muscle cell.

Abnormal values of arterial oxygen pressure (P_{aO_2})

There are various conditions when the partial pressure of oxygen in arterial blood may be higher or lower than the normal value of 13.3 kPa (100 mmHg). The most obvious condition for low arterial oxygen partial pressure is living or exercising at altitude. Barometric pressure falls with increasing altitude and has a direct effect on the oxygen capacity of the blood.

Exercise 3.4

Calculate the oxygen content and capacity of a litre of blood with a normal haemoglobin level at an altitude of about 5000 m (barometric pressure of $\sim$ 50 kPa ($\sim$ 380 mmHg)).

There are two other conditions when arterial oxygen partial pressure can be below normal. The first is the reduction of the diffusing capacity of the lungs (D_L) at the level of alveolar–capillary membrane. Even under normal conditions the membrane *appears* to present a barrier to diffusion. The oxygen molecule first has to pass through the fluid lining the alveoli and the squamous epithelial cells that make up the alveoli walls. It has to cross the interstitial fluid barrier between the alveoli and the capillaries. It then has to penetrate the inner and outer faces of capillary walls before entering the plasma. The final hurdle is crossing the membrane of the erythrocyte. The distance between alveoli and blood cell ranges between 0.3 and 5 μm, but the fact that we can still perform strenuous exercise tells us that, normally, these barriers to diffusion are not sufficient to affect oxygen transfer and carriage in the blood.

Lung disease

However, any additional barrier can lead to a reduction in oxygen transfer. Chronic bronchitis is one condition affecting oxygen transfer in this way. It is a condition often brought about by addictive smoking. Tobacco smoke irritates the bronchial passages and results in excessive activity of the mucous cells that line the bronchi. The increased amount of mucus produced overwhelms the normal lung clearing mechanism, and drains into the small airways forming mucus plugs that interfere with gas exchange. Individuals with severe chronic bronchitis have reduced lung function, low arterial oxygen pressure, and carbon dioxide retention (hypercapnia); their exercise tolerance is very limited and simply climbing the stairs often represents a test of maximal exertion.

Acute bronchitis, linked to colds and influenza, also interferes transiently with gas transfer and will diminish oxygen transfer and exercise tolerance until recovery is complete. A maximal oxygen uptake test within 14 days of any chest infection would be unwise, and a high white blood cell count would lead to postponement of the test. An acute episode lasting longer than a fortnight would almost certainly result in a de-training effect, and lower than expected maximal oxygen uptake values.

Another form of airflow limitation occurs during an asthma attack. Here the barriers to oxygen transfer may include, singly or in combination, contraction of the smooth muscle of the bronchi (bronchospasm), swollen bronchial mucosa, secretion of mucus, and the formation of mucus plugs. This reduces forced expiratory volume in one second (FEV_1), and peak expiratory flow (PEF). Exercise-induced asthma is generally relieved by inhalation of a bronchodilator taken in aerosol form.

Erythrocyte transit time through the pulmonary capillary bed

The second condition relates to the time taken for the red blood cell to pass through the alveolar network. The microstructure of the pulmonary circulation is very complex and transit times vary greatly. At rest the range lies between 0.5 s to 8 s, but the average transit time for a single erythrocyte is 1.5 s. As haemoglobin combines rapidly with oxygen, it becomes almost fully saturated in about 0.3 s. The very small difference between alveolar and arterial partial pressures $(P_{AO_2}-P_{aO_2})$ – namely 13.7 kPa (103 mmHg) and 13.3 kPa (100 mmHg) respectively – reveals the efficiency of the entire oxygen transfer system at pulmonary level. During exercise, the transit time for erythrocytes is reduced, but even under these conditions, oxygen transfer for the majority of us is still complete during erythrocyte transit time. However, in some elite endurance athletes maximal cardiac output reaches as much as $40 \, L \cdot min^{-1}$, and at such high flow rates there is evidence that oxygen saturation of arterial blood (S_{aO_2}) falls below 90 per cent and oxygen content is lowered. We revisit this issue when we look at the factors that may limit maximal oxygen uptake in Chapter 10.

Hyperoxia

Higher than normal arterial oxygen partial pressure occurs when breathing air to which oxygen has been added; this is called a hyperoxic gas mixture. It occurs routinely following serious surgical operations and in the treatment of chronic lung disease; tourists now climb Everest with the aid of supplemental oxygen; and we perform laboratory experiments to study the effects of hyper-oxic gas mixtures on exercise tolerance. It is interesting to look at the possible effects of such gas mixtures on the oxygen capacity of blood.

Let us take the example of breathing pure oxygen ($F_{IO_2} = 1.0$ (100 per cent) at standard pressure (101 kPa (760 mmHg)) and a normal haemoglobin value of 150 gHb $\cdot L_{bl}^{-1}$. Having cleared the lungs of nitrogen, and taken the partial pressure of water (P_{H_2O}) into account, the partial pressure of oxygen in the conductive airways is now 94.8 kPa (713 mmHg). We saw earlier that haemo-globin is fully saturated at 20 kPa (150 mmHg); so the nearly fivefold increase in pressure will not increase the *chemically* bound oxygen beyond the pre-viously calculated maximal value of 210 $mLO_2 \cdot L_{bl}^{-1}$. The only increase can come from *dissolved* oxygen. We discovered earlier that at normal arterial partial pressure of 13.3 kPa (100 mmHg) the amount carried in solution was 2.7 $mLO_2 \cdot L_{bl}^{-1}$. We calculate the amount carried when breathing pure oxygen as follows:

$$\text{Volume in solution} = \frac{0.0209 \cdot 100}{101.1} \cdot 89.5 \text{ kPa} = 18.5 \text{ } mLO_2 \cdot L_{bl}^{-1}$$

$$= \frac{0.0209 \cdot 100}{760} \cdot 673 \text{ mmHg} = 18.5 \text{ } mLO_2 \cdot L_{bl}^{-1}$$

The oxygen capacity now is 228.5 $mLO_2 \cdot L_{bl}^{-1}$ rather than the 207.7 found under normoxic conditions. The additional oxygen made available is important for medical conditions, and is known to improve exercise tolerance when administered in the laboratory. Supplemental oxygen also assists performance during breath-holding events, but is of little physiological benefit when used to aid recovery from exercise.

Key points

- Blood is an alkaline fluid consisting of liquids and solids.

- Its main functions are transporting oxygen, nutrients and hormones, removing waste products, regulating body temperature, providing protec-tion against infectious diseases, and maintaining fluid and salt balance.

- The liquid compartment is the plasma, a pale straw-coloured fluid.

- It contains water and dissolved materials – proteins, glucose, lipids, vitamins, enzymes, hormones, immune bodies and inorganic materials such as sodium, potassium, calcium and phosphate.

- Red blood cells (erythrocytes), white cells (between 5 and 10 thousand per microlitre (μL)) and platelets are suspended in the plasma.

- Men have between 5.0 and 5.5 million and women between 4.5 and 5.0 million erythrocytes per microlitre (μL) of blood.

- Erythrocytes are flexible discs with concave surfaces about 7 μm in diameter able to pass through the capillaries of the circulatory system.

- The hormone erythropoietin (EPO) stimulates erythrocyte production in the bone marrow of large flat bones (skull, pelvis) and of long bones (femur).

- The haematocrit (Hct) is the proportion of erythrocytes to plasma.

- Values for men lie between 42 and 52 per cent, and for women between 36 and 46 per cent.

- The main constituent of the erythrocyte is the main oxygen carrier haemoglobin (Hb).

- The normal value for men ranges between 140 and 170 g $\cdot$ L_{bl}^{-1}, and for women between 120 and 150 g $\cdot$ L_{bl}^{-1}.

- The relationship between oxygen and haemoglobin is S-shaped or sigmoid.

- Arterial blood carries 2.7 m$LO_2 \cdot L_{bl}^{-1}$ in solution and 204.7 m$LO_2 \cdot L_{bl}^{-1}$ in chemical combination with haemoglobin.

- The oxyhaemoglobin curve is not fixed and shifts to the left or the right as the result of changes in the partial pressure of carbon dioxide in the blood (P_{CO_2}), the acidity (pH) of the blood, body temperature, and the level of 2,3-diphosphoglycerate (2,3-DPG).

Answers to questions in the text

Question 3.1

The measure of acidity/alkalinity of a solution is called its pH. It is the negative logarithm of the hydrogen ion concentration in that solution, i.e. $pH = \log_{10}(1/[H^+])$. A pH = 7 is neutral; more than 7 indicates the solution is alkaline, below 7 it is acid. Resting blood pH = 7.4; the pH of gastric juices in the stomach reach pH = 3.

Question 3.2

In each microlitre of blood there are about 5 200 000 red blood cells. There are 1000 μL in a millilitre, and 1000 mL in a litre. Men have total blood volume of about 5500 mL. The total number (5 200 000 × 1000 × 5500) of circulating RBCs is about 29 trillion (2.9×10^{13}). Women have a slightly smaller total blood volume of about 5000 mL; the total number of circulating RBCs is thus about 26 trillion (2.6×10^{13}). About two and a half million red blood cells need to be produced every second to replace those being destroyed.

Question 3.3

The short answer is anaemia. There are two dietary deficiencies – iron, leading to a lack of haemoglobin, and vitamin B_{12}, leading to immature red cell formation – that are invariably followed by reduced levels of red blood cells.

One would be following a sudden loss of blood, as in a haemorrhage or blood donation. Another would be the illegal use of synthetic erythropoietin (EPO), often used by unscrupulous endurance athletes to boost performance. Another would be living at altitude. Another would be training at altitude.

Question 3.4

As altitude increases barometric pressure falls, and with it the partial pressure of oxygen in the atmosphere. This affects the oxygen content of arterial blood. If the oxyhaemoglobin dissociation curve were rectilinear, rather than sigmoid, in shape, the fall in oxygen content would be considerably greater than it actually is. Thus, the plateau acts as a protective mechanism against the hypoxia of high altitude. The partial pressure of oxygen in the alveoli can fall to about 8 kPa (60 mmHg) with only an 11 per cent fall in oxygen saturation and a similar loss in oxygen content of the blood. This means that those living at 8000 feet or below, for example, can go about their daily business without any problems. Exercise, however, is a different matter; no Olympic records were broken in endurance events at the 1968 Mexico Olympic Games and times were slower than at Games held at sea level.

Question 3.5

The amount of oxygen combined with haemoglobin at 5.3 kPa (40 mmHg) is

$150 \ mLO_2 \cdot L_{bl}^{-1}$; the blood is still 75 per cent saturated. When the curve shifts to the right, as it does when blood is warmer or more acidic, a greater amount of oxygen is released from haemoglobin at the same partial pressure. For example, at 5.3 kPa (40 mmHg) a core temperature of 45°C or pH = 7.2 results in saturation levels of 40 and 55 per cent respectively. The reverse applies when the curve shifts to the left, which is does when core temperature falls or blood becomes more alkaline. Given the same partial pressure the saturation level at pH = 7.2 rises to 80 per cent and less oxygen is released. One of the features of people suffering from hypothermia is confusion as less oxygen is released to the brain.

Answers to exercises in the text

Exercise 3.1
Subject 1 is a normal male. Subject 2 is a trained male endurance athlete. Subject 3 is a normal female.

Exercise 3.2
The amount dissolved in the plasma is given by the equation

$$\text{Volume} = \frac{\alpha \cdot 100}{P_B} \cdot P_{O_2}$$

where α is the solubility coefficient; for oxygen this is 0.0209. Thus, breathing air at sea level at standard pressure of 101.1 kPa (760 mmHg) and an alveolar partial pressure of oxygen of 13.3 kPa (100 mmHg), only 2.76 millilitres of oxygen is carried in a litre of blood ($mLO_2 \cdot L_{bl}^{-1}$) as dissolved oxygen. The total, with a whole body blood volume of 5 L, is only 13.8 mLO_2.

Breathing pure oxygen at sea level increases the amount of oxygen carried in solution in the plasma. Providing time is allowed for the nitrogen in the lung to be washed out the oxygen partial pressure in the alveoli is

$$P_B - P_{H_2O} \cdot F_{IO_2} = 101.1 - 6.3 \cdot 1.0 \text{ kPa} \quad (760 - 47 \cdot 1.0 \text{ mmHg})$$

$$= 94.8 \text{ kPa} \qquad\qquad (713 \text{ mmHg})$$

The amount carried in solution is therefore

$$\text{Volume} = \frac{0.0244 \cdot 100}{101.1} \cdot 94.8 \text{ kPa} \quad \frac{0.0244 \cdot 100}{760} \cdot 713 \text{ mmHg}$$

$$= 23 \ mLO_2 \cdot L^{-1}$$

or about 115 mL in total.

Breathing pure oxygen in a high-pressure chamber at three times the pressure at sea level is a tactic used when someone suffers from carbon monoxide poisoning. Carbon monoxide attaches itself to the haemoglobin molecule even more avidly than oxygen. In severe cases, there is insufficient oxygen to sustain even basal functions and death ensues. This hyperbaric oxygen treatment provides enough oxygen carried in solution to maintain minimal bodily function until the carbon monoxide is excreted. Here's how.

The partial pressure of oxygen in the alveoli is the total pressure minus the water vapour tension at body temperature, 6.3 kPa (47 mmHg), and the partial pressure of alveolar carbon dioxide, 5.3 kPa (40 mmHg)

4 Oxygen Delivery and the Heart

Learning Objectives

By the end of this chapter, you should be able to

- outline the main anatomical features of the heart

- describe the sequence of events that sends blood from the venae cavae to the aorta

- describe the sequence of electrical activity leading to ventricular contraction

- label a typical ECG wave and match the electrical and mechanical events of the cardiac cycle

- outline the changes in pressure, ventricular volume, and blood flow of the left side of the heart during each phase of the cardiac cycle

- differentiate between cardiac function in untrained subjects and elite endurance athletes

- explain the Frank–Starling law as an intrinsic control mechanism of cardiac function

- differentiate between the actions of the sympathetic and parasympathetic divisions of the autonomic nervous system

- explain the actions of acetylcholine and the hormones adrenaline and noradrenaline on cardiac function

Exercise Physiology: A Thematic Approach Tudor Hale
© John Wiley & Sons, Ltd   ISBN: 0 470 84682 8 (cloth), ISBN 0 470 84683 6 (pbk)

Objective test

Say whether the following answers are true (T) or false (F). If you do not know, say so (D) – not knowing is not an academic crime, but not finding out is. Try not to look at the answers until you have worked your way through the chapter and completed the test a second time. In this way you can monitor your progress.

	Pre-test			Post-test		
	T	F	D	T	F	D
1. The heart lies within the pericardial sac						
2. The heart consists of smooth muscle						
3. The heart consists of four chambers, two atria and two ventricles						
4. The atria are larger and more muscular than the ventricles						
5. The right ventricle sends blood around the systemic circulation						
6. The septum divides the left and right sides of the heart						
7. The mitral valve divides the right atrium and ventricle						
8. The chordae tendinae prevent back-flow of blood into the atria						
9. The left ventricular wall is much thinner than the right						
10. Semilunar valves guard the exit of the left and right ventricles						
11. The left ventricle pumps deoxygenated blood around the body						
12. The contraction phase of the heart beat is called the diastole						
13. The SA node is the primary pacemaker for the heart						
14. The bundle of His transmits impulses from atria to ventricles						

	Pre-test			Post-test		
	T	F	D	T	F	D
15. The record of the electrical impulse is known as the ECG						
16. The ECG comprises 5 phases labelled P–Q–R–S–T						
17. The period from P-wave to P-wave is called the cardiac cycle						
18. Peak pressure generated by the right ventricle at rest is 120 mmHg						
19. At rest 120 mL of blood is ejected per beat from the ventricles						
20. A typical resting cardiac output in young adults is about 5 $L \cdot min^{-1}$						
21. Maximal cardiac output in trained athletes can exceed 40 $L \cdot min^{-1}$						
22. Estimated maximum heart rates can be derived from $220 - age$						
23. Maximum heart rate is always lower in trained endurance athletes						
24. Maximum stroke volume is lower in trained endurance athletes						
25. The sympathetic nervous system inhibits cardiac function						
26. Sympathetic nerve fibres release adrenaline and noradrenaline						
27. The vagal nerve releases acetylcholine						
28. The vagal nerve increases heart rate and myocardial contractility						
29. β_1 receptors are found in the peripheral blood vessels						
30. The myocardium contains α and β_2 receptors only						

Symbols, abbreviations and units of measurement

aorta	ao	
atrio-ventricular	AV	
blood pressure – diastolic	P_{dia}	mmHg
blood pressure – systolic	P_{sys}	mmHg
blood volume	V_{bl}	$L; mL$
capillary	c	
cardiac output, whole body flow	$\dot{Q}_C$	$L \cdot min^{-1}$
cardiac output (resting)	$\dot{Q}_{Crest}$	$L \cdot min^{-1}$
cardiac output (maximal)	$\dot{Q}_{Cmax}$	$L \cdot min^{-1}$
electrocardiogram	ECG	
end-diastolic volume	EDV	mL
end-systolic volume	ESV	mL
heart rate, cardiac frequency	f_C	$bt \cdot min^{-1}$
sino-atrial	SA	
stroke volume	V_S	$mL \cdot bt^{-1}$

Introduction

The red cell is now loaded with oxygen and is in need of a distribution network that connects the lungs with the skeletal muscle cell, and a means of delivery around the network. The heart is the driving force behind oxygen delivery whilst the arteries and veins direct that oxygen to regions of greatest need. In explaining the structure and function of this distributive network, it is easier to consider the heart and the systemic circulation as two separate mechanisms, so that the particular processes in each system are clearly laid out and accessible. What we lose in physical reality we gain in ease of understanding.

To put the process into the context of maximal oxygen uptake, we should look at some delivery data derived from a maximal test. These data show changes in cardiac output ($\dot{Q}_C$ $L \cdot min^{-1}$), heart rate (f_C $bt \cdot min^{-1}$), mean stroke volume ($\bar{V}_S$ $mL \cdot bt^{-1}$), and systolic and diastolic blood pressures (P_{sys} and P_{dia} mmHg) as we go from rest to maximum exercise (Figure 4.1).

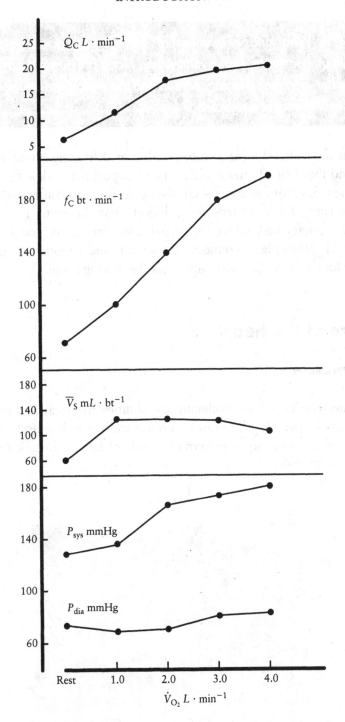

Figure 4.1 Graph showing the relationship between oxygen uptake ($\dot{V}_{O_2}$) and cardiac output ($\dot{Q}_C$), heart rate (f_C), mean stroke volume ($\overline{V}_S$), and systolic and diastolic blood pressure (P_{sys} and P_{dia})

Question 4.1 *What kinds of relationships exist between power output and cardiac output, heart rate, stroke volume and blood pressure? What are the differences between the sedentary person and the endurance athlete? How might these differences be explained?*

The heart is a parallel double pump, capable of delivering blood to and from the lungs and the skeletal muscle cells. The transport network – the pulmonary and systemic circulatory systems – consists of a one-way traffic system; arteries provide the route for outward-bound blood, and the veins for the inward-bound. The capillary bed, where the actual unloading of oxygen and uptake of carbon dioxide takes place, connects the arterial and venous networks. In this chapter, we look at how the heart generates the driving force.

Structure of the heart

Cardiac muscle

The heart derives its power-producing capabilities from cardiac muscle. Seen under a microscope, cardiac muscle, unlike the smooth muscle seen in the bronchioles of the lung, shows alternate bands of light and dark material and many nuclei (Figure 4.2).

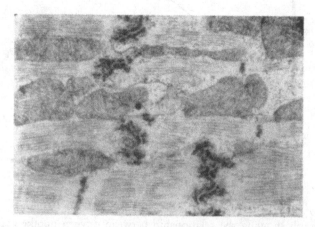

Figure 4.2 Striated cardiac muscle. (Reproduced with permission of Philip Harris Education, Ashby-de-la-Zouch)

Although the individual muscle fibres are self-contained entities, they connect to adjacent fibres through structures called intercalated discs. It is through these discs that the electrical impulses, which produce the contraction of the individual cells, are transmitted across the entire myocardium (from the Greek for muscle, *myos*, and heart, *kardia*). This means that the heart obeys the 'all-or-none law'. This law states that if a stimulus is above a certain threshold the entire myocardium contracts as a single unit; but if the stimulus is below this threshold, the muscle does not contract at all.

Atria and ventricles

The heart is an electrically driven mechanical pump. It lies in the thorax within a tough, fluid-lined, membranous bag called the pericardial sac, and consists of a fibrous skeleton around which are built four chambers. The two smallest are the left and right auricles, known colloquially as 'dead men's ears' because of their appearance, but now universally referred to as the right and left atria – from the Latin *atrium* for a Roman entrance hall. The larger chambers are the left and right ventricles. Atrial and ventricular septa divide the heart into its left and right sides. Blood enters the thin-walled atria. Venous blood, coming from the body tissues via the vena cavae, pours into the right atrium; the right ventricle pumps the blood through the pulmonary circulation where it picks up more oxygen. The oxygenated blood, coming from the lungs via the pulmonary vein, pours into the left atrium and ventricle and is despatched around the body via the systemic circulation.

Between the atria and ventricles, there are fibrous sheets that make up the atrio-ventricular valves; the tricuspid valve in the right heart has three flaps, and the bicuspid, or mitral, valve in the left has two. Attached to the free borders of these flaps are thin, strong fibrous chords called the chordae tendinae; these in turn are attached to the papillary muscle in the wall of the ventricle. When contraction occurs the increased pressure in the ventricles causes the valves shut to prevent blood being forced back into the atria.

Question 4.2 *What functions do the papillary muscle and chordae tendinae perform during the contraction of the heart muscle?*

The outer walls of the two ventricles are also much thicker than the atria, and the left ventricle is thicker than the right. Two further sets of valves, called the semilunar valves, lie between the left ventricle and the aorta, and the right ventricle and the pulmonary artery. The right ventricle pumps the venous blood into the adjacent low-pressure pulmonary circulation. Oxygenated blood is forced out of the left ventricle into the high-pressure systemic circulation servicing body tissues as far apart as the head and the feet.

Question 4.3   *Why is the left ventricular wall thicker than the right?*

The opening and closing of the four sets of valves occurs solely as the result of the changes in pressure as the heart muscle contracts and relaxes. The contraction phase is the systole, and the relaxation and recovery phase is the diastole.

Thus, the heart consists of two pumps working in parallel and their actions are synchronized. This means that the volume of blood pumped to the lungs is the same as that sent around the rest of the body. Unlike ordinary transport systems, the oxygen delivery process cannot tolerate congestion, tailbacks, and standstills, and blood keeps on the move through a variety of control mechanisms. Occasionally the system fails; the pooling of blood in the lower limbs after strenuous exercise such as the Wingate test is an example. When this happens, we may faint; in these circumstances, we can assist venous return to the heart by raising the person's legs. The last thing we should do is to haul the person upright!

Exercise 4.1

Given the information provided above list the features of the anatomy of the heart labelled A to L in Figure 4.3.

The electrical activity of the heart

Cardiac muscle contracts as the result of an electrical impulse originating in specialized tissue found in the right atrium close to the entrance of the superior vena cava. This area of tissue is called the sino-atrial node (SA node) and is the primary pacemaker for the heart. Because of the specialized structure of cardiac muscle, particularly the intercalated discs, the electrical impulse spreads across

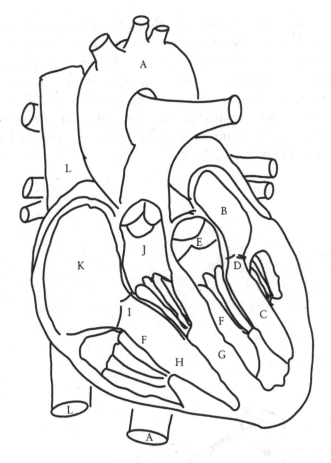

Figure 4.3 Schematic cross-section of the heart and major blood vessels

both atria producing atrial contraction. The fibrous skeleton of the heart prevents the electrical impulse from the SA node from progressing directly to the ventricles.

Question 4.4 *There is a good reason why the impulse should not flow directly to the ventricles. Can you say what it is?*

However, a second area of specialized tissue – the atrio-ventricular node (AV node) lying near the atrial septum and the tricuspid valve – picks up the impulse and transmits it through the fibrous skeleton via a bundle of fibres called the bundle of His. This bundle enters the ventricular septum and immediately divides into the right and left bundle branches. The branches extend down each side of the septum carrying the impulse to the apex of the heart before spreading through the walls of the ventricles via specialized tissue called the Purkinje fibres. This arrangement results in the contraction of the intra-ventricular septum, followed by the ventricular walls from the apex and towards the arterial blood vessels leaving the heart.

Exercise 4.2

Name the features labelled A to E in Figure 4.4.

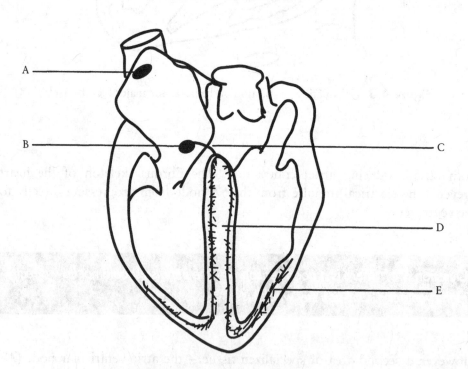

Figure 4.4   The electrical pathways of the heart

The electrocardiogram

Summarizing the entire mechanical process, we have atrial contraction, followed by a slight pause whilst the impulse passes through the bundle of His, leading to contraction of the septum and then the outer walls of the ventricles. The electrical activity associated with these actions can be recorded from electrodes placed on the chest; the signal received is called the electrocardiogram (ECG). A typical recording of this, shown in Figure 4.5, gives a picture of the events occurring during a single cardiac cycle. The P-wave indicates the contraction of the atria; the amplitude of the wave is small because of the relatively small muscle mass involved. The P–Q interval represents the time taken for the impulse to reach the atrio-ventricular node and pass through the bundle of His to the left and right bundle branches. The Q–R–S complex indicates the contraction of ventricles; the amplitude of this wave mirrors the greater muscle mass involved. The recovery phase of the atria is hidden by Q–R–S complex; the T-wave represents the recovery phase of the ventricles. The T-P interval is the resting period between contractions. The period from P-wave to P-wave is the cardiac cycle, and the typical resting heart rate (fc_R) of an adult is about 70 bt · min^{-1}.

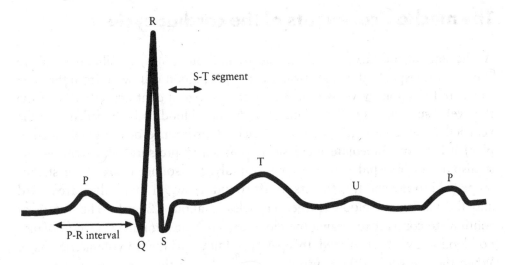

Figure 4.5　A typical electrocardiogram trace

The recording is important in two ways. Firstly, the sharp peak of the R-wave enables heart rate to be counted easily, either directly from chart recorder traces or by miniaturized computers such as the Polar heart rate monitor. Secondly, the number, rhythm and shape of the waves help to diagnose abnormal heart function due to coronary heart disease. Unlike intense, short-term exercise in skeletal muscle, cardiac muscle cannot function effectively when deprived of adequate supplies of oxygen.

Abnormal electrocardiograms

In patients suffering from insufficient blood supply brought about by narrowing of the coronary arteries, we see changes in the appearance of the electrocardiogram during a stress test that are sometimes accompanied by chest pain called angina pectoris – literally 'pang in the chest'. For example, a common feature seen during exercise tests of such individuals is depression of the S–T segment below the base line and inversion of the T-wave. There is evidence that maximal exercise in trained athletes also produces similar S–T segment and T-wave changes in the wave formation. Unlike the patient with angina, these abnormalities are short-lived and disappear rapidly during recovery, but they do indicate the kinds of demands placed on the heart during severe exercise.

The mechanical events of the cardiac cycle

At the start of the cardiac cycle the aortic and pulmonary semilunar vales are shut, but tricuspid and bicuspid valves are open; blood is flowing from the vena cavae and pulmonary veins into the ventricles. Atrial contraction (start of the P-wave) results in a small amount of additional blood to be expelled into the ventricles. The contraction of the ventricles (appearance of the Q–R–S complex) brings an immediate increase in ventricular pressure which causes the tricuspid and bicuspid valves to close rapidly; the sound, heard via a stethoscope held to the chest, is the first heart sound. Now, all four valves are closed and the volume of blood in the ventricles is about 120 mL. The ventricles continue to contract squeezing the blood towards the semilunar valves; because no blood has yet been ejected, this period is known as the iso-volumetric phase. When the pressure in the ventricles exceeds that in the aorta and pulmonary artery – about 10.6 kPa (80 mmHg) on the left side of the heart, but only a third of that for the right side – the semilunar valves are forced open and there is rapid ejection of blood into the two arteries. Ventricular contraction continues until the left ventricle reaches its peak, or systolic, pressure; at rest this is typically about 16 kPa (120 mmHg), but for the right ventricle, it is only 4.7 kPa or 35 mmHg. The ventricles begin their recovery (the onset of the T-wave) and the pressure begins to fall; blood is still flowing into the arteries, but at a reduced rate. When the ventricular pressure drops below that found in the two arteries, the semilunar valves close creating the second heart sound. Only ~70 mL of the original ventricular volume, called the stroke volume (V_S mL $\cdot$ bt^{-1}), has been ejected; but even this amount causes the elastic tissues of the aorta to stretch to accommodate it. The elastic rebound that follows sets up the pulsatile flow; we feel this at the wrists (the radial pulse), and on either side of the trachea (the carotid pulse). Now all four valves are closed again as the ventricles continue to relax. This period of the cycle is the iso-volumetric relaxation phase.

During ventricular contraction, venous blood has been pouring into the atria, producing a small rise in atrial pressure. When the atrial pressure exceeds the pressure in the relaxing ventricles, the tricuspid and bicuspid valves open, introducing periods of rapid, and then reduced, ventricular filling. The initiation of the P-wave begins the cycle again. The cardiac output at rest ($\dot{Q}_{Crest}$) is the sum of the stroke volumes of about 70 cardiac cycles each minute.

Question 4.5 *Using the above information what is a typical value for $\dot{Q}_{Crest}$?*

The major features of the cardiac cycle are summarized in Figure 4.6.

Cardiac output during exercise

Cardiac output ($\dot{Q}_C$) is the total amount of blood ejected from the ventricles in one minute and is described by the simple equation

$$\dot{Q}_C \; L \cdot min^{-1} = f_c \; bt \cdot min^{-1} \cdot \overline{V}_S \; mL \cdot bt^{-1}$$

where f_c bt $\cdot$ min^{-1} is heart rate and $\overline{V}_S$ mL $\cdot$ bt^{-1} is mean stroke volume. The increased oxygen supply demanded by muscles during exercise is met by increased cardiac output resulting from a faster heart rate and larger stroke volumes. In the normal young, untrained adult, the maximal cardiac output ($\dot{Q}_{Cmax}$) is about 15–20 $L \cdot min^{-1}$. Maximal heart rate (f_{Cmax}) is variable, but a good guide ($\pm$ 10 per cent) is given by subtracting age from 220.

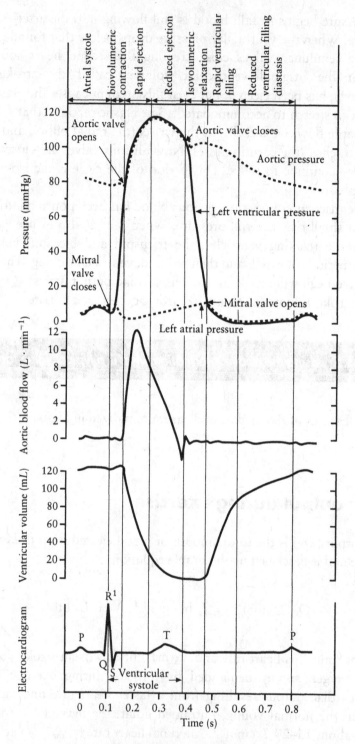

Figure 4.6 The cardiac cycle. (Reproduced with permission of CV Mosby Company from the original by Berne and Levy (1967))

Question 4.6   What is the effect of age on cardiac output?

The maximal heart rate for a 20-year-old normal adult therefore is in the region of 200 bt · min^{-1}. At a cardiac output of 20 L · min^{-1} this gives an average stroke volume of 100 mL · bt^{-1}; however, this figure is an average not the maximum. Stroke volume does increase with exercise intensity until it reaches about 120 mL · bt^{-1}; it then levels off, but finally falls as heart rates increase towards maximum.

Question 4.7   Can you explain this inverted-U-shaped relationship?

Cardiac output in endurance athletes

In highly trained endurance athletes the figures are very different. Studies performed on elite Swedish cross-country skiers by Ekblom and Hermansen in 1966 show that the resting cardiac output is similar to untrained adults, but the maximum values can exceed 40 L · min^{-1}; maximum heart rates reach 200 bt · min^{-1}, and stroke volume exceeds 200 mL · bt^{-1}. To grasp the scale of the changes in cardiac output during maximal exercise we need to relate these figures to an everyday event – such as beer-drinking in the Union bar. Reverting for a moment to Imperial measures, one pint of beer is just over half a litre (568 mL). At rest, about eight and a half pints (~5 L) of blood are being pumped around the body each minute. At maximal exercise for the untrained student, this grows to 35 pints a minute; for the elite endurance athlete it is a barely imaginable 70 pints a minute. Picture 70 pints of beer on the bar counter – that represents the amount of blood pumped around the body of an elite endurance athlete in *1 minute*. For the more sophisticated, it represents 56 bottles – nearly five cases – of wine delivered in *1 minute*. The next section explains the main intrinsic and extrinsic mechanisms that bring about this astonishing phenomenon.

Intrinsic and extrinsic control of cardiac function

The Frank–Starling law

The most important intrinsic control mechanism resides in the elastic properties of cardiac muscle itself. Within limits, the more elastic tissue is stretched, the more powerful is its recoil, and it is this relationship which provides the basis for the Frank–Starling law of the heart. The elastic nature of cardiac muscle of the atria and ventricles plays a key role in maintaining a balance between the volume of blood returning to the heart and the volume being pumped out. This occurs through changes in stroke volume.

During diastole – the recovery period of the cardiac cycle – blood is pouring into the atria, through the open atrio-ventricular valves, and into the ventricles; now blood has weight (mass), and is accelerating under the force of gravity. The product of mass and acceleration is force; this stretches the elastic elements of cardiac muscle. The degree of stretch depends on three factors. The first, and most important, is the amount of blood in the ventricles at the end of diastole – the end-diastolic volume (EDV). The greater the volume, the more extensive the stretch; this leads to a more powerful contraction of ventricular muscle, a more forceful ejection of blood, a lower end-systolic volume (ESV), and a greater stroke volume. The second is the diastolic filling time. If all other factors remain constant, a faster heart rate leads to a shorter filling time, smaller end-diastolic volume and a reduced stroke volume. The third factor, the rate of venous return, is important here. If this rate is not increased and the filling time is reduced, stroke volume will fall in line with smaller end-diastolic volume. Venous return does increase with exercise and, in the short term at least, compensates for the shorter diastole. However, at high heart rates, especially in the untrained individual, this compensatory mechanism breaks down and explains the inverted-U relationship between rate and stroke volume. Indeed, at maximum heart rates, cardiac output may fall and thus fail to deliver sufficient oxygen for exercise to continue.

Autonomic nervous control

The Frank–Starling law is not the only mechanism controlling cardiac function. Although an isolated heart provided with a suitably warm, nutritious, fluid environment will continue to beat without the intervention of external nerves, under everyday circumstances nerves and chemicals have a profound influence on cardiac function, particularly during exercise. The subconscious mechanisms involved are part of the autonomic nervous system (ANS) that controls all bodily functions except skeletal muscle contraction. There are two divisions of the autonomic nervous system – the sympathetic and the parasympathetic (Figure 4.7). The two systems generally oppose each other, the sympathetic tending to excite (the accelerator) and the parasympathetic to inhibit (the brake); but they do work in harmony. An increase in heart rate is achieved through reduced parasympathetic inhibition (foot *off* the brake) and increased sympathetic activity (foot *on* the accelerator); reduced heart rate sees the reverse, that is, foot on the brake and off the accelerator. Both divisions modify the Frank–Starling response by affecting heart rate and cardiac muscle contractility.

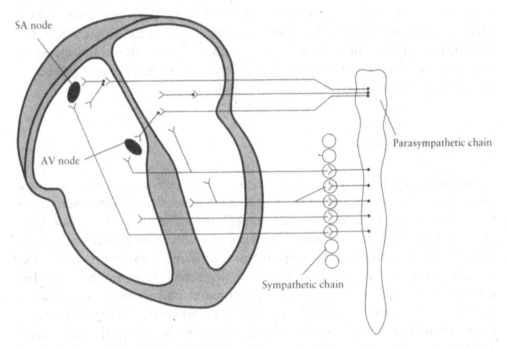

Figure 4.7   The innervation of the heart by the autonomic nervous system. (Reproduced by permission of AstraZeneca UK Limited)

The parasympathetic division

As far as heart rate is concerned, the parasympathetic division is the more influential. The left and right vagus nerves, running down each side of the neck close to the carotid artery, are the principal carriers of parasympathetic activity to the heart. The right vagus affects mainly the sino-atrial node, whilst the left influences the firing of the atrio-ventricular node; but there is no direct parasympathetic nerve effect on the ventricles. Thus, the vagus affects heart rate but has no effect on contractility of ventricular muscle.

The mechanism involved is a neurochemical secretion from nerve endings. At the vagus nerve endings are synaptic knobs, with a small gap, the synaptic cleft, between the synaptic knob and the cells of the sino-atrial and atrio-ventricular nodes. Within the synaptic knobs are vesicles containing the neural transmitter acetylcholine (ACh). A nerve impulse sent down the nerve fibres causes the vesicles to release the acetylcholine which floods the gap and stimulates receptors in the cell membranes of the two nodes. These receptors are described as cholinergic receptors. The effect is a slowing of heart rate; the greater the stimulation the slower the heart rate. Endurance athletes with very low resting heart rates, 35 bt·min^{-1} for example, are said to exhibit vagal tone. Indeed, excessive experimental stimulation of the vagus can lead to cardiac arrest. On the other hand, less stimulation leads to reduced vagal control and increased heart rate. Blocking vagal control, by injection of atropine for example, leads to a small rise – 10 to 15 bt·min^{-1} – in resting heart rate.

The sympathetic division

On the other hand, the sympathetic division affects both heart rate and muscle contractility, largely through the effects of the two neurotransmitters adrenaline (epinephrine) and noradrenaline (norepinephrine). The sympathetic side initiates the 'fight or flight' response. The receptor cells for both forms of sympathetic transmitters are the adrenergic receptors. There are two types involved in oxygen transport – alpha (α) and beta (β), with the β receptors being further divided into β_1 and β_2. The myocardium contains only β_1 receptors, whilst α and β_2 receptors are found in the peripheral blood vessels. Sympathetic nerve fibres abound in the myocardium and influence the sino-atrial and atrio-ventricular nodes as well as the atrial and ventricular musculature. The sympathetic neurochemical transmitter mainly responsible is noradrenaline.

However, there is also a second mechanism, involving the adrenal glands, that supplements the activity of the sympathetic nerve fibres via a different process. The adrenal glands lie on top of the kidneys and contain two types of chromaffin cells, so called because of they contain granules that are stained brown by chrome salts. When stimulated by sympathetic nerves, about 80–85 per cent of the cells secrete adrenaline directly into the blood stream, whilst the remaining 15–20 per cent secrete noradrenaline. The circulating blood carries both neurotransmitters to the coronary blood vessels, reinforcing the sympathetic activity in the myocardium. This two-pronged approach produces two responses – an increased heart rate and a more forceful ventricular ejection. Thus, cardiac output is raised not only by faster beats but also by greater stroke volumes.

The sympathetic division provides an important defence and survival mechanism. When attacked we can either stand and fight or turn and flee; the sympathetic division prepares us for both possibilities. Our heart rate increases immediately and rapidly; ventricles contract more strongly and raise blood pressure; blood is diverted from the skin and the gut to the muscle bed and we become pale; our airways dilate ensuring greater lung ventilation; insulin secretion moves glucose from the blood into the muscle cells. These primeval characteristics, very necessary for our survival, are also very helpful in our battles in the boxing ring, and on the athletics track and sports pitches.

To complete the story of oxygen delivery we now need some knowledge of the structure, function, and autonomic control of the circulatory system. This is covered in the next chapter.

Key points

- The heart lies in the pericardial sac.

- It is an electrically driven, four-chambered, mechanical pump consisting of striated cardiac muscle.

- It pumps blood around the body through two separate one-way systems.

- Atrio-ventricular and semilunar valves control blood movement in the heart.

- The right side of the heart sends venous blood through the pulmonary circulation.

- The left side of the heart sends oxygenated blood through the systemic circulation.

- The sino-atrial node generates electrical impulses that initiate the cardiac cycle.

- The impulses spread via the atria, the atrio-ventricular node, the bundle of His, the left and right bundle branches in the septum, and the Purkinje fibres in the outer ventricular walls.

- An electrocardiogram (ECG) is a record of the passage of the impulses.

- The cardiac cycle consists of seven phases: atrial systole, iso-volumetric contraction, rapid ejection, reduced ejection, iso-volumetric relaxation, rapid filling, and diastasis.

- Left ventricular systolic and diastolic pressures at rest are typically 16 kPa and 10.6 kPa (120 and 80 mmHg) respectively.

- Right ventricular pressure is about 4.7 kPa (35 mmHg).

- Cardiac output ($\dot{Q}_C$) is the product of heart rate (f_C) and mean stroke volume ($\overline{V}_S$) and is size-related.

- Maximum heart rates can be estimated from 220 − age.

- Resting cardiac output in a 70 kg male adult is about 5 $L \cdot min^{-1}$.

- Maximum cardiac output in untrained male adults is about 20 $L \cdot min^{-1}$, but can exceed 40 $L \cdot min^{-1}$ in highly trained male endurance athletes.

- The main differences between trained and untrained subjects lie in resting heart rates, and resting and maximum stroke volumes.

- Women have lower values, reflecting their generally smaller stature.

- Cardiac function is controlled by the Frank–Starling law – the larger the end-diastolic volume the greater the stroke volume.

- The autonomic nervous system (ANS) consists of two divisions.

- The parasympathetic division inhibits cardiac function via stimulation of the vagus nerve and release of acetylcholine leading to a reduction in heart rate.

- The sympathetic division excites cardiac function by stimulation of the sympathetic nerves and the release of noradrenaline that increases the rate of sino-atrial node firing, and ventricular muscle contractility.

- The adrenal glands on top of the kidneys secrete mainly adrenaline directly into the blood stream that also increases heart rate and muscle contractility.

Answers to questions in the text

Question 4.1
At sub-maximal exercise, the heart rate and cardiac output relationships are rectilinear, but the rates of increase begin to slow down as maximal power output approaches; the technical term for this is an asymptote. Stroke volume, on the other hand, follows an inverted-U curve. In healthy untrained subjects, as heart rate increases, stroke volume rises to about $120 \, mL \cdot bt^{-1}$ in response to greater contractility of the ventricular muscle. As heart rate continues to increase, volume plateaus as end-diastolic volume and ejection fraction are matched; but as heart rate continues to increase, stroke volume actually declines because of the reduced filling time and end-diastolic volume. The combination of an asymptotic heart rate increase and reduced stroke volume inevitably lead to reduced cardiac output. Systolic blood pressure also increases initially but reaches a clear plateau at sub-maximal exercise; diastolic pressure remains unchanged, although some studies have shown a gradual but small decline, indicating a fall in peripheral resistance.

Question 4.2
The chordae tendinae, attached to the outer rim of the atrio-ventricular valve flaps, act like guy-ropes and prevent eversion of the valves and regurgitation of blood back into the atria. The chords grow out of the papillary muscle of the ventricular walls. When the electrical impulse reaches the ventricles, the papillary muscles contract; this provides a firm foundation for the chords enabling them to resist the forces pushing against the closed valve flaps.

Question 4.3
The left ventricle has to deliver enough force to send the blood around body tissues located as far apart as the foot and the head. This means pushing against the force of gravity in arteries leading to the brain, and veins leading from the feet. The ventricular wall consists largely of cardiac muscle; the muscle fibres, like skeletal muscle fibres, respond to harder work by becoming thicker and stronger. The right ventricle, however, has to push blood into the pulmonary circulation against very low pressures. Right ventricular thickening occurs in those living at altitude, and those suffering from chronic lung disease, where hypoxia – a shortage of oxygen – is present.

Question 4.4

The two major arteries – the pulmonary and aorta – lie at the superior surface of the heart. The electrical impulse for each heart beat originates in the sino-atrial node, which is also in the upper part of the heart. If the impulse were allowed to move directly over the ventricles, blood would be squeezed in the opposite direction to that needed. The specialized tissue pathways conduct the impulse to the apex of the heart via the atrio-ventricular node and the bundle of His, down the septum separating the ventricles, and on to the Purkinje fibres that invade the lower regions of the ventricles. The contraction begins in the septum which provides a firm base against which the rest of the ventricular muscle mass can contract. Stimulation by the Purkinje fibres ensures that the ventricles contract from the apex of the heart, squeezing the blood upwards and into the two major arteries.

Question 4.5

Typical resting cardiac output of both trained and untrained is similar – about $5 \; L \cdot \text{min}^{-1}$. In the case of the untrained, it is given by the equation

$$\dot{Q}_C = f_C \; \text{bt} \cdot \text{min}^{-1} \cdot \overline{V}_S \; \text{mL} \cdot \text{bt}^{-1}$$

$$= 72 \cdot 70$$

$$= 5.04 \; L \cdot \text{min}^{-1}$$

In the trained endurance athlete however, the picture is very different

$$\dot{Q}_C = f_C \; \text{bt} \cdot \text{min}^{-1} \cdot \overline{V}_s \; \text{mL} \cdot \text{bt}^{-1}$$

$$= 35 \cdot 144$$

$$= 5.04 \; L \cdot \text{min}^{-1}$$

Question 4.6

Maximum cardiac output is reduced. The reason is that heart rate falls with age: at 20 years of age the maximum heart rate is about 200 $\text{bt} \cdot \text{min}^{-1}$; at 60 the maximum heart rate is about 160 $\text{bt} \cdot \text{min}^{-1}$. Maximum cardiac output must fall.

Question 4.7

At rest, a typical left ventricular end-diastolic volume is about 120 mL. At a heart rate of 70 $\text{bt} \cdot \text{min}^{-1}$, the volume ejected per beat (the ejection fraction) is about 70 $\text{mL} \cdot \text{bt}^{-1}$ and the cardiac output is $\sim 5 \; L \cdot \text{min}^{-1}$. As we begin to exercise, three things happen. First, heart rate increases. Second, the contraction of the left ventricle becomes more forceful and the ejection fraction increases. This results in increased stroke volume and cardiac output. Third, the rate of venous return also increases to match output and so we maintain end-diastolic volume and stroke volume. However, a point is reached where the heart rate is fast enough to reduce ventricular filling, and therefore end-diastolic volume, during diastasis. Because of the Frank–Starling mechanism, the lower end-diastolic volume results in a smaller ejection fraction and reduced stroke volume.

Answers to exercises

Exercise 4.1

A = aorta; B = left atrium; C = left ventricle; D = mitral valve; E = aortic semilunar valve; F = chordae tendinae; G = septum; H = right ventricle; I = tricuspid valve; J = pulmonary artery semilunar valve; K = right atrium; L = vena cava.

Exercise 4.2

A = sino-atrial node; B = atrio-ventricular node; C = bundle of His; D = left and right bundle branches; E = Purkinje fibres.

5 Oxygen Distribution and the Circulation

Learning Objectives

By the end of this chapter, you should be able to

- state typical resting systolic and diastolic blood pressures in the healthy adult, and describe the effects of exercise on both measures

- describe the principles of blood pressure measurement

- outline the structure of the systemic circulatory system

- link the detailed anatomical structure of the various blood vessels with the function they perform

- describe the changes in cross-sectional area, pressure and flow as blood travels from the aorta to the right atrium

- outline the mechanisms responsible for maintaining venous return

- indicate the way blood is redistributed from the resting state to strenuous exercise

- explain the mechanisms that interact to maintain arterial vascular tone

- describe the relationship between blood distribution and body temperature

- list the factors that affect blood flow in arterioles and capillaries

- describe briefly the mechanisms that regulate blood pressure.

Exercise Physiology: A Thematic Approach Tudor Hale
© John Wiley & Sons, Ltd ISBN: 0 470 84682 8 (cloth), ISBN 0 470 84683 6 (pbk)

Objective test

Say whether the following answers are true (T) or false (F). If you do not know, say so (D) – not knowing is not an academic crime, but not finding out is. Try not to look at the answers until you have worked your way through the chapter and completed the test a second time. In this way, you can monitor your progress.

	Pre-test			Post-test		
	T	F	D	T	F	D
1. The systemic circulation feeds the lungs						
2. Blood is carried to the heart by arteries, away from it by veins						
3. Vessels called capillaries connect the arterial and venous systems						
4. Blood moves around the body by the force generated by the heart						
5. Recording blood pressure requires turbulent blood flow						
6. A typical resting systolic pressure is about 80 mmHg						
7. Diastolic pressure reflects the resistance of peripheral vessels						
8. During exercise systolic blood pressure is raised						
9. The wall of the aorta is thinner than that of the vena cava						
10. The diameter of the vena cava is greater than that of the aorta						
11. The combined cross-sectional area of the capillaries is about 3000 cm^2						
12. Blood velocity is greatest in the capillaries						
13. The venous system is a low-pressure system						
14. Valves in lower limb arteries prevent back-flow of blood						

	Pre-test			Post-test		
	T	F	D	T	F	D
15. The venous side provides an important storage reservoir of blood						
16. At rest the veins store about 60% of total blood volume						
17. Diameter changes in arterioles affect skeletal muscle blood flow						
18. Noradrenaline acts on α receptors to produce vasodilatation						
19. Noradrenaline acts on β_1 receptors to produce vasoconstriction						
20. CO_2, lactate, & ADP constrict arterioles & pre-capillary sphincters						
21. Capillary flow depends on tube length, radius, pressure & viscosity						
22. Flow in blood vessels is either laminar or turbulent						
23. Turbulent flow is defined by the Hagen–Poiseuille law						
24. Reynolds number defines flow rate						
25. Reducing the radius of a vessel by half increases flow $\times$ 16						
26. Neural, chemical and hormonal mechanisms control blood pressure						
27. The cardiac control centre is found in the cerebral cortex						
28. Stretch receptors are found in the aortic arch and carotid sinus						
29. Chemically driven vasodilatation reverses low blood pressure						
30. Renin release produces angiotensin II which lowers blood pressure						

Symbols, abbreviations and units of measurement

adenosine triphosphate	ATP	
carbon dioxide	CO_2	
cardiac output, whole body flow	$\dot{Q}_C$	$L \cdot min^{-1}$;
hydrogen ion	H^+	
lactate	La	$mmol \cdot L^{-1}$; mM
maximal oxygen uptake	$\dot{V}_{O_2max}$	$L \cdot min^{-1}$; $mL \cdot min^{-1}$
maximal voluntary contraction	MVC	
micrometre, previously called micron	μm	

Greek symbols

alpha	α
beta	β
eta	η
pi	π
rho	ρ
nu	ν

The circulatory system

The circulatory system is a distribution network comprising the arteries, the capillaries, and veins. Arteries transport blood from the heart, veins return blood to it; the capillaries connect the two. We saw in Chapter 4 that the pulmonary circulation feeds the lungs. The systemic circulation feeds the rest of the body and we concentrate on this system in this chapter.

We start by describing blood pressure measurement, and describe the effect of exercise on systolic and diastolic blood pressures measured during exercise. We go on to uncover the complex relationships that exist between blood vessel structure, blood vessel function, the autonomic nervous system, and blood flow.

Question 5.1   *What do you think happens to systolic and diastolic pressures during progressive exercise?*

Blood pressure measurement

Blood pressure measurement is a common procedure whenever we visit our doctor. There are now electronic devices that do the job quickly, but we get a much better understanding of what is happening in the artery if we use the traditional mercury sphygmomanometer and stethoscope. The principle that underpins blood pressure measurement is that turbulent flow produces sounds detectable via the stethoscope. Under normal circumstances peripheral arterial blood flow generates no little sound. However, if we constrict the artery in some way blood flowing past that constriction accelerates, resulting in greater turbulence and detectable noise. A blood pressure cuff – a cloth bag containing a balloon – is wrapped around the upper arm, level with the heart. A hand-held pump inflates the balloon until the mercury column reaches about 180 mmHg. (Note: blood pressure is the only physiological measure that is not converted into the SI unit for pressure.) This pressure exerted on the upper arm is sufficient to obstruct the brachial artery so that no blood flows past the obstruction; therefore, there is no noise. The stethoscope is placed over the brachial artery just below the cuff. We release the air in the cuff slowly thus lowering the pressure and causing the height of the mercury column to fall. When the pressure generated by the left ventricle *just* exceeds the restraining pressure in the cuff a spurt of blood is forced past the obstruction; turbulent flow, and therefore noise, is produced and detected through the stethoscope. The height of the mercury column coinciding with this first sound is registered as the systolic pressure. As the air continues to leak from the cuff the pressure falls further and the sound becomes more muffled and faint until it finally disappears altogether. The point at which this disappearance occurs is registered as the diastolic pressure. The procedure is accomplished reliably on resting subjects. There are difficulties in detecting the appropriate sounds during exercise, particularly maximal exertion on the treadmill, because of extraneous sounds resulting from increased upper body movements. Under these circumstances, systolic pressure can be determined by palpating the radial pulse. Whilst the cuff pressure exceeds systolic pressure, the radial pulse is absent, but reappears as soon as the systolic pressure exceeds that of the cuff. It is impossible to detect diastolic pressure by this method, however. The mechanisms that regulate blood pressure are covered at the end of the chapter. (See Figure 5.1.)

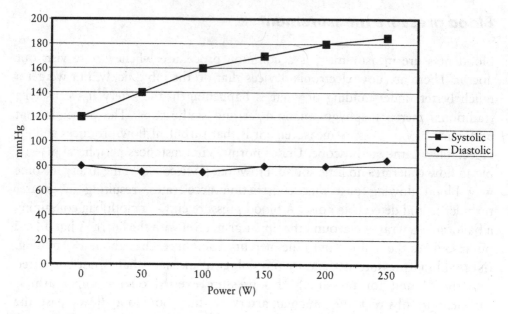

Figure 5.1 Schematic representation of systolic and diastolic blood pressure responses to progressive exercise

The systemic circulation

Just as the national road transport network consists of different kinds of roads serving different purposes – motorways, A roads, B roads, country lanes, and city streets – so the circulatory system consists of blood vessels – the aorta, arteries, arterioles, pre-capillary sphincters, capillaries, venules, veins and the venae cavae – that differ in detailed structure and function. Many of the major blood vessels mimic a motorway where the two carriageways, the arteries and veins, are separate and carry material in opposite directions. (See Figure 5.2.)

Blood vessel structure

The walls of the blood vessels are constructed from three different tissue layers. The innermost layer – the intima – consists of endothelial cells; the middle layer – the media – consists of a combination of elastic tissue and smooth muscle; the outer layer – the adventitia – consists of fibrous connective tissue, invaded by nerves and small blood vessels. The proportions of these particular tissues in the vessels walls change as we move from the heart to the periphery of the system and back again(Figure 5.3).

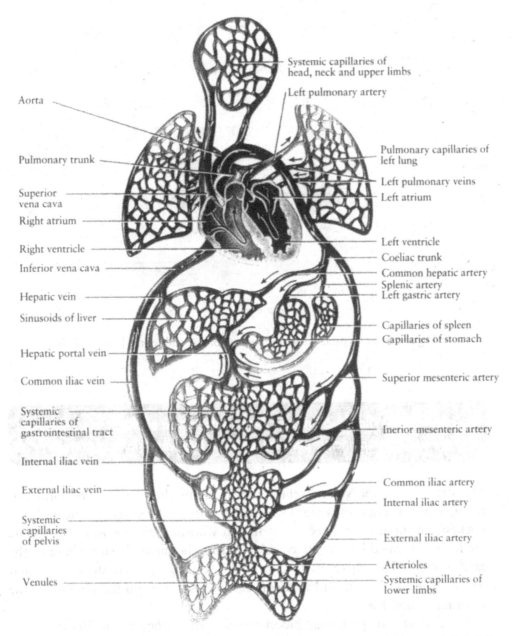

Figure 5.2 Schematic representation of the circulatory system. (With permission John Wiley & Sons, Ltd. from the original in Tortura, GJ & Grabowski, SR (2003))

Guarding the entrance to the capillary bed are pre-capillary sphincters that contain the highest percentage of smooth muscle. Some capillaries, called 'thoroughfare capillaries' make a direct link from arteriole to venule, and contain a small amount of smooth muscle in their walls.

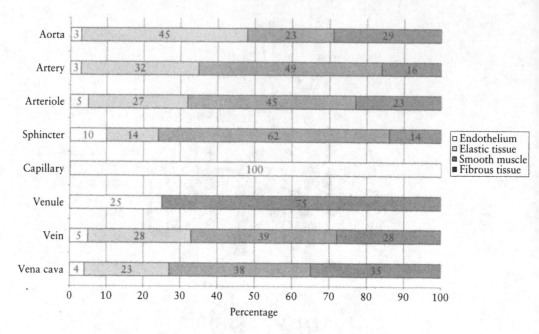

Figure 5.3 Typical tissue components of the walls of the blood vessels

Question 5.2 *What function does the smooth muscle of the arteries, arterioles and pre-capillary sphincters perform when an individual starts to exercise?*

The structure of the vessels reflect the functions they have to perform; for example, the arterial walls are thicker than those of the veins. The aorta is the thickest, at about 2 mm, because it has to withstand the pressure created by the force generated by the left ventricle during the rapid ejection phase of the cardiac cycle. The capillary wall, at only 1 μm thick, is the thinnest so that oxygen, carbon dioxide and nutrients can pass freely from the blood into the working tissues (Figure 5.4).

The diameter of particular blood vessels varies from about 30 mm in the main vein, the vena cava, to 7 to 8 μm in the capillaries. The cross-sectional area of the aorta is about 5 cm^2. By comparison, the combined cross-sectional area of the capillaries is about 4500 cm^2, enough to cover a quarter of a full-sized soccer pitch. This dramatic difference affects the pressure of blood and its velocity as it passes through the various regions of the systemic circulation. Pressure and velocity are greatest in the aorta; mean resting values are about 100 mmHg and 50 cm $\cdot$ s^{-1} respectively. There is a sharp drop in both values as

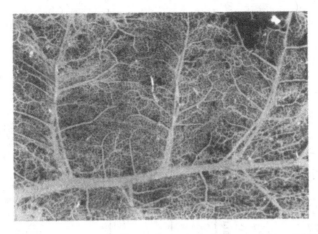

Figure 5.4   A micrograph of a capillary network. (With permission Philip Harris Education, Ashby-de-la-Zouch)

the arterioles are reached because of the sudden increase in the number of blood vessels. Although the resistance to flow in individual capillaries is high, their number is so great that their combined resistance is low – resting mean pressure now is about 20 mmHg, and velocity has dropped to 0.1 cm · s^{-1} or less. This allows time for adequate exchange of oxygen, nutrients and metabolites.

On the venous side, the cross-sectional area diminishes as we move from the capillaries through the venules and veins to the great veins, and the area of the vena cava near the entrance to the right atrium is about 700 mm^2. The blood leaves the capillary bed at a pressure of about 15 mmHg, but the venous side presents very little resistance to flow. So even at this relatively low pressure, the blood is able to reach the heart although its velocity of about 40 cm · s^{-1} is 10 cm · s^{-1} slower than that seen in the aorta and arteries. The resting values of mean pressure, cross-sectional area, and blood velocity of the principal blood vessels appear in Table 5.1.

Maintenance of venous return

The volume of venous return must match the initial volume pumped out by the left ventricle to sustain cardiac output. In addition to the 15 mmHg of venous pressure, three other mechanisms maintain venous blood flow back to the heart. The first consists of valves in the veins that prevent back-flow; the second is the negative pressure found in the thoracic cage which acts as a vacuum pump;

Table 5.1 Typical resting mean pressure, cross-sectional area, and blood velocity within the major divisions of the circulatory system

	Aorta	Large arteries	Small arteries	Arterioles	Capillaries	Venules	Small veins	Large veins	Venae cavae
Mean pressure (mmHg)	100	98	95	65	20	10	5	3	0
Cross-sectional area (cm^2)	5	175–225	475–525	~2600	~4500	~3500	1000	175	7
Blood velocity (cm · s^{-1})	48	46	45	17	0.1	1	10	35	40

finally, intra-abdominal pressure brought about by the flattening of the diaphragm during inspiration squeezes abdominal veins and speeds up blood flow.

Blood volume and its distribution

The distribution of the resting cardiac output of about 5 litres differs between the various regions of the circulatory system, and responds to the metabolic needs of particular tissues. The heart and the pulmonary circulation hold about 20 per cent, the arteries, arterioles and capillaries about 20 per cent, with the remaining 60 per cent stored in the veins and venules. Thus, the venous side performs an important function as a storage reservoir of blood that can be called upon in time of need such as exercise.

Blood flow distribution during exercise

The response of the systemic circulation to exercise is an example of the evolutionary 'fight or flight' mechanism. The autonomic nervous system controls this survival mechanism, and Figure 5.5 shows the effects on blood distribution. When faced with danger, the survival options are to stand and

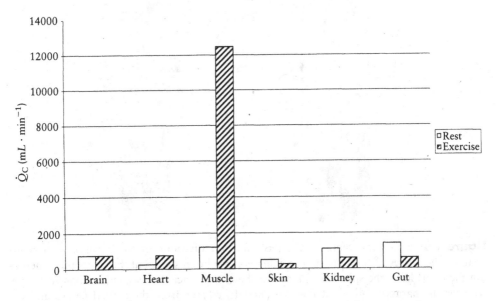

Figure 5.5   Distribution of blood volume at rest and during exercise

fight or to turn and flee; either option requires preparation for strenuous exercise. All body systems require oxygen in order to function, but in extreme situations, most systems can operate at a maintenance level whilst the maximum amount of blood that can be spared is re-directed to the muscles involved in survival activity. For example, irrespective of exercise intensity, blood flow to the brain is maintained or even increased slightly. This seems an appropriate safeguard; reduced oxygen supply to the brain resulting in impaired function may be fatal. The oxygen supply to the heart actually increases during exercise because of the increased work of the heart. However, blood flow to the viscera and the skin is restricted at the onset of exercise; the latter is seen when our face suddenly pales when faced with danger. The reservoir of blood in the venous system, together with the blood spared from the viscera and skin, can be redirected to the skeletal muscle tissue engaged in fighting or fleeing.

The autonomic nervous system and blood distribution

Several mechanisms combine to bring about the changes seen in Figure 5.5. These include the sympathetic division of the autonomic nervous system (see Figure 5.6), locally produced metabolites, temperature, and pressure. They

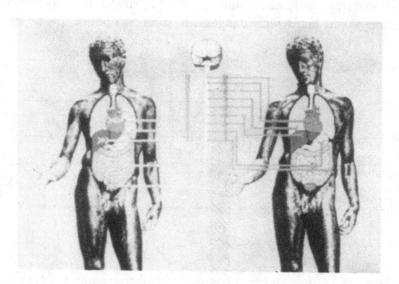

Figure 5.6 Schematic representation of the two divisions of the autonomic nervous system. The nerves of both divisions originate in the brain stem, but the sympathetic nerves (on the right) leave the spinal cord between the first thoracic and second lumbar vertebrae, whereas the parasympathetic nerves (on the left) emerge from the cranial nerves and the sacral vertebrae. (Reproduced by permission of Astra Zeneca plc)

regulate vascular tone to ensure skeletal muscle receives the maximum amount of blood possible without totally depriving other body systems of their vital oxygen.

Nor-adrenaline

The first of these mechanisms is the interaction between the sympathetic fibres of the autonomic nervous system innervating arteries and veins and activating the α and β_2 receptors. The profusion of sympathetic α receptors found in the arterioles of the skin, the viscera (the gut, the liver, the spleen and the kidneys) are stimulated by the release of noradrenaline. This release triggers an adrenergic response, namely, vasoconstriction and a marked reduction in blood flow.

Question 5.3   *Why is eating immediately before exercise a bad idea?*

However, the plentiful supply of β_2 receptors found in the arterioles and pre-capillary sphincters of skeletal muscle respond differently to noradrenaline: the general effect is vasodilatation but the response is rather moderate.

Adrenaline

This is not the case as far as adrenaline, the other sympathetic hormone, is concerned. This catecholamine preferentially stimulates the two forms of β receptors – β_1 found in the heart, and β_2 in skeletal muscle–that results in a cholinergic response, namely vasodilatation and increased blood flow. But adrenaline also has a vasoconstrictor effect on the α receptors of the peripheral circulation. For example, a weak solution of adrenaline is applied to cuts to the eyebrow received during professional boxing contests to constrict the exposed blood vessels and staunch blood flow.

Local metabolites

Another mechanism is the result of the by-products of metabolic activity in particular tissues. Metabolites such as carbon dioxide, lactate (La), and adenosine diphosphate (ADP) result from the breakdown (catabolism) of carbohydrates and fats. All of these by products are potent local vasodilators that directly affect the smooth muscle of the arterioles and pre-capillary sphincters. The presence of small quantities of such metabolites in all tissues, even at rest, ensures automatic regulation of blood supply and therefore oxygen. During strenuous exercise, the effects are magnified because of the increased production of all three metabolites. The metabolites form the principal autoregulatory mechanism, and in skeletal muscle overrides the slight vasoconstrictor effect of noradrenaline.

Temperature

Temperature also affects blood distribution. Core body temperature is 37°C, but exercise increases temperature because of the relative inefficiency of muscular activity; between 75 and 80 per cent of mechanical work is degraded into heat. Physical performance is adversely affected if core temperature increases significantly from normal. Various regulatory mechanisms exist to maintain temperature within acceptable boundaries. One mechanism reverses the initial vasoconstriction of blood vessels in the skin that can result in pallor; blood is shunted to the surface of the skin so that cooling can take place by conduction and sweat evaporation. This mechanism competes with those seeking to direct blood to the skeletal muscles and presents a physiological dilemma for the long-distance runner competing in hot humid conditions. Many sporting activities take place in cold environments – cross-channel swimming probably presents the most serious long-term challenge. The immediate reaction to cold exposure is constriction of the peripheral blood vessels, even when artificial insulation is introduced by applying grease to the body; women, who are the better competitors in this kind of event, already have an advantage because of their greater body fat. Here, physical performance is hampered by two mechanisms. The first is the withdrawal of blood from the periphery to the core, thus diverting blood away from skeletal muscle. Under extreme conditions such as mountaineering and trans-polar treks, prolonged flow restrictions to the extremities, particularly the feet, can result in death of tissue and loss of fingers or toes. The second is the temperature at which shivering – the body's reflex response designed to generate heat and raise core temperature – is triggered. In cold water immersion tests, reflex shivering, in an attempt to stave off hypothermia, can result in as much as 50 per cent of maximal oxygen uptake ($\dot{V}_{O_2max}$) being utilized. Clearly, the need to keep body temperature within narrow limits takes precedence over, and is detrimental to, physical performance.

Pressure

Finally, contraction of muscle fibres exerts pressure on blood vessels and interferes with capillary blood flow. For example, sustained isometric contractions as low as 20 per cent of maximal voluntary contraction (MVC) result in restricted blood flow to the muscle group concerned, and lead to a progressive fall in the force generated. Myocardial blood flow is interrupted during systole because of pressure on capillaries as the myocardium contracts. Flow occurs largely during diastole, and in normal circumstances is sufficient to meet the increased demand. During severe exercise S–T-segment depression and T-wave inversion are indicators of myocardial embarrassment sometimes seen in trained athletes, and frequently observed in patients with coronary heart disease undergoing diagnostic exercise stress tests.

Conversely, on the venous side of the systemic circulation, the consequences of rhythmical pressure generated by muscles of the lower limbs are beneficial. Because of the arrangement of valves in the veins of the limbs, the contractions, known as the muscle pump, squeeze venous blood vessels, pushing venous blood towards the heart thus augmenting venous return. You can repeat William Harvey's experiment to confirm this. Harvey was an English physician who described the links between the heart and the blood vessels in 1628. He put a tourniquet around an artery and then a vein in his arm; he saw that blood built up on the heart side of the artery, but on the side away from the heart in the vein. He then squeezed the blood out of the occluded vein, and saw that blood did not flow back into it. He came to two conclusions; first, that the veins must carry blood to the heart, and second that there must be valves within the blood vessel preventing blood from flowing back into the vein.

The Hagen–Poiseuille equation

All of the mechanisms described above share one feature, namely a change in the diameter of the blood vessel. Jean Poiseuille, a French physician and physiologist, studied the flow of blood in the arteries. In 1849, he reported that the volume of a fluid flowing through a capillary depended on

(a) the *radius* and *length* of the vessel;

(b) the driving *pressure*;

(c) and the *viscosity* of the fluid.

Flow is directly proportional to pressure and diameter, and inversely proportional to length and viscosity. The relationship, which only applies to laminar flow, was called Poiseuille's law until it was realized that a German engineer interested in hydraulics, Gotthilff Hagen, had discovered the relationship a year earlier. The Hagen–Poiseuille equation, as it is now known, is

$$Q = \frac{\pi PR^4}{8L\eta}$$

where π (pi) equals 3.147, P is pressure, R is the radius of the tube, L is its length and η (eta) is the fluid viscosity.

Let us see how exercise affects each of the elements of this relationship. Pi is a constant: greater driving pressure increases flow, the increased length of the tube, brought about by vasodilatation of previously closed capillaries, reduces flow; a greater viscosity (stickiness of the blood) results in increased resistance to flow and reduces it. Thus far, the changes appear to have a net disadvantage for blood flow to skeletal muscle. However, the key factor lies in the expression R^4, that is $(R \cdot R \cdot R \cdot R)$. Suppose the original flow rate is $1000 \ \text{mL} \cdot \text{min}^{-1}$; *doubling* the radius – a vasodilator effect – increases flow by 16 times $(2 \cdot 2 \cdot 2 \cdot 2)$ its original rate, i.e. it would increase to $16\,000 \ \text{mL} \cdot \text{min}^{-1}$. Vasodilator responses are at work on arterioles and pre-capillary sphincters. *Halving* the radius would reduce flow to $62.5 \ \text{mL} \cdot \text{min}^{-1}$ – a sixteenth of its original rate. The vasoconstrictor response is at work in the skin, viscera, and kidneys, reducing blood flow to a minimum and allowing delivery of a greater proportion of the total blood volume to skeletal muscle. Clearly, the *radius* of a blood vessel has a dramatic effect on blood flow, and the interaction of vasoconstriction and vasodilatation is responsible for the redistribution of blood seen in Figure 5.5 above.

This holds provided flow in the blood vessels is laminar. Flow can be crudely described as either laminar (streamlined) or turbulent. The difference between the two forms appears in Figure 5.7.

Reynolds number

A second equation, the dimensionless Reynolds number (R_e), derived by the Irish engineer Osborne Reynolds, indicates the point at which laminar flow becomes turbulent. The equation is

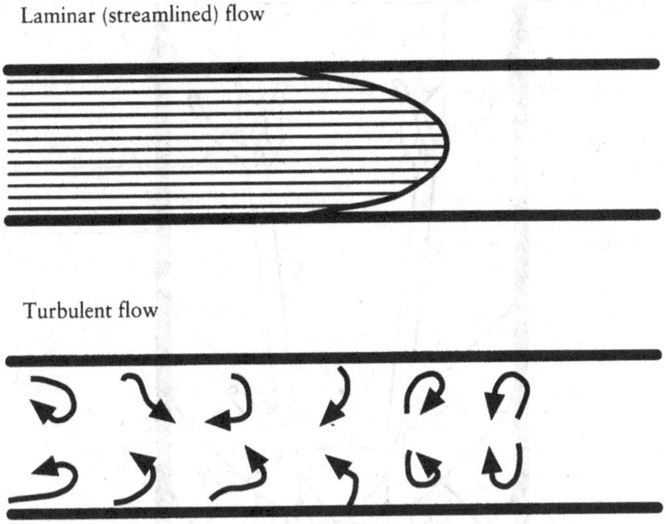

Laminar (streamlined) flow

Turbulent flow

Figure 5.7 Laminar and turbulent flow profiles

$$R_e = \frac{d\rho v}{\eta}$$

where d is the diameter of the tube, ρ (rho) is the density of the fluid, η (eta) its viscosity, and v (nu) its velocity. Below 2000 the flow is generally laminar, above 2000 flow is generally turbulent. Turbulence is likely if blood velocity is high and pulsatile, and the vessel diameter large.

Question 5.4 *Where in the systemic circulation would turbulent flow be most likely?*

Regulation of arterial blood pressure

The maintenance of blood pressure requires the interaction of neural, chemical and hormonal mechanisms. We find stretch receptors, often called baroreceptors (Figure 5.8), in the venae cavae, the right atrium, the aortic arch, and the carotid sinus. If the pressure from blood flowing past these receptors is too high, signals are sent to the cardiac centres in the medulla oblongata. Both sides of the autonomic nervous system become involved. Parasympathetic activity is stimulated and impulses from the vagus nerve slow heart rate; sympathetic

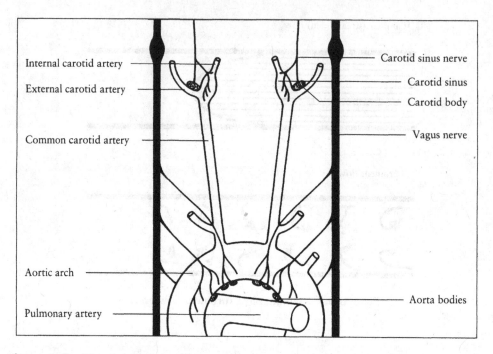

Internal carotid artery

External carotid artery

Common carotid artery

Aortic arch

Pulmonary artery

Carotid sinus nerve

Carotid sinus

Carotid body

Vagus nerve

Aorta bodies

Figure 5.8   The distribution of baroreceptors and chemoreceptors of the aorta, carotid sinus and carotid bodies. (With permission of Astra Zeneca plc)

activity is inhibited so arteries dilate and venous return falls. Both actions lead to a reduced cardiac output and lowered blood pressure. If blood pressure is too low, the opposite set of responses is provoked.

Question 5.5   *There is a quick, effective, but illegal, way of winning a wrestling competition. What might it be?*

Chemoreceptors in the aortic and carotid bodies are also involved. Low pressure results in sluggish flow and slow removal of metabolites such as carbon dioxide, and hydrogen ions (H^+). These conditions are detected by the receptors and transmitted to the medulla; sympathetic stimulation occurs, leading to vasoconstriction, and pressure is raised. Hormones belonging to the group known as angiotensins also play a part in regulating blood pressure. When blood pressure is low in the kidney, it releases the hormone renin; this stimulates the production of angiotensin II, a powerful arteriolar vasoconstrictor, which reinforces other regulatory mechanisms and raises blood pressure.

The oxygen molecules are now on the threshold of the skeletal muscle cells. Before we consider the mechanisms that drive oxygen consumption during skeletal muscle contraction, we need to look at the structure of skeletal muscle and how contraction can take place. This is the topic for the next chapter.

Key points

- The systemic circulatory system consists of the aorta, arteries and arterioles to carry blood away from the heart, whilst venules, veins and the venae cavae return blood to the heart.

- A network of capillaries invading body tissues connects the two sides.

- Resting systolic and diastolic pressures in young adults are typically 120 and 80 mmHg respectively.

- During sub-maximal, steady-state exercise, systolic pressure rises initially and then plateaus.

- During continuous, progressive exercise, systolic pressure rises in line with heart rate.

- Diastolic pressure hardly changes, and during steady-state exercise may fall fractionally.

- The walls of the arteries and veins consist of an inner layer of cells (the intima), a middle layer of elastic tissue and smooth muscle (the media), and an outer layer of connective tissue (the adventitia).

- The capillaries consist of a single layer of endothelial cells.

- The walls of the arteries are thicker than the veins and contain more elastic tissue and smooth muscle.

- The velocity of blood is lowest in the capillaries, thus ensuring adequate time for exchange of materials.

- At rest most of the total blood volume goes to the viscera – the gut, the liver, the spleen and the kidneys – and skin.

- During exercise most of the blood is redirected to the working skeletal muscles.

- This redistribution is achieved (a) by autonomic nervous system release of noradrenaline that constricts blood vessels leading to the viscera and skin, and (b) by increased production of carbon dioxide, lactate, and adenosine diphosphate by skeletal muscle that act as vasodilators on the smooth muscle of the pre-capillary sphincters.

- Body temperature also affects peripheral blood vessels.

- A low temperature drives blood to the core of the body to retain heat; a high temperature diverts blood to the skin to lose heat.

- When flow is laminar – that is, has a Reynolds number less than 2000 – the Hagen–Poiseuille equation governs flow in tubes.

- Changes in the radius of the capillary change flow by the fourth power of the radius.

- Halving the radius reduces flow to one-sixteenth of its original volume; doubling the radius increases flow by a factor of 16.

- Blood pressure is regulated by stretch receptors and chemoreceptors in the aortic arch and carotid sinus, stretch receptors in the vena cava and right atrium, and autonomic nervous activity of both sympathetic and parasympathetic systems.

- The cardiac control centre in the medulla oblongata responds to low or high blood pressure by increasing or reducing cardiac output.

Answers to questions in the text

Question 5.1

In response to continuous, progressive exercise, systolic pressure rises in line with cardiac output; at maximal exercise, pressures may exceed 200 mmHg. In sub-maximal, steady-state exercise, the pressure rises to a plateau; in progressive, steady state exercise, the plateaus appear at higher levels until a steady state cannot be maintained. Diastolic pressure generally changes little, about 5 to 10 mmHg increase at maximal exercise; in sub-maximal, steadystate diastolic pressure can fall slightly in response to peripheral vasodilatation.

Question 5.2

Smooth muscle is under the control of the autonomic nervous system and responds to local metabolic vasodilators such as carbon dioxide, lactate, and adenosine diphosphate. During exercise, the smooth muscle in the arterioles and particularly the pre-capillary sphincters leading to skeletal muscles dilate, enhancing blood flow. Conversely, the smooth muscle in vessels leading to the viscera and the skin contract, thus restricting blood flow. Applying the Hagen–Poiseuille equation indicates the extent of the change in vessel radius on blood flow.

Question 5.3

In response to intake of food, blood flow to the stomach and intestines increases to cope with the digestive process. During exercise, the blood is shunted away from the gut to meet the more important demands of skeletal muscles. Thus, there is competition between the two needs. The needs of the muscle are paramount, so blood flow to the gut is minimized and that interferes with the digestion.

Question 5.4

Turbulent flow is most likely where velocity is high; it is highest in the aorta and falls dramatically as blood approaches the arterioles. Laminar flow is most likely in the capillaries.

Question 5.5

The carotid sinuses situated on either side of the larynx can be stimulated by external pressure. Excessive stimulation can lead to a dramatic fall in blood pressure and blood flow, particularly to the brain; this leads to a momentary loss of consciousness. A rule forbidding wrestlers to apply pressure on the sinuses prevents victory in a competition using this tactic.

6

Oxygen Consumption – the Structure and Contraction of Skeletal Muscle

Learning Objectives

By the end of this chapter, you should be able to

♦ name the three types of muscle fibre and describe their main characteristics

♦ describe the major constituents of intracellular and extracellular fluid

♦ explain the presence of the resting membrane potential

♦ explain the formation of an action potential and its subsequent propagation

♦ provide a definition of the 'all-or-none law' in relation to muscle fibre contraction

♦ label the major features of the sarcomere

♦ describe the constituent features of myofilaments

♦ explain the importance of calcium in the contraction process

♦ describe the sliding filament mechanism

♦ explain the part played by adenosine triphosphate in the contraction and relaxation process

Exercise Physiology: A Thematic Approach   Tudor Hale
© John Wiley & Sons, Ltd   ISBN: 0 470 84682 8 (cloth), ISBN 0 470 84683 6 (pbk)

Objective test

Say whether the following answers are true (T) or false (F). If you do not know, say so (D) – not knowing is not an academic crime, but not finding out is. Try not to look at the answers until you have worked your way through the chapter and completed the test a second time. In this way, you can monitor your progress.

	Pre-test			Post-test		
	T	F	D	T	F	D
1. Type I fibres are fast-twitch fibres						
2. The Type I fibres contain little myoglobin and few mitochondria						
3. The main source of ATP for Type I fibres is anaerobic glycolysis						
4. Type IIb fibres exert large forces and fatigue quickly						
5. Type IIb fibres rely on oxidative phosphorylation for their ATP						
6. Type IIa fibres are fast-twitch oxidative						
7. The extracellular fluid contains high levels of sodium						
8. The intracellular fluid is low in potassium						
9. The outside of a cell membrane is negative in relation to the inside						
10. The resting membrane potential is ~ -75 mV						
11. When stimulated, a nerve fibre produces an action potential						
12. An action potential makes the membrane permeable to sodium						
13. When stimulated the membrane potential becomes positive						
14. The 'all-or-none law' applies only to single muscle fibres						

	Pre-test			Post-test		
	T	F	D	T	F	D
15. The 'all-or-none law' states that any stimulus produces a contraction						
16. Skeletal muscle is smooth and involuntary						
17. The basic contractile unit of skeletal muscle fibres is the sarcomere						
18. Thousands of sarcomeres stacked end-to-end make up a myofibril						
19. The membrane of the sarcomere is called the neuro-lemma						
20. The membrane restrains a gel-like mixture called the sarcoplasm						
21. Embedded in the sarcoplasm are protein filaments						
22. The thin filaments are made up from the protein myosin						
23. The thick filaments are made up from the protein actin						
24. The thin filaments consist of a double helix of globular molecules						
25. The thick filaments contain troponin and tropomyosin						
26. Muscle contracts when thin filaments slide between thick filaments						
27. Contraction is triggered by release of Ca^{2+}						
28. The sarcoplasm contains high levels of Ca^{2+}						
29. The Ca^{2+} interacts with the myosin filament to produce contraction						
30. ADP is the primary energy source for muscle contraction						

Symbols, abbreviations and units of measurement

acetylcholine	ACh	
adenosine diphosphate	ADP	
adenosine triphosphate	ATP	
adenosine triphosphatase	*ATPase*	
calcium	Ca^{2+}	
chloride	Cl^-	
creatine kinase	*CK*	
electromyography	EMG	
fibre type – slow oxidative	Type I; SO	
fibre type – fast oxidative glycolytic	Type IIa; FOG	
fibre type – fast glycolitic	Type IIb; FG	
hydrogen carbonate, bicarbonate	HCO_3^-	
inorganic phosphate	P_i	
magnesium	Mg^+	
maximal voluntary contraction	MVC	
millivolts	mV	
myoglobin	Mgb	
phosphate	PO_4^{3-}	
potassium	K^+	
sodium	Na^+	
velocity	v	$m \cdot s^{-1}$

Introduction

At the simplest level, skeletal muscle contraction is nothing more than a succession of electrical, chemical and mechanical events, all of which use adenosine triphosphate (ATP) as fuel. The process begins with an electrical impulse from the brain, called an action potential. This initiates a chain of biochemical reactions that ends in the burning of adenosine triphosphate, the fuel for muscle contraction. Its use results in the forces that move the limbs and generate heat. Electrodes attached to a muscle group record the electrical activity accompanying contraction; the name of this recording process is electromyography (EMG).

Question 6.1 *You have already seen an example of a similar kind of recording when looking at the heart action. What was it called, and what did it represent?*

Electromyography

There are three major muscle actions – isometric, concentric and eccentric – performed by skeletal muscle; all three forms occur during the actions seen in sport and exercise performance. Isometric (from the Greek *isos* = equal and *metron* = measure) action occurs when an athlete tries to leg-press a heavy load by flexing the quadriceps muscles, but cannot move the weight-stack in spite of a maximum effort. The muscle produces force, but it is insufficient to overcome the mass of the weight-stack; hence, the overall muscle length does not shorten. Concentric action occurs when a muscle is active and shortening; for example, during the biceps curl the biceps shorten and exert enough force to lift the barbell. Eccentric action occurs when a muscle is active and shortening; for example, when lowering the barbell the biceps exert force to ensure the movement is controlled. The typical electrical activity produced during the three actions is shown in Figure 6.1.

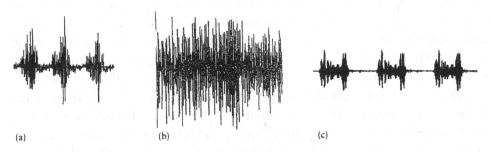

(a)   (b)   (c)

Figure 6.1 Electromyographic output showing responses to concentric, eccentric and isometric muscle actions. (See the answer to Question 6.2 for further information)

Question 6.2 *Which EMG trace reflects which action?*

The origins of contraction

It is important to recall that skeletal muscle, unlike the smooth and cardiac varieties, is under voluntary control. We decide whether we want to stretch out an arm to switch off the alarm, get out of bed, make a cup of coffee, lift a pen, or run a marathon. Thus, the contraction process starts in the motor cortex of the brain. A change in the chemistry of the brain cells leads to an electrical impulse called an action potential. This impulse travels swiftly down the motor nerves of the pyramidal tract in the spinal cord and then to the motor end-plates attached to a particular group of muscle fibres. The impulse crosses the gap between the end-plate and the membrane of the muscle fibre by means of a neurotransmitter.

> **Question 6.3**   *Can you remember what this gap is called, and how the nerve impulses cross it?*

This stimulates the muscle cell to release its stored calcium (Ca^{2+}) which results in a shortening of the contractile units of the sarcomere and the production of force.

Intracellular and extracellular fluids

To gain some understanding of the initiation and propagation of the action potential we need to look at the electrochemical nature of nerve and muscle fibres and their membranes. All cells, including nerve and muscle cells, contain an intracellular fluid (ICF). In nerves, the fluid is axoplasm; in muscles, it is sarcoplasm. An extracellular fluid (ECF), called the interstitial fluid, bathes the tissues. The critical feature of these two fluids is that they have different chemical compositions. The intracellular fluid contains high levels of potassium (K^+), phosphate (PO_4^{3-}) and proteins. The extracellular fluid consists mainly of sodium (Na^+), chloride (Cl^-), and hydrogen carbonate (HCO_3^-), also known as bicarbonate, but no protein.

The resting membrane potential

The membranes of the nerve and muscle cells – the neurolemma, and the sarcolemma, respectively – consist of a double layer of lipid (fat) and protein molecules known as phospholipids; this double layer is the plasma membrane. Some materials can pass through the membrane easily – water and oxygen, for example – but others, e.g. large protein molecules, cannot. When this state of affairs exists, the membrane is said to be *selectively* permeable. As we have seen earlier, there is an imbalance in the levels of sodium and potassium between the intracellular and extracellular fluids. This results in the potassium diffusing *out* of the fibre easily; but the sodium diffuses *into* the muscle cell much more slowly. This leads to an ionic (electrical) imbalance between the two fluids. However, the electrical charges of each fluid compartment strive to maintain electrical neutrality. To ensure that this happens the sodium ions are actively pumped out of the cell and the potassium ions actively pumped in; the mechanism, fuelled by adenosine triphosphate, is an ionic pump. The major anion in the sarcoplasm, i.e. protein, cannot diffuse across the membrane and so escape from the ICF. This makes the inner layer of the membrane negatively charged in relation to the outer layer; thus, the membrane is polarized. The negative electrical difference between the inside and outside – the resting membrane potential – is about −90 millivolts (mV) (Figure 6.2).

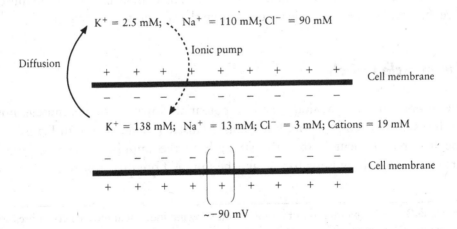

Figure 6.2   The chemical composition of intracellular and extracellular fluids that results in the development of the resting membrane potential of about −90 mV. The intracellular potassium level of ∼138 mM is maintained by active transport of the ions across the selectively permeable cell membrane

The action potential and transmission of the nerve impulse

An easy way of understanding the action potential and transmission of the nerve impulse is to look at a motor unit (Figure 6.3). This consists of three parts: first, a motor nerve; second, the myoneural (muscle–nerve) junction consisting of a complex of several motor end-plates; and, third, a bundle of myofibrils.

The decision to perform a movement begins in the motor cortex of the brain. This impulse, providing it is above a certain threshold, produces a local disturbance that transiently changes the permeability of the neurolemma of the motor neuron. Sodium moves into the nerve cells, and reverses the polarity of the membrane to positive inside and negative outside. The process is depolarization that results in an action potential (Figure 6.4).

Once one cell is depolarized, it then affects its neighbour *ad infinitum*. The wave of depolarization travels down the motor nerve quickly – between 60 and 120 m · s^{-1} – in a 'domino effect' until the action potential reaches the motor end-plate. However, the analogy of the 'domino-effect' is only partly useful. Once knocked over, dominoes stay down, but as the wave of depolarization moves on to the adjoining parts of the fibre, the ionic pump rapidly restores the resting membrane potential; this process is repolarization, and the membrane is now ready for the next stimulus. When the action potential reaches the end of the nerve fibre it crosses the gap between nerve and muscle, and passes along the muscle fibre at a speed of about 5 m · s^{-1}. The depolarization of the muscle fibre membrane leads to a release of calcium that triggers contraction.

The muscle twitch

The propagation of a single action potential down a single muscle fibre produces a single contraction, known as a muscle twitch, shown in Figure 6.5. The first requirement is that the strength of the impulse exceeds a certain threshold. If the impulse is too weak, the muscle fibre does not respond at all;

Figure 6.3 (a) A micrograph of a motor unit showing individual motor nerve fibres and the myoneural junction. (The tissue has been damaged slightly during the preparation of the slide.) (a) (Reproduced by permission of Philip Harris Education, Ashby-de-la-Zouch) (b) A schematic representation of the link between the central nervous system and the motor unit. Supra-threshold stimulation of the motor unit leads to all muscle fibres contracting, illustrating the 'all-or-none' law

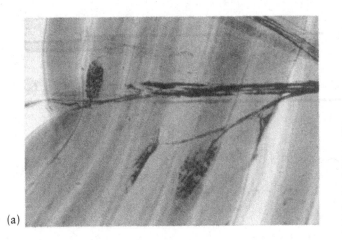

(a)

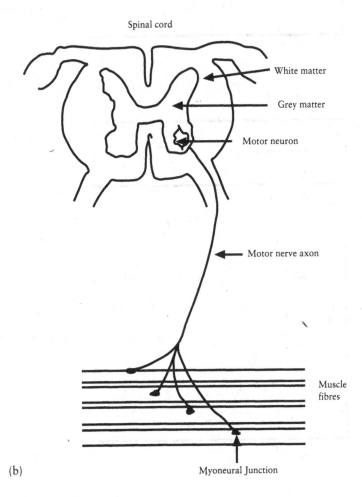

Spinal cord

White matter

Grey matter

Motor neuron

Motor nerve axon

Muscle
fibres

Myoneural Junction

(b)

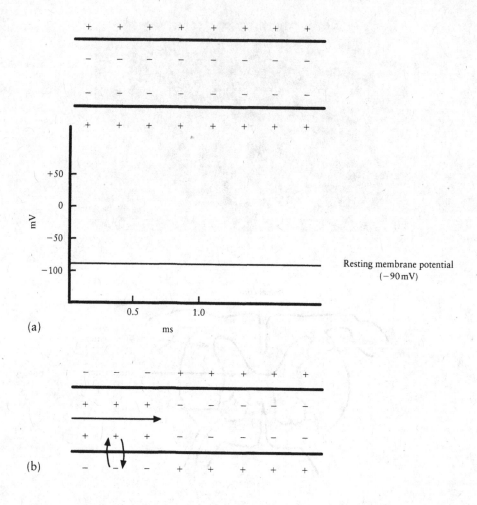

Resting membrane potential
(−90 mV)

(a)

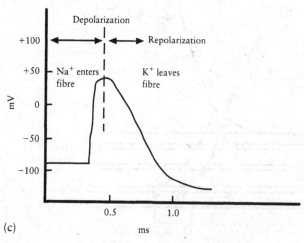

(b)

(c)

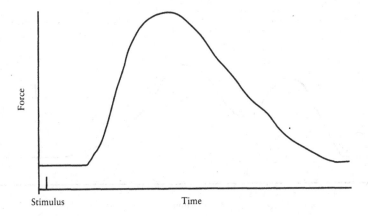

Figure 6.5 A muscle twitch: the response of a single muscle fibre to a single supra-threshold stimulus showing the latent period between stimulus and response and the force generated

but if the impulse is strong enough to exceed the threshold, the muscle responds fully, irrespective of the strength of the stimulus received. This is the 'all-or-none law'. The outcome of the response is a muscle twitch consisting of three phases. The first, which occurs between the arrival of the action potential and the start of the response, is the latent, or refractory, phase. During this refractory phase, the muscle cannot respond to any further stimulation. The second phase sees the development of tension. The final stage is the relaxation phase.

Summation and tetanus

If a second stimulus develops *after* the refractory phase, the muscle can respond with another twitch response, and will develop greater force; this is summation. Multiple stimuli result in tetanus, a phase of prolonged contraction, that generates greater force and is one of the mechanisms involved in the production of smooth, coordinated muscle actions seen in everyday activities. The other

Figure 6.4 The development of an action potential: (a) the polarized membrane at rest; the positive potassium ions leaking out of the nerve fibre lead to the negatively charged inner surface and the resting membrane potential at about $-90mV$; (b) a stimulus makes the membrane permeable to sodium, causing the inner surface becoming positively charged; this is depolarization of the cell membrane; (c) the resultant action potential and repolarization as the ionic pump restores the resting membrane potential

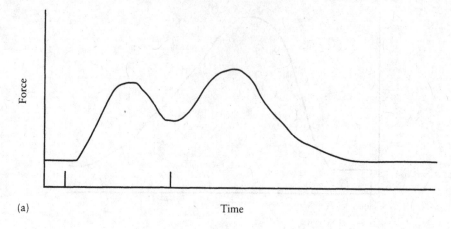

(a)   Time

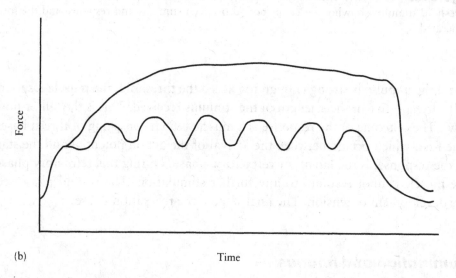

(b)   Time

Figure 6.6   The response of a single muscle fibre to (a) two, and (b) multiple supra-threshold stimuli. The former is called 'summation', the latter 'tetany'. The lower trace is unfused tetany, the upper trace is fused tetany. Note the increased force generated by increasingly frequent stimuli

mechanism arises from the fact that motor units fire at different times, and muscles vary in the time taken to contract and relax.

The grading of muscle response

The motor axon leaving the spinal cord contains many individual nerve fibres serving a number of end-plates. A single nerve fibre, with its end-plates attached to several muscle fibres, is a motor unit. Once a motor unit is stimulated, all of the fibres in that unit are depolarized and contract. The number of motor units in any particular muscle group varies with the functions to be performed.

Question 6.4   *Can you think of two factors needed for the generation of maximum force of a muscle group?*

The number of fibres per motor unit is low where fine movements are required, such as those performed by the fingers, and for fast movements required to focus the eyes. In slower, gross movements, such as those involving the legs, fewer nerve fibres serve hundreds of muscle fibres.

The force generated by the muscles is a function of the rate of stimulation and the number of motor units involved. Theoretically, a maximum voluntary contraction (MVC) entails a stimulus rate of about $50-60$ s^{-1} and engagement of all motor units. However, untrained subjects do not engage all units. An example of this occurs during an attempted maximum voluntary isometric contraction of the quadriceps muscle. External electrical stimulation of the femoral nerve produces greater tension than that seen under voluntary effort, suggesting engagement of more motor units. Supra-maximal stimulation, however, can be dangerous and may lead to a catastrophic rupture of the patellar tendon.

Muscle fibre types

Humans exhibit a range of muscle actions whilst taking part in exercise and sports. Consider the differences between the slow, precise control of the cue when playing a delicate shot in snooker and the slow withdrawal of the drawstring of a bow in archery, where precision is just as important but where the load placed on the muscles is much greater. Compare the delicacy of a controlled lay-off in soccer, to the power of a goal kick. Look at the power generated by the 100-m runner compared with that of a 10 000-m runner. In terms of survival, our muscles have had to respond to all of these kinds of demands. It is hardly surprising, then, that the natural selection at work during our evolutionary past responded to these varying demands by selecting those of our ancestors who developed a range of at least three kinds of muscle fibres to cater for different needs.

We can illustrate this by looking at track and field athletes. Sprinters and throwers do not often compete in marathons, long-distance runners do not often excel at hammer throwing, shot-putters do not excel at the high jump. One of the factors involved in their choice of event is the fact that all skeletal muscle consists of two main types of muscle fibres: (Type I) slow-twitch, or slow oxidative (SO), and fast-twitch (Type II). The latter type subdivides into (IIa): fast oxidative glycolytic (FOG), and (IIb) fast glycolitic (FG). Evolution has given us a mixture of all three types in varying proportions mainly laid down at conception, but partially adapted to usage. These proportions, together with other social and environmental factors, largely determine whether we have the capacity to develop into a sprinter, thrower, high jumper, marathon runner, or decathlete.

The Type I fibres are the thinnest of the three types, contract relatively slowly, and generate relatively low forces. Their red colour arises from the presence of large quantities of stored myoglobin (Mgb). They are aerobic fibres and more resistant to fatigue; they are richly supplied with capillaries and mitochondria so that oxygen is readily accessible and available for oxidative phosphorylation. Type IIb fibres are the complete opposite of Type I. They are the thickest fibres, and generate large forces quickly. They contain very little myoglobin and so are very pale, and have few mitochondria. They are dependent for their adenosine triphosphate on the glycolitic pathway, and so fatigue relatively quickly. The characteristics of the Type IIa fibres lie between the two extremes, and their main advantages are that they contract quickly and forcefully, and can call on both glycolytic and oxidative pathways for their adenosine triphosphate supply.

Exercise 6.1

What proportions of the Type I, IIa and IIb fibres are likely to be present in the quadriceps muscle group used to create power during the activities of the five kinds of athlete listed at the end of the previous paragraph but one? What about soccer players?

The ultra-structure of muscle fibres

The sarcomere

The basic building block of skeletal muscle is the sarcomere (from the Greek *sarkos* for flesh). The sarcomere is the smallest unit of striated skeletal muscle that is capable of independent contraction. A membrane, called the sarcolemma, holds the sarcomere together. This membrane separates the intracellular fluid – sarcoplasm – from the extracellular, or interstitial, fluid. Sarcoplasm is a 'physiological soup' consisting of water, enzymes that speed up chemical reactions, nutrients such as carbohydrate (glycogen) and fat (triglycerides), many nuclei, and the mitochondria, often referred to as the powerhouse of the cell. Also present are electrically charged atoms and molecules called ions that have the potential to act as physiological electric batteries. Ions carry positive (cations) or negative (anions) charges. Within the intracellular fluid the main cations, are potassium, nearly 80 per cent, and magnesium (Mg^+); there is very little sodium. The main anions are organic phosphates, about 68 per cent, and protein 26 per cent, with very small amounts of chloride, and hydrogen carbonate. The main cation of the extracellular fluid is sodium, about 95 per cent; the major anions are chloride, about 75 per cent, and hydrogen carbonate about 20 per cent.

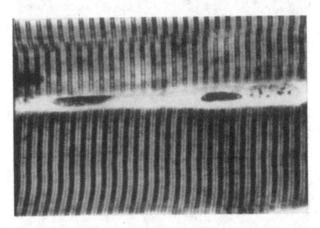

Figure 6.7 Micrograph of skeletal muscle clearly showing the characteristic striations (Reproduced by permission of Philip Harris Education Ashby-de-la-Zouch.)

Myofilaments

Embedded in the sarcoplasm are strands of protein known as myofilaments. There are thick myofilaments, about 12 nanometres (nm) – one thousand millionth of a metre – in diameter, containing mainly myosin. In the middle of the myosin filament is the M line; this contains M filaments that provide structural support, and hold the enzyme *creatine kinase* (CK). Actin is another protein, crucial for muscle contraction; this protein takes the form of thin filaments about 6 nm in diameter.

The thick and thin myofilaments overlap giving rise to the pattern of light and dark bands, zones and lines that result in their striated appearance. This light pattern is given a series of letters – A and I bands, the H zone, and M and Z lines – as shown in Figure 6.8.

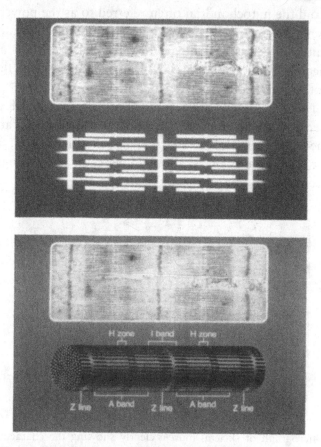

Figure 6.8   The relationship between the striations and the bands, zones and lines of the sarcomere. The H zone is bisected by the M line which supports the myosin filaments. (Reproduced by permission of Astra Zeneca plc)

Question 6.5   *Define the following features of the sarcomere: Z discs; I band; A band; H zone; M line.*

The structure lying between two Z lines, or more properly Z discs, constitutes the sarcomere (Figure 6.9).

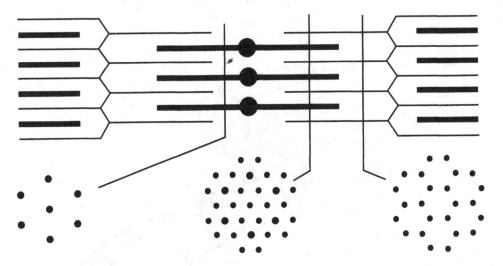

Figure 6.9 The arrangement of filaments at different sections of the sarcomere. (Reproduced by permission of Astra Zeneca plc)

Connective tissues

The sarcolemma consists of three sections. The innermost layer is made up from lipids and proteins and is called the plasma membrane; this is supported by a basement membrane. The final layer is a network of connective tissue in the form of very fine collagen fibres. Many sarcomeres stacked end-to-end form a myofibril with a diameter of about 1 μm. Many myofibrils make up the individual muscle fibre and may stretch its entire length. Three connective tissues give strength to the muscle. The endomysium supports the fibre, along with its supply of nerves and blood vessels. The perimysium encloses large numbers of fibres. The final capsule, the epimysium, surrounds a major muscle group like the biceps and quadriceps. Each successive layer of connective tissue is important because they all fuse together at each end of the muscle fibre to make up the muscle tendon. Attached to bones, the tendons transmit the force generated by muscle activation to stabilize or produce movements at the joints (see Figure 6.10).

The mechanics of the sliding filament theory

Muscle contraction is the result of the actin filaments sliding between the myosin filaments, thus bringing the two Z discs closer together. This process is

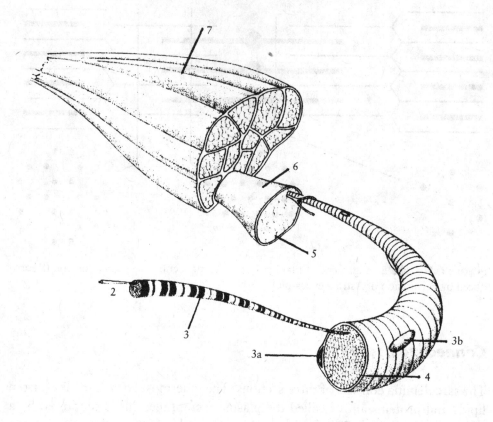

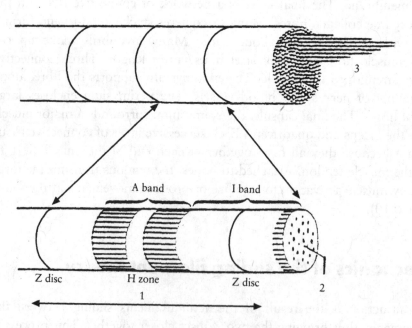

the 'sliding filament theory' of muscle contraction, proposed separately, but coincidentally, in 1954 by the unrelated H. E. Huxley and A. F. Huxley.

Question 6.6 *What disappears as the filaments slide past each other?*

Let us look at the sequence of events involved in a single muscle contraction.

Actin and myosin filaments

If we make a cross-section of the I band of a myofibril we can see that the actin filaments, attached to the Z discs, form a hexagonal pattern. If we do the same at the H zone, actin is absent but the myosin filaments form a similar pattern. A section across the A band shows myosin filaments in the centre of the hexagonal framework of actin, and actin filaments in the centre of equilateral triangles of myosin (Figures 6.9 and 6.11). The thick filaments consist of myosin molecules in the form of a collection of hinged rods to which are attached protein heads; at rest, the rods lie horizontally, with the heads protruding slightly. The myosin heads hold an enzyme, *adenosine triphosphatase* (*ATPase*), which breaks down adenosine triphosphate into adenosine diphosphate and inorganic phosphate (P_i).

The thin filaments consist of spherical actin molecules twisted together to form a thread-like structure called an alpha (α) helix. Short strands of the protein tropomyosin lie in the groove of the α helix and conceal sites that are capable of interacting with the myosin heads. Troponin, which consists of three regulatory proteins, occurs at regular intervals along the α helix. One of the proteins is attached to the actin globule; the second is attached to the strand of tropomyosin; the third, is capable of taking up calcium. An action potential

Figure 6.10 The sub-units of a muscle group. The basic building block is the sarcomere (1) containing myofilaments of actin and myosin (2) embedded in sarcoplasm. Sarcomeres stacked end-to-end make up the myofibril (3). Collections of myofibrils, together with their nuclei (3a), and mitochondria (3b) contained by the sarcolemma (4) make up muscle fibres (5) supported by connective tissue called the endomysium. Bundles of fibres surrounded by the perimysium (6) make up the muscle group enclosed by the epimysium (7). The connective tissues eventually fuse together to make up the tendons attached to bones. (Based on Tortora and Grabowski, John Wiley, New York, 2003)

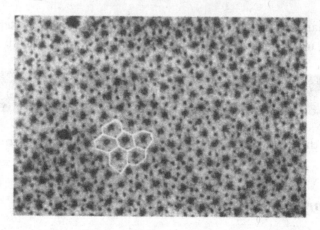

Figure 6.11   Cross-section through the A band of a muscle fibre showing the myosin filament surrounded by six actin filaments. (Reproduced by permission of Astra Zeneca plc)

stimulates the release of calcium from storage reservoirs; this combines with the third troponin protein and causes the tropomyosin strands to sink deeper into the actin α helix, thus exposing the actomyosin binding sites.

The sarcoplasmic reticulum

The sarcoplasm contains very little free calcium, so other mechanisms are involved in the release of calcium ions from their storage reservoir. This release involves three structures. The first is a sleeve of longitudinal microtubules wrapped around the muscle cell called the sarcoplasmic (or endoplasmic) reticulum. The second structure consists of deep invaginations of the fibre called the transverse or T-tubules (Figure 6.12). These tubules lie near the junctions of the A and I bands of the sarcomere; they resemble blind passageways and convey the action potential deep into the muscle fibres. The final element consists of two calcium storage vessels at the outer edges of the longitudinal tubules called the cisternae. The cisternae are in very close proximity to the T-tubules. This suggests that the T-tubule carries the action potential to the very heart of the myofibrils and ensures the triggering of calcium release. Ionic pumps, fuelled by adenosine triphosphate, return the calcium to the storage vessels ready for the next action potential.

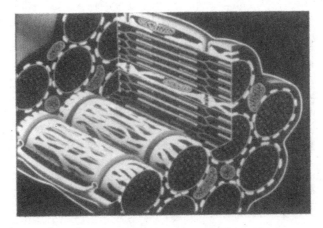

Figure 6.12 The longitudinal tubules and T-tubules of the sarcoplasmic reticulum. (Reproduced by permission of AstraZeneca plc)

Adenosine triphosphate

Contraction can only occur when both calcium and adenosine triphosphate are present. The presence of the calcium exposes the actin binding sites, and, together with magnesium, activates the enzyme *adenosine triphosphatase* stored in the myosin heads.

Adenosine triphosphate performs two functions. First, one phosphate bond is split off (it is dephosphorylated) to form adenosine diphosphate and inorganic phosphate; in doing so, the splitting provides the energy for contraction. The hinged myosin rods allow the heads to swing away from the body of the filament, rather like the oars of a rowing boat. The myosin heads, representing the blade of the oars, engage with the exposed binding sites on the actin α-helix, rather similar to oars catching the water (Figure 6.13). The myosin heads then drag the actin filaments, similar to dragging the boat past the oars. The sarcomere shortens, pulling the Z discs closer together, and the H zone disappears (Figure 6.14). Thus, the energy from the dephosphorylation of adenosine triphosphate fuels the rowing action.

Second, adenosine triphosphate binds to the myosin heads causing them to disengage from the actin-binding sites, and the entire process of hydrolysis, attachment and power stroke begins again. As the wave of polarization spreads along the entire fibre, countless numbers of sarcomeres shorten, thus pulling on the tendons attached to the bones. Finally, additional adenosine triphosphate provides the energy needed for the ionic pump to return the calcium to the sarcoplasmic reticulum. Without the continual supply of adenosine triphosphate via the phosphagen system, aerobic glycolysis, the Krebs cycle and the

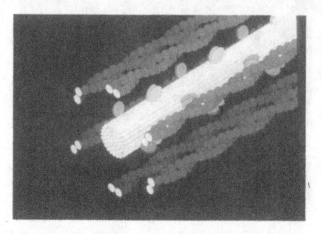

Figure 6.13   The location of a myosin filament, with its protruding heads, and the six actin filaments in a hexagonal arrangement. The heads of the myosin filament swing out and attach themselves to the actin filaments during the power stroke of contraction, resulting in the filaments sliding past each other. (Reproduced by permission of Astra Zeneca plc)

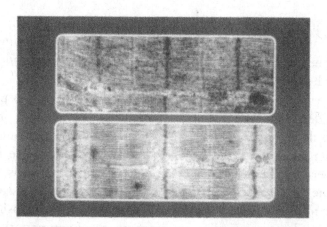

Figure 6.14   Relaxed (lower) and contracted (upper) striated muscle. Note the disappearance of the I band and H zone as the filaments slide past each other. (Reproduced by permission of Astra Zeneca plc)

electron transfer chain, muscle contraction cannot take place. The mechanisms that maintain this supply are the subjects of the next chapter.

Key points

- Skeletal muscle is under voluntary control.

- Skeletal muscle performs three basic actions – isometric (force production without movement), concentric (force production during shortening) and eccentric (force production during lengthening).

- Contraction results from the passage of an action potential via motor nerves, across the myoneural junction, and along the muscle fibre.

- The composition of the fluids across nerve fibre membranes differ, resulting in a resting membrane potential difference of about –70 mV, with the outside positive in relation to the inside; therefore the membrane is polarized.

- The action potential temporarily reverses this polarity, and the fibre is depolarized.

- Depolarization releases calcium from its storage in the cisternae of the sarcoplasmic reticulum, and opens the way for contraction of the muscle fibre.

- The electrical stimulus must exceed a minimal threshold before contraction can take place; if the threshold is breached the fibre contracts fully.

- This is the 'all-or-none law'.

- A stimulus acting on a single muscle fibre leads to a muscle twitch; repeated stimuli lead to summation or tetanus.

- A single motor nerve serves several muscle fibres and is a motor unit.

- The more motor units involved, the greater the force generated.

- Three types of muscle fibre provide the force for contraction.

- Type I (slow oxidative) fibres are the thinnest, contract slowly, and generate low forces, but can do so over long periods and are predominant in long-distance runners.

- Type IIb (fast glycolitic) fibres are the complete opposite and are found in high proportions in sprinters and power athletes.

- An intermediate fibre, Type IIa (fast oxidative glycolitic), is found in high proportions in 800-m and 1500-m athletes.

- The basic unit of all muscle fibres is the sarcomere.

- It consists of two overlapping protein filaments – thin ones containing actin are attached to the sarcomere end-plates or Z discs, and thick ones contain myosin and interdigitate between the actin strands.

- The overlapping of the filaments gives the striated appearance of skeletal muscle.

- Many hundreds of sarcomeres stacked end-to-end and constrained by a membrane called the sarcolemma make up a single muscle cell or myofibril.

- Connective tissue called the endomysium supports the myofibril, together with its nerve supply and blood vessels.

- The perimysium binds groups of fibres, and the epimysium provides the final capsule for muscle groups like the quadriceps.

- All of these connective tissues coalesce to form the muscle tendon that transmits the force generated during contraction to the bones.

- Contraction occurs when the action potential, via the transverse tubules and the sarcoplasmic reticulum, stimulates the release of calcium from the cisternae.

- The calcium interacts with the actin filaments, uncovering sites to which the myosin heads can bind and pull the actin filaments and Z discs closer together, thereby shortening the sarcomere.

- *Adenosine triphosphatase* stored in myosin heads catalyses the reaction.

- Rephosphorylation of the adenosine diphosphate produced releases the myosin heads so that they can re-attach to new binding sites.

Answers to question in the text

Question 6.1

The electro-cardiogram (ECG). This gave a picture of the electrical activity of cardiac muscle during a single heart beat.

Question 6.2

(a) Concentric action – note the intermittent appearance of electrical activity as the muscle contracts and relaxes. This is a recording of a cyclist pedalling at a moderate exercise load.

(b) Isometric action – note maintenance of maximal contraction. This is a recording of a sailor performing the hiking manoeuvre.

(c) Eccentric action – bit of a cheat this! This is a recording of an athlete performing a biceps-curl. Note (i) the electrical activity associated with the concentric action of lifting the weight, followed by (ii) a short reduction of activity as the weight reaches shoulder level, and (iii) the eccentric activity as the weight is lowered.

Question 6.3

The gap, or synaptic cleft, between the presynaptic knob of the motor neuron and the postsynaptic membrane of the muscle fibre is the known as the myoneural junction. The action potential crosses this gap through the release of the neurotransmitter acetylcholine (ACh); the acetylcholine binds to receptors in the sarcolemma and passes on the action potential. The acetylcholine is then neutralized by cholinesterase to make way for the next action potential.

Question 6.4

Maximum action potential firing rate is necessary for maximal voluntary contraction; in addition, all motor units must be engaged. Untrained subjects seem to be unable to engage all motor units available; after specific strength training, part of any improvement in voluntary maximal contraction arises from the training of the neuromuscular system to maximize motor unit involvement.

Question 6.5

The Z discs provide the boundary of the sarcomere and anchor the actin filaments. The I band is the region consisting only of actin filaments; it is the band lying between the Z discs and the outer ends of the myosin filaments. The A band is that part of the sarcomere where the actin and myosin filaments overlap. The H zone is the area that contains only myosin filaments. The M line contains M filaments that support the myosin filaments.

Question 6.6

The H zone disappears when the actin filaments and Z discs draw closer together as contraction occurs.

Answer to exercise in the text

Exercise 6.1

It is difficult to be precise. Everyone has a mixture of the three fibre types; the proportion of each type is genetically driven, and probably determines what kind of athlete we are likely to become. Furthermore, specific training enhances performance of particular fibre types. Aerobic training enhances both Type I slow-twitch fibres and Type IIa fast-twitch oxidative fibres; power training enhances Type IIb fast-twitch glycolytic fibres. Sprinters, throwers and high jumpers are likely to have a high proportion, ~60 per cent of Type IIb fibres; marathon runners will have up to 80 per cent, Type I fibres; decathletes will probably have a preponderance of Type IIa and IIb. Outfield soccer players are likely to have Types I and IIa; goalkeepers are more likely to have plenty of Types IIa and IIb.

7

Oxygen Consumption in the Muscle Cell

Learning Objectives

By the end of this chapter, you should be able to

♦ explain mechanisms by which oxygenated blood is directed to working muscles

♦ describe the effects of changes in the internal environment on the oxyhaemoglobin dissociation curve

♦ explain the importance of myoglobin in providing oxygen to working muscle

♦ calculate oxygen consumption using the Fick equation

♦ distinguish between substrate-level phosphorylation and oxidative phosphorylation

♦ list the mechanisms that resynthesize ATP from carbohydrate and fats, and describe the main features of each mechanism

♦ state the theoretical amount of ATP derived from oxidative phosphorylation of glucose, glycogen, and lipids

♦ present arguments which offer alternative accounts of ATP production via the electron transfer chain

♦ say how knowledge of the RER indicates which fuel is being broken down during steady state exercise

Exercise Physiology: A Thematic Approach   Tudor Hale
© John Wiley & Sons, Ltd   ISBN: 0 470 84682 8 (cloth), ISBN 0 470 84683 6 (pbk)

Objective test

Say whether the following answers are true (T) or false (F). If you do not know, say so (D) – not knowing is not an academic crime, but not finding out is. Try not to look at the answers until you have worked your way through the chapter and completed the test a second time. In this way you can monitor your progress.

	Pre-test			Post-test		
	T	F	D	T	F	D
1. At rest, many skeletal muscle pre-capillary sphincters are closed						
2. During exercise blood is shunted away from muscle capillary beds						
3. ADP, P_{CO_2} and lactate are constrictors of pre-capillary sphincters						
4. Increased temperature, acidity and P_{CO_2} releases more O_2 from Hb						
5. Myoglobin is an important store of O_2 in skeletal muscle						
6. Aerobic metabolism is a biochemical reaction in the presence of O_2						
7. ADP is the symbol for adenosine triphosphate						
8. ADP is the immediate energy source for muscle contraction						
9. Muscle stores contain large amounts of ATP						
10. The phosphagen cycle resynthesizes ATP						
11. The phosphagen cycle is ATP $\leftrightarrow$ ADP + PCr						
12. The phosphagen cycle takes place in the mitochondria of the cell						
13. The phosphagen cycle supplies enough ATP for about a 60 m dash						

	Pre-test			Post-test		
	T	F	D	T	F	D
14. The breakdown of glucose is called glycolysis						
15. Glycolysis cannot proceed without oxygen being present						
16. $ADP + P_i = ATP$ is an example of substrate-level phosphorylation						
17. Glycolysis produces three molecules of ATP per molecule of glucose						
18. Glycolysis in the presence of O_2 results in lactic acid production						
19. Glycogen is the stored form of glucose						
20. Glycogen is the preferred fuel for strenuous exercise						
21. Glycogen stores become depleted after 2 hours hard exercise						
22. Aerobically a molecule of glycogen provides 38 molecules of ATP						
23. The end product of aerobic glycolysis is pyruvate						
24. The TCA-cycle produces large quantities of ATP directly						
25. The main function of the TCA-cycle is dehydrogenation						
26. The loss of a hydrogen atom is called reduction						
27. O_2 is the final electron acceptor of the electron transfer chain						
28. The final products of aerobic metabolism are CO_2, H_2O, and ATP						
29. Fats provide less energy per gram than carbohydrates						
30. Fats are the preferred fuel for short-term strenuous activity						

Symbols, abbreviations and units of measurement

adenosine diphosphate	ADP	
adenosine triphosphate	ATP	
arterial oxygen content	C_{aO_2}	$mLO_2 \cdot L_{bl}^{-1}$
arterial oxygen saturation	S_{aO_2}	%
arterio-venous oxygen difference	C_{a-vO_2}	$mL_2 \cdot L_{bl}^{-1}$
blood lactate concentration	$[La_{bl}]$	$mmol \cdot L^{-1}; mM$
body mass	bm	kg_{bm}
cardiac output, whole body flow	$\dot{Q}_C$	$L \cdot min^{-1};$ $mL \cdot min^{-1}$
electron	e^-	
electron transfer chain	ETC	
flavin adenine dinucleotide	FAD	
flavin adenine dinucleotide – reduced	$FADH_2$	
guanosine triphosphate	GTP	
hydrogen ion, proton	H^+	
inorganic phosphate	P_i	
iron atom	Fe	
iron atom – ferric form	Fe^{3+}	
iron atom – ferrous form	Fe^{2+}	
maximal oxygen uptake	$\dot{V}_{O_2max}$	$L \cdot min^{-1};$ $mL \cdot min^{-1}$
muscle blood flow	Q_M	
myoglobin	Mgb	
nicotinamide adenine dinucleotide	NAD^+	
nicotinamide adenine dinucleotide – reduced	$NADH + H^+$	
oxymyoglobin	$MgbO_2$	
partial pressure of oxygen	P_{O_2}	kPa (mmHg)
partial pressure of carbon dioxide	P_{CO_2}	kPa (mmHg)
partial pressure of oxygen in arterial blood	P_{aO_2}	kPa (mmHg)
partial pressure of oxygen in venous blood	P_{vO_2}	kPa (mmHg)
partial pressure oxygen in the tissues	P_{tiO_2}	kPa (mmHg)
phosphocreatine (creatine phosphate)	PCr	
power in watts	W	$J \cdot s^{-1}; kg \cdot m \cdot s^{-1};$ $N \cdot m \cdot s^{-1}$
respiratory exchange ratio ($\dot{V}_{CO_2} / \dot{V}_{O_2}$)	RER	

tricarboxylic acid (citric acid/Krebs) cycle	TCA	
venous oxygen content	C_{vO_2}	$mLO_2 \cdot L_{bl}^{-1}$
volume of carbon dioxide excreted	$\dot{V}_{CO_2}$	$L \cdot min^{-1}$;
		$mL \cdot min^{-1}$
volume of oxygen consumed	$\dot{V}_{O_2}$	$L \cdot min^{-1}$;
		$mL \cdot min^{-1}$

Introduction

The oxygen transported in the blood and distributed via the arterial network has now arrived in the capillary bed of the skeletal muscle tissue. How much of the oxygen the muscle cells consume depends on an individual's level of physical activity. The shape of the oxygen-uptake and exercise intensity graph, beginning at rest and moving progressively towards volitional exhaustion, takes the form of a sigmoid curve (Figure 7.1). At rest, the metabolic activities involved in maintaining a stable internal environment lead to a background consumption of about a quarter of a litre of oxygen per minute or about 3 to

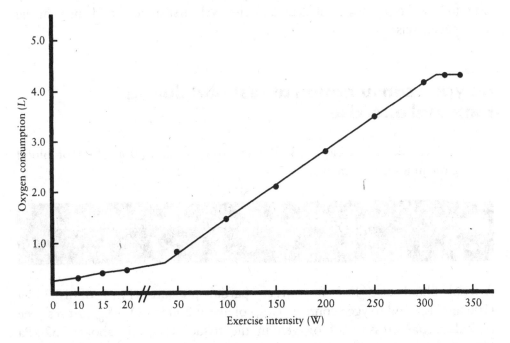

Figure 7.1 Schematic representation of the relationship between oxygen consumption and exercise intensity

4 $mLO_2 \cdot kg_{bm} \cdot min^{-1}$ in the average 70-kg adult man. Cycling at very low loads, e.g. 0–25 W, or slow walking on a flat treadmill, result in only small increases in oxygen demand. Thus, the graph is almost flat at this point. When the activities performed are sufficiently taxing to raise heart rates to about 120 $bt \cdot min^{-1}$ the oxygen uptake curve enters an increasing, linear phase. The gradient of this line depends on factors such as age and habitual physical activity patterns. Trained endurance runners and cyclists, for example, tend to be economic in their use of oxygen for any given level of exercise, and their linear phase tends to be less steep than that of untrained subjects. We use this linear phase to estimate oxygen consumption of various activities. As the subjects approach their maximum, the final section of the curve begins to flatten again, and becomes asymptotic. In some cases, the characteristic oxygen plateau occurs, indicating that we have reached our maximal oxygen uptake ($\dot{V}_{O_2max}$), but this plateau is not always present at volitional exhaustion.

The volume of oxygen consumed reflects a combination of the degree of perfusion of the muscle with arterial blood – that is muscle blood flow (Q_M), and the rate at which the muscle fibres extract the oxygen delivered. The measure that reveals the extent of this oxygen extraction is the difference between the oxygen content of blood entering the capillary bed – arterial content – a and that leaving the capillary bed – venous content – i.e (C_{a-vO_2}). Let's follow the process at skeletal muscle level, first at rest, and then during maximal exercise.

Oxygen consumption at rest and during maximal exercise

You may recall from Chapter 3 that the oxygen saturation (S_{O_2}) of blood leaving the lungs is very high.

Question 7.1   *Assuming standard pressure can you remember the actual S_{aO_2}?*

Arterial blood also has an oxygen partial pressure (P_{aO_2}) of 13.3 kPa (100 mmHg), and oxygen content (C_{aO_2}) of about 200 $mLO_2 \cdot L_{bl}^{-1}$. At rest, the typical partial pressure of oxygen in the tissues (P_{tiO_2}) is about 5.32 kPa (40 mmHg), and oxygen diffuses down the large pressure gradient – about 8 kPa (60 mmHg) – that exists between the arterial blood and the cells. At rest, many of the pre-capillary sphincters that guard the entrances to the true capillaries remain closed. Much of the blood, and thus the oxygen it carries, bypasses the muscle cells via the 'thoroughfare capillaries' – rather like a ring road around a town – and returns by way of the veins to the right side of the heart and thence to the lungs. Thus, when we measure the oxygen content of the resting venous blood arriving back at the lungs via an indwelling catheter, we find that it is about $150 \ mLO_2 \cdot L_{bl}^{-1}$. In other words, the arterio-mixed venous oxygen *difference* is only $50 \ mLO_2 \cdot L_{bl}^{-1}$, and three-quarters of the oxygen originally carried by arterial blood returns unused to the lungs.

Question 7.2 *Explain how this occurs (hint: look at the shape of the oxyhaemoglobin dissociation curve), and say whether this reserve is a useful evolutionary strategy or not.*

Now using the above data, and assuming a resting cardiac output of $5 \ L \cdot min^{-1}$ and a typical haemoglobin level of $150 \ g \cdot L_{bl}^{-1}$, we can calculate the oxygen consumption at rest via the Fick equation, as shown below.

$$\dot{V}_{O_2} \ L \cdot min^{-1} = \dot{Q}_C \ L \cdot min^{-1} \cdot C_{a-\bar{v}O_2} \ mLO_2 \cdot L_{bl}^{-1}$$

$$5 \cdot 200 - 150$$

$$5 \cdot 50$$

$$= 250 \ mL \cdot min^{-1} \ or \ 0.250 \ L \cdot min^{-1}$$

As we exercise, the position changes. Firstly, cardiac output increases delivering more blood to the muscles per minute. Secondly, blood is shunted away from non-essential areas, such as the viscera and, temporarily, the skin, towards the exercising muscles. Thirdly, the exercising muscles produce adenosine diphosphate, carbon dioxide and lactate; each of these substances is a vasodilator that acts on the smooth muscle of the pre-capillary sphincters causing them to relax and allow blood to flood the true capillaries of the muscle bed. In keeping with our analogy of a road traffic system, the true capillaries are the streets and alleys of the town. This mechanism ensures an optimum supply of oxygen to the working muscle.

> **Question 7.3**   *Can you remember how flow changes if the pre-capillary sphincter doubles its radius? Can you remember the equation used to calculate flow rate in tubes?*

Oxyhaemoglobin and myoglobin dissociation curves

There are two other important factors affecting oxygen availability that we need to consider here. The first is the mobility of the oxyhaemoglobin dissociation curve. It is not a fixed curve, but responds to changes in the internal environment of the muscle cells. You may remember from Chapter 3 that increases in the partial pressure of carbon dioxide (the Bohr effect), acidity (the Henderson effect), or blood temperature drive the curve downwards and to the right. The result of all three conditions is that more oxygen dissociates from the haemoglobin molecule to the working muscle cell. Figure 7.2 shows the general effect of this kind of response.

> **Question 7.4**   *How do increases in P_{CO_2}, acidity and blood temperature affect oxygen availability to the muscle cells? Hint: compare oxygen saturation (S_{aO_2}) values at a P_{aO_2} of 3.3 kPa (25 mmHg) at temperatures of 37 and 43°C. Can you work out the difference between arterial oxygen contents (C_{aO_2}) at these two temperatures?*

The second factor is the presence of myoglobin (Mgb) in skeletal muscle. Myoglobin is the other form of oxygen-carrying molecule, and is the red pigment that distinguishes the dark meat of the leg from the white meat of the breast of the Christmas turkey. Myoglobin combines with oxygen, but its structure is very different to haemoglobin as there is only one atom of iron per molecule of myoglobin.

$$Mgb + O_2 = MgbO_2$$

Figure 7.2   Effects of changes in carbon dioxide levels, pH, and blood temperature on the oxyhaemoglobin dissociation curve

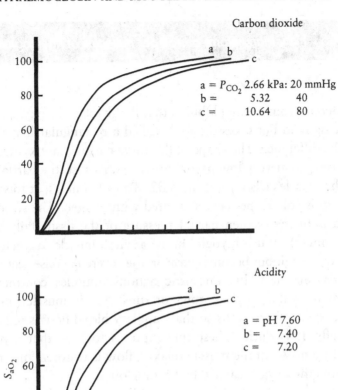

Carbon dioxide

a = P_{CO_2} 2.66 kPa: 20 mmHg
b =   5.32   40
c =   10.64   80

Acidity

a = pH 7.60
b =   7.40
c =   7.20

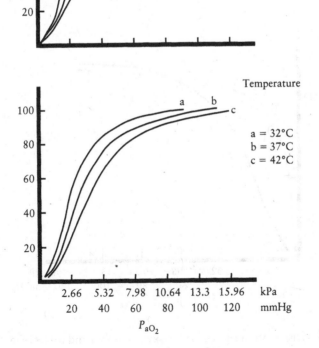

Temperature

a = 32°C
b = 37°C
c = 42°C

2.66	5.32	7.98	10.64	13.3	15.96	kPa	
20	40	60	80	100	120	mmHg	

P_{aO_2}

Question 7.5   *How many atoms of iron per molecule of haemoglobin?*

It is also different from haemoglobin in that the shape of its oxygen dissociation curve is not sigmoid but takes the form called a rectangular hyperbola. Figure 7.3 shows the difference. The shape of the curve means that oxymyoglobin only gives up its oxygen at very low partial pressures. At rest, the partial pressure of oxygen in the muscle cells is typically 5.32 kPa (40 mmHg); at this pressure the oxymyoglobin is still 95 per cent saturated with oxygen. The stored oxygen is not released until the oxygen partial pressure of the tissue falls below about 0.7 kPa (5 mmHg); thus, myoglobin is a vital muscle oxygen store. The importance of myoglobin becomes clear in the severe exercise seen towards the end of a maximal test. In concentric actions, muscles contract and relax repeatedly as the subject cycles, rows or runs. As the muscle fibres contract, they squeeze the capillary walls so that capillary blood flow is reduced or even stopped briefly. It is during these interruptions to flow that myoglobin can release its oxygen. When the muscle relaxes, flow is restored and myoglobin is recharged from the oxygen carried by haemoglobin.

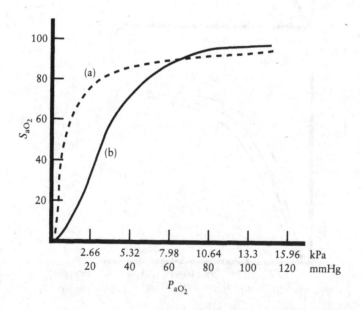

Figure 7.3   Dissociation curves for (a) oxymyoglobin and (b) oxyhaemoglobin

Exercise 7.1

Assume that C_{aO_2} remains constant at $200\ mLO_2 \cdot L_{bl}^{-1}$, but $C_{\bar{v}O_2}$ is now $50\ mLO_2 \cdot L_{bl}^{-1}$, and cardiac output is $40\ L \cdot min^{-1}$, use the Fick equation to calculate the oxygen consumption at maximal exercise.

In this example, there has been a 24-fold increase in oxygen consumption between the rest and maximal effort. The next section introduces the mechanisms that lead to such large increases in oxygen consumption.

An overview of adenosine triphosphate production

At rest when the demand for oxygen is low, fatty acids, together with some blood-borne glucose, provide the main source of fuel to drive the body's maintenance systems. As exercise intensity increases, the energy source switches increasingly to the stored form of glucose called glycogen, stored as granules within the muscle cell itself. When glycogen stores are depleted, blood-borne glucose can be used; but unless supplemental glucose is provided in the form of carbohydrate drinks, for example, the energy source switches to fats as the main energy source.

The 6 litres of oxygen, released from the haemoglobin and myoglobin molecules during maximal exercise in elite endurance athletes, take part in the oxidation of carbohydrate and fats to maintain adenosine triphosphate (ATP) levels. This process is critical. Every cell in the body requires adenosine triphosphate; without it, none of the body's functions, including muscle contraction, can operate. Figure 7.4 gives the simplest model of adenosine triphosphate resynthesis. This model shows that protein can also be a source of adenosine triphosphate production through breakdown of amino acids, but its contribution to exercise is relatively small and will not be considered further.

Phosphorylation

As adenosine triphosphate is essential for muscle contraction, we could be forgiven for expecting large stores of it to be held in the muscle cells. This is not the case; indeed, there is very little adenosine triphosphate present in the muscle

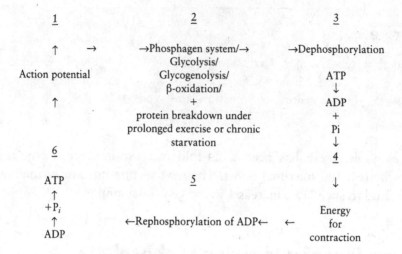

Figure 7.4   A simplified model of the resynthesis of ATP

cell, so it follows that there must be a mechanism, or a series of mechanisms, by which it is replaced as fast as it is being used. In fact, there are two mechanisms involved in adenosine triphosphate production; they are substrate-level phosphorylation, and oxidative phosphorylation. Substrate-level phosphorylation, is the conversion of adenosine *di*phosphate (ADP) to adenosine *tri*phosphate (ATP) *without* the intervention of oxygen – in other words, it is an *anaerobic* process. Oxidative phosphorylation, on the other hand, requires oxygen for the transfer of phosphate from a high-energy phosphate compound to phosphorylate adenosine diphosphate to its triphosphate form, and is thus an *aerobic* process. As we saw in the Introduction to the book, we can subdivide the two fundamental phosphorylating mechanisms into four processes. They are

(a) the phosphagen system,

(b) glycolysis,

(c) the Krebs or tricarboxylic acid cycle, and

(d) the electron transfer chain.

It is important to note that the first two processes take place within the sarcoplasm of the muscle cells, the second two within the mitochondria, often called the powerhouses of the cells.

Although the general principles underpinning the processes of adenosine triphosphate production have been established for some time and are reasonably well understood, there is still some debate regarding the actual amount produced by oxidative phosphorylation.

The phosphagen system, discovered by the American scientist Fritz Lipmann in 1941, is the immediate source of energy for muscle contraction. Three main phosphagens – adenosine triphosphate, adenosine diphosphate, and phosphocreatine (PCr) – are involved. To enable muscle contraction to take place, adenosine triphosphate loses one of its phosphate bonds – in other words, it is dephosphorylated to adenosine diphosphate – to provide the energy for the contraction. The availability of the phosphocreatine stored in the muscle cell allows the immediate resynthesis of adenosine triphosphate. The phosphate bond from phosphocreatine is split off; it phosphorylates adenosine diphosphate, thereby allowing further muscle contraction to take place. However, because of the limited stores of both adenosine triphosphate and phosphocreatine, the phosphagen system serves only as a short-term mechanism for adenosine triphosphate resynthesis, and longer bouts of activity need other processes.

The next process is concerned with the breakdown of carbohydrate in the form of glucose or glycogen. Each molecule of glucose is broken down to produce two molecules of pyruvate in a series of reactions called *glycolysis*, or the Embden–Meyerhof pathway after its German discoverers. The breakdown process (catabolism) starts by consuming *two* molecules of adenosine triphosphate but ends by producing *four* molecules.

> **Question 7.6   *What is the net gain in ATP molecules from glycolysis at this stage?***

Glycogenolysis is the breakdown of *glycogen* to pyruvate. The process is almost identical to glycolysis, but it consumes only *one* molecule initially whilst still producing *four* molecules of adenine triphosphate during the reactions.

> **Question 7.7   *What is the net gain in ATP molecules from glycogenolysis?***

Both sets of reactions are examples of substrate-level phosphorylation, and therefore do not need oxygen; but the amount of adenosine triphosphate generated is relatively small.

However, if sufficient oxygen is available to the muscle cell during glycolysis, oxidative phosphorylation takes over, and dramatically increases the amount of adenosine triphosphate produced. First, the way is cleared for pyruvate to be broken down to a very active coenzyme, coenzyme A, also discovered by Fritz Lipmann. This coenzyme then opens up the second stage, the tricarboxylic acid (TCA) or Krebs cycle, so called after its main discoverer, the English scientist, Hans Krebs. Finally, hydrogen atoms enter an electron transfer chain, a process first suggested by the English biochemist, Peter Mitchell. Lipmann, Krebs and Mitchell were all awarded Nobel Prizes for their work.

Although the carbon, hydrogen and oxygen atoms that make up glycogen interact to form carbon dioxide and water as part of the reactions of the Krebs cycle, it is only at the final electron transfer stage that oxygen from the atmosphere is used as the final hydrogen acceptor that leads to adenosine triphosphate production. It is the use of the oxygen available that gives the entire sequence of events its description of *aerobic* metabolism. A shortened version of the main steps in the production of adenosine triphosphate during aerobic glycolysis is shown in Figure 7.5.

The reactions occurring via the Krebs cycle and the electron transfer chain take place in one of the organelles of the muscle cell called the mitochondrion (Figure 7.6). This important structure is the powerhouse of the muscle cell, and our genes and our environment influence their number. Endurance athletes, for example, have more mitochondria per muscle fibre than do power athletes, reflecting that both our genetic make-up and the type of training we may undertake determine our maximal oxygen uptake. Genetically, our mitochondria come directly from the female line; so, if you want to be an elite endurance athlete it is necessary to choose your mother carefully.

The rest of this chapter sets out in more detail the series of reactions that take place during hydrolysis of adenosine triphosphate and the consumption of oxygen. We also examine the uncertainty regarding the actual number of molecules of adenosine triphosphate produced from each fuel source.

The phosphagen system

To provide the energy required for muscle contraction, a molecule of adenosine triphosphate interacts with water, a process known as hydrolysis, and splits into adenosine diphosphate and inorganic phosphate.

$$ATP - actinomyosinATPase \rightarrow ADP + P_i$$

This splitting, which is driven (catalysed) by the enzyme *actinomyosinATPase*,

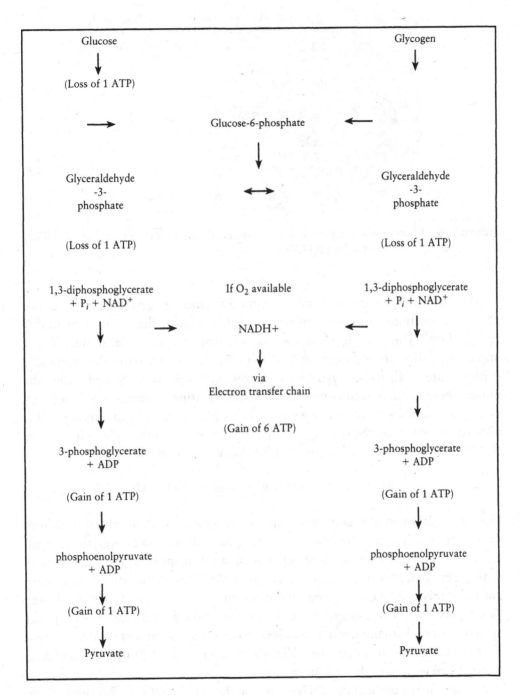

Figure 7.5 A brief outline of aerobic glycolysis leading to the synthesis of eight molecules of adenosine triphosphate

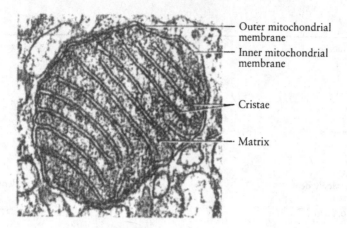

Outer mitochondrial membrane

Inner mitochondrial membrane

Cristae

Matrix

Figure 7.6 Micrograph of a mitochondrion. (Reproduced with permission of John Wiley & Sons) Inc, Tortura and Grabowski (2003)

provides the energy for muscle contraction. Enzymes are generally restricted to particular reactions and can be recognized easily because their names invariably end in 'ase'. High levels of adenosine diphosphate in skeletal muscle are important indicators of fatigue and impair contraction. To avoid this adenosine triphosphate needs to be resynthesized as quickly as possible. Stored within the muscle there is the critical compound phosphocreatine, sometimes also referred to as creatine phosphate. The presence of this phosphagen in the muscle cell is important; driven by the enzyme *creatine kinase*, it rephosphorylates adenosine diphosphate to produce adenosine triphosphate and creatine.

$$ADP + PCr — \textit{creatine kinase} \rightarrow ATP + Cr$$

However, although the concentration of phosphocreatine is about 10 times greater than adenosine triphosphate, phosphocreatine stores are still limited. Put into context, if your survival depends on a 60-m sprint to safety then there is about enough phosphocreatine stores to achieve this. A hint of the short-term nature of this system can be seen on the velocity graph of an elite 100-m runner. (See Figure 7.7.) There is rapid acceleration over the first 30 m; velocity peaks at about 50 m, is maintained at this level for another 30 m, before decelerating over the last 20 m. It is often said that the winner of the 100-m is the one who slows down least over the last 30 m or so.

As there is no immediate mechanism for the rephosphorylation of creatine, stores are quickly depleted in an all-out effort such as the 100-m. The resynthesis of phosphocreatine occurs during recovery when adenosine triphosphate becomes more available. If a more sustained effort – say anything from 60 to

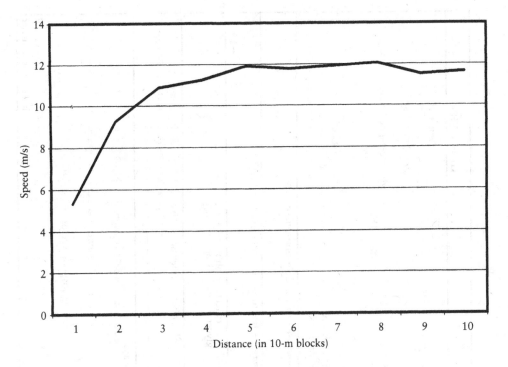

Figure 7.7 The velocity–distance curve of an elite 100-m runner

800 m – is needed, then a combination of the other three mechanisms, that is glycogenolysis, the Krebs cycle, and electron transfer, is necessary.

Glycolysis and glycogenolysis

The oxidation of glucose and glycogen is virtually identical. However, a small but important difference occurs at the start of the process. Glucose is transported by the blood and enters the muscle cell under the influence of insulin; here, it is stored in the form of granules made up from long strings of individual glucose molecules. In this stored form it is called glycogen. During glycogenolysis, the glucose molecules have to be detached from the long strings and broken down to glucose-6-phosphate. This requires two reactions, shown as Steps 1a and 1b in Figure 7.8; importantly, the process consumes no adenosine triphosphate. On the other hand, free glucose completes its breakdown to glucose-6-phosphate in a single step (Step 1 in Figure 7.8). However, that single step does require energy from adenosine triphosphate to drive the reaction. Thus, because its breakdown is slightly more efficient, glycogen becomes the preferred fuel for

GLUCOSE	GLYCOGEN
Step 1	**Step 1a** Glycogen + P_i
Glucose + ATP	$\rightarrow$ *phosphorylase*
$\rightarrow$ *hexokinase* $\rightarrow \rightarrow \rightarrow \rightarrow \rightarrow \rightarrow$	glucose-1-phosphate
glucose-6-phosphate + ADP	**Step 1b** $\rightarrow$ *phosphoglucomutase*
−1ATP	glucose-6-phosphate **−1ATP**

**Common Glycolytic Pathway
(Embden–Meyerhof Pathway)**

Step 2

glucose-6-phosphate — *phosphoglucoisomerase* $\rightarrow$ fructose-6-phosphate

$\rightarrow$

Step 3   **−1ATP**

fructose-6-phosphate + ATP — *phosphofructokinase* $\rightarrow$ fructose-1,6-disphosphate + ADP

$\rightarrow$

Step 4

fructose-1,6-diphosphate — *aldolase* $\rightarrow$ dihydroxyacetone phosphate + glyceraldehyde-3-phosphate

$\rightarrow$

Step 5

dihydroxyacetone phosphate + glyceraldehyde-3-phosphate — *triose phosphate isomerase* $\rightarrow$ glyceraldehyde-3-phosphate + glyceraldehyde-3-phosphate

$\rightarrow$

Step 6   **Parallel Pathways**

glyceraldehyde-3-phosphate + NAD^+ + P_i	glyceraldehyde-3-phosphate + NAD^+ + P_i
$\rightarrow$ *glyceraldehyde-3-phosphate dehydrogenase*	$\rightarrow$ *glyceraldehyde-3-phosphate dehydrogenase*
1,3 diphosphoglycerate + NADH + H^+	1,3 diphosphoglycerate + NADH + H^+
$\rightarrow$	$\rightarrow$
1,3 diphosphoglycerate	1,3 diphosphoglycerate

+3 ATP
via electron transfer   **+3 ATP** via electron transfer

Step 7	1,3 diphosphoglycerate + ADP + P_i ↓ *phosphoglycerate kinase* ↓ 3-phosphoglycerate + ATP	1,3 diphosphoglycerate + ADP + P_i ↓ *phosphoglycerate kinase* ↓ 3-phosphoglycerate + ATP
+1 ATP **via substrate-level phosphorylation**		**+1 ATP** **via substrate-level phosphorylation**
Step 8	3-phosphoglycerate ↓ *phosphoglyceromutase* ↓ 2-phosphoglycerate ↓	3-phosphoglycerate ↓ *phosphoglyceromutatse* ↓ 2-phosphoglycerate ↓
Step 9	2-phosphoglycerate ↓ *enolase* ↓ phosphoenolpyruvate ↓	2-phosphoglycerate ↓ *enolase* ↓ phosphoenolpyruvate ↓
Step 10	phosphoenolpyruvate ↓ *pyruvate phosphokinase* ↓ pyruvate + ATP ↓	phosphoenolpyruvate ↓ *pyruvate phosphokinase* ↓ pyruvate + ATP ↓
+1 ATP **via substrate-level phosphorylation**	↓	**+1 ATP** **via substrate-level phosphorylation** ↓
	↓ **Tricarboxylic acid cycle** **(Krebs cycle)** ↓	↓ **Tricarboxylic acid cycle** **(Krebs cycle)** ↓
	Electron transfer chain + O_2	**Electron transfer chain + O_2**

Figure 7.8 Aerobic pathways of glycolysis and glycogenolysis

strenuous exercise. To give the complete picture, the rest of this section describes the breakdown of both glucose and glycogen; see Figure 7.8 for the full pathway.

As we have seen, the initial stages of glycolysis and glycogenolysis lead to the creation of a molecule of glucose-6-phosphate, but by slightly different routes. Starting with glycogen, the first move (Step 1a) is to detach a single molecule of glucose from the glycogen chain. This involves the enzyme *glycogen phosphorylase*, which together with a molecule of inorganic phosphate (P_i), gives glucose-1-phosphate. The glucose-1-phosphate molecule is then transformed into glucose-6-phosphate by *phosphoglucomutase* (Step 1b). Glucose, driven by the enzyme *hexokinase*, is also broken down to glucose-6-phosphate, but in one step. The most significant difference is that the glucose → glucose-6-phosphate step requires the phosphorylation of the glucose molecule by adenosine triphosphate, whereas the two steps taken in the initial breakdown of glycogen do not.

This means that, paradoxically, the quest for the *production* of adenosine triphosphate by glycolysis begins with the *loss* of a molecule of it. The situation appears to be getting worse, because after the conversion of glucose-6-phosphate to fructose-6-phosphate (Step 3), we lose another molecule of adenosine triphosphate during the phosphorylation of fructose-6-phosphate to fructose-1,6-diphosphate. Thus far, glycogenolysis leads to the loss of one molecule of adenosine triphosphate, and glycolysis to the loss of two.

We have now reached a critical point (Step 4). The enzyme *aldolase* splits fructose-1,6-diphosphate, a *six*-carbon molecule, into two separate *three*-carbon compounds that have the same composition but different structures; in technical terms, they are isomeric. In this instance, the two isomers are glyceraldehyde-3-phosphate, and dihydroxyacetone-phosphate. Under the influence of the enzyme *triose phosphate isomerase*, the dihydroxyacetone-phosphate is converted into a second molecule of glyceraldehyde-3-phosphate at Step 5. From this point, all subsequent reactions involve both molecules in parallel pathways as shown in Figure 7.8, but we shall return to Step 6 at the end of this description of glycolysis. Step 7 produces *two* molecules of adenosine triphosphate from the interaction between 1,3-diphosphoglycerate and adenosine diphosphate, driven by *phosphoglycerate kinase*, to give 3-phosphoglycerate and adenosine triphosphate. The next two steps (8 and 9) lead to phosphoenolpyruvate. This is catalysed by *pyruvate phosphokinase* to pyruvate and a further *two* molecules of adenosine triphosphate (Step 10). Thus, the total production of adenosine triphosphate via glycolysis and glycogenolysis is *four* molecules. However, some reactions consume adenosine triphosphate, so the net gain is *two* molecules from glucose and *three* from glycogen. The fate of pyruvate is described in the next section, but before that we must return to Step 6 in the glycolitic pathway.

This chapter is concerned with *oxygen* consumption, and in this section, we have been dealing with the breakdown of glycogen in the presence of oxygen – i.e. *aerobic* metabolism. However, it is worth noting that thus far there has been no direct involvement of oxygen in any of the reactions described; in other words the mechanism involved is substrate phosphorylation which can take place in the absence of oxygen – i.e. *anaerobically*. This is a very important process, and is a topic we shall discuss further in Chapter 8.

However, at Step 6 of the glycolytic pathway we see the first example of oxidative phosphorylation. To explain this oxidative process we require a short digression.

Oxidation

Oxidation can take three forms. The most obvious is to add an oxygen atom to a substance; the second form removes a hydrogen atom from a substance; the third form removes an electron. However, oxidation cannot take place without an accompanying reduction; the two processes, called reduction-oxidation (redox) reactions, go together. The obverse of oxidation is the removal of oxygen, or the addition of a hydrogen atom or an electron. For example, in the first two equations below, substance A is *oxidized* by adding oxygen or removing hydrogen. These reactions automatically *reduce* substance B by removing oxygen or adding hydrogen. In the third equation, A is oxidized by the removal of an electron.

$$A + BO_2 \rightarrow AO_2 + B$$

$$AH + B \rightarrow A + BH$$

$$A^{2+} \rightarrow A^{3+} + e^-$$

All three processes are involved in oxidative phosphorylation in the muscle, but the order in which they occur is as follows:

(a) removing hydrogen (dehydrogenation); this also requires the presence of a hydrogen carrier;

(b) splitting hydrogen into a proton (H^+) and an electron (e^-) and transferring the electrons down a series of reactions

(c) molecular oxygen acting as the final electron acceptor, combines with the protons and electrons to give water.

The result is adenosine triphosphate, carbon dioxide and water.

If sufficient oxygen is available, we see these reactions at work at Step 6 of the glycolytic pathway. Each molecule of glyceraldehyde-3-phosphate interacts with the hydrogen carrier nicotinamide adenine dinucleotide (NAD^+) and inorganic phosphate (P_i) via *glyceraldehyde-3-phosphate dehydrogenase*; this gives 1,3-diphosphoglycerate and the reduced form of nicotinamide adenine dinucleotide, usually written $NADH + H^+$. The reduced form then takes part in a series of redox reactions that make up the electron transfer chain (ETC), at the end of which is oxygen, an avid electron acceptor. This chain of reactions produces many more molecules of adenosine triphosphate than anaerobic glycolysis, but the actual amount is subject to debate.

The current view is that each of the two molecules of glyceraldehyde-3-phosphate produces *three* molecules of adenosine triphosphate, making *six* in total. Under this process, aerobic glycolysis produces *eight* molecules of adenosine triphosphate from glucose and *nine* from glycogen. However, we shall return to this issue later in the chapter.

Question 7.8. *Where have the extra two and three molecules come from?*

Ignoring any uncertainty for the moment, the benefits of oxidative phosphorylation over substrate-level phosphorylation should be obvious. It will become even more obvious as we follow the fate of pyruvate under the aerobic conditions necessary for entry in the Krebs cycle.

The Krebs cycle (The Krebs cycle is also known as the tri-carboxylic acid, or citric acid cycle.)

For continuous strenuous exercise, lasting between one and two hours, the oxidation of mainly glycogen to carbon dioxide and water provides the continuous supply of adenosine triphosphate. More than two hours of hard exercise depletes the glycogen stores, so for events lasting longer than this fats (lipids) are the likeliest source of energy. However, both glycogen and fat have to pass around the Krebs cycle. We will follow the fate of glycogen first, starting at the end of the glycolitic pathway with the production of two molecules of pyruvate from one molecule of glucose-6-phosphate.

At its simplest level, pyruvate in the presence of adequate oxygen supplies, is oxidized to carbon dioxide and water, and produces 30 molecules of adenosine triphosphate.

> **Question 7.9** *What is the combined number of ATP molecules produced from the aerobic breakdown of a) glucose and b) glycogen via the Embden–Meyerhof pathway and Krebs cycle?*

The Krebs cycle converts pyruvate to carbon dioxide, reduced nicotinamide adenine dinucleotide ($NADH + H^+$) and flavin adenine dinucleotide ($FADH_2$), and adenosine triphosphate. The process requires hydrogen carriers and enzymes called *dehydrogenases*. The carriers are the coenzymes nicotinamide adenine dinucleotide, flavin mononucleotide (FMN), flavin adenine dinucleotide (FAD), ubiquinone (Q), also known as coenzyme Q, and iron-bearing proteins called cytochromes. The driver of the Krebs cycle is also a coenzyme – acetyl coenzymeA (written acetyl CoA). This is produced when pyruvate, interacting with the enzyme *pyruvate dehydrogenase*, loses carbon, in the form of carbon dioxide, and hydrogen to the carrier nicotinamide adenine dinucleotide (Step 11). The reduced form of nicotinamide adenine dinucleotide enters the electron transfer chain to give *three* molecules of adenosine triphosphate. Acetyl CoA now starts the cyclical process by interacting with oxaloacetate to give citrate (Step 12). The enzyme responsible is *citrate synthetase*. Step 13 sees citrate converted to isocitrate via *aconitase*. Isocitrate then loses carbon dioxide, and is dehydrogenated to become α-ketoglutarate, catalysed by *isocitrate dehydrogenase*. The result is *three* more molecules of adenosine triphosphate. A similar process occurs at Step 14 when α-ketoglutarate converts to succinate, via an intermediary succinyl CoA; this releases more carbon dioxide, and *three* more molecules of adenosine triphosphate. Step 15 sees the only example of substrate-level phosphorylation during the Krebs cycle reactions. Succinyl CoA interacts with water, guanosine triphosphate (GTP) and adenosine diphosphate; the guanosine triphosphate donates one of its phosphate bonds to adenosine diphosphate to produce succinate and *one* molecule of adenosine triphosphate. In Step 16 *succinate dehydrogenase* strips hydrogen from succinate to give fumarate; the hydrogen carrier here is flavin adenine dinucleotide, which is reduced by the addition of hydrogen, giving *two* molecules of adenosine triphosphate. Fumarate then converts to malate (Step 17); this in turn is dehydrogenated to give oxaloacetate (Step 18), and produces *three* more molecules of adenosine triphosphate. The oxaloacetate is available to start the cycle all over again.

Figure 7.9 shows the whole process. It is very important to remember that glycolysis results in two molecules of pyruvate, so the sequence shown in Figure 7.9 represents only half of the ATP production from the aerobic breakdown of glycogen.

Exercise 7.2

The electron transfer chain is brought into action on six occasions during the breakdown of glycogen to carbon dioxide and water with the production of 34 molecules of ATP. Using Figures 7.9 and 7.10 say where these dehydrogenating steps take place.

The electron transfer chain

Before we can understand the basic processes entailed in the electron transfer chain we need to know some details of the make-up of a mitochondrion. There are four structures (Figure 7.10):

(a) the inner space called the matrix;

(b) the folded inner membrane along which the electron transfer chain is located;

(c) the inter-membrane space;

(d) the outer membrane dividing the mitochondrion from the sarcoplasm of the muscle cell.

Figure 7.9 Schematic representation of the Krebs/citric acid/tricarboxylic acid cycle, following on from Step 10 of the Embden–Meyerhof pathway.

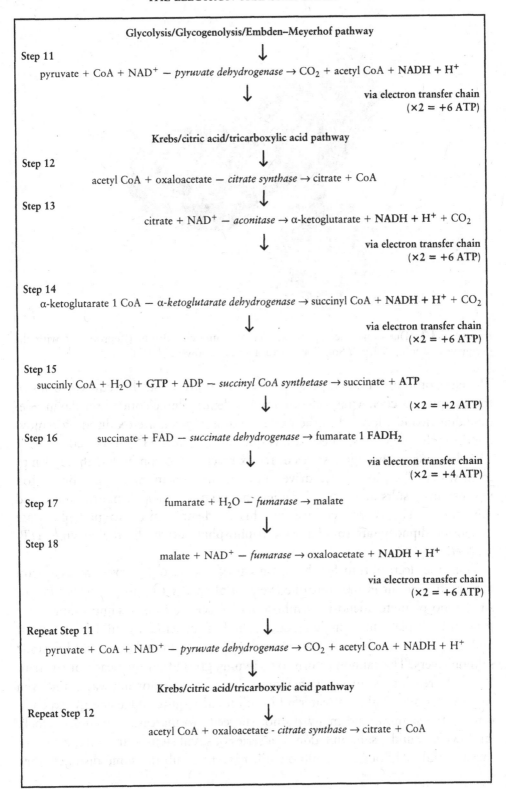

Glycolysis/Glycogenolysis/Embden–Meyerhof pathway

Step 11

$\downarrow$

pyruvate + CoA + NAD^+ — *pyruvate dehydrogenase* $\rightarrow$ CO_2 + acetyl CoA + **NADH + H^+**

$\downarrow$ via electron transfer chain
($\times 2$ = +6 ATP)

Krebs/citric acid/tricarboxylic acid pathway

Step 12

$\downarrow$

acetyl CoA + oxaloacetate — *citrate synthase* $\rightarrow$ citrate + CoA

Step 13

$\downarrow$

citrate + NAD^+ — *aconitase* $\rightarrow$ α-ketoglutarate + **NADH + H^+** + CO_2

$\downarrow$ via electron transfer chain
($\times 2$ = +6 ATP)

Step 14

α-ketoglutarate 1 CoA — *α-ketoglutarate dehydrogenase* $\rightarrow$ succinyl CoA + **NADH + H^+** + CO_2

$\downarrow$ via electron transfer chain
($\times 2$ = +6 ATP)

Step 15

succinly CoA + H_2O + **GTP** + ADP — *succinyl CoA synthetase* $\rightarrow$ succinate + **ATP**

$\downarrow$ ($\times 2$ = +2 ATP)

Step 16 succinate + FAD — *succinate dehydrogenase* $\rightarrow$ fumarate 1 **FADH$_2$**

$\downarrow$ via electron transfer chain
($\times 2$ = +4 ATP)

Step 17 fumarate + H_2O — *fumarase* $\rightarrow$ malate

$\downarrow$

Step 18

malate + NAD^+ — *fumarase* $\rightarrow$ oxaloacetate + **NADH + H^+**

via electron transfer chain
($\times 2$ = +6 ATP)

Repeat Step 11 $\downarrow$

pyruvate + CoA + NAD^+ — *pyruvate dehydrogenase* $\rightarrow$ CO_2 + acetyl CoA + **NADH + H^+**

$\downarrow$

Krebs/citric acid/tricarboxylic acid pathway

Repeat Step 12

$\downarrow$

acetyl CoA + oxaloacetate - *citrate synthase* $\rightarrow$ citrate + CoA

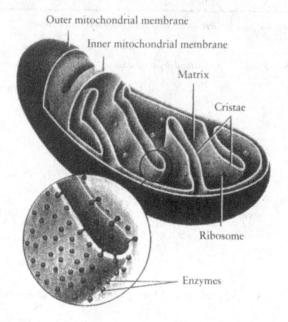

Figure 7.10 Diagrammatic representation of a mitochondrion. (Reproduced with the permission of John Wiley & Sons Inc, Tortura and Grabowski (2003))

The electron transfer chain performs five functions. First, the reduced forms of the energy-rich coenzymes, nicotinamide adenine dinucleotide and flavin adenine dinucleotide, located in the mitochondrial matrix, are oxidized by removing the hydrogen atoms. These atoms split into protons (H^+) and electrons (e^-). The electrons go through a series of redox reactions to combine with oxygen to form water. The protons are driven into the inter-membrane space by proton pumps; this results in a proton gradient between the inter-membrane space and the matrix. The energy created by this gradient is used to phosphorylate adenosine diphosphate to adenosine triphosphate driven by the enzyme *ATP-synthetase*.

Thus, the electron transfer chain consists of a series of hydrogen and electron carriers that result in the controlled release of energy to phosphorylate adenosine *di*phosphate to adenosine *tri*phosphate. A series of steps is important; if the process took place in a single reaction, the heat generated would be too great and would damage the cell. A good analogy is the 'salmon ladder' used in some salmon rivers. The salmon return to spawning grounds at the heads of rivers to breed. To reach these grounds they must overcome fast-flowing water and even small waterfalls. Scaling a waterfall in full flood requires huge energy expenditure by the salmon, and many do not succeed. To increase the salmon stock, landowners build a salmon ladder – a series of small steps – around the edge of the waterfall. Although the salmon still have to climb the same distance, they do so in a series of small steps rather than in one gigantic leap; the small steps use energy in smaller and more accessible packets. The electron transfer chain does a similar thing in reverse. Figure 7.11 shows a simplified version of the processes involved. For ease of understanding, the description that follows deals separately with the oxidation of the reduced forms of nicotinamide adenine dinucleotide ($NADH + H^+$) and flavin adenine dinucleotide ($FADH_2$).

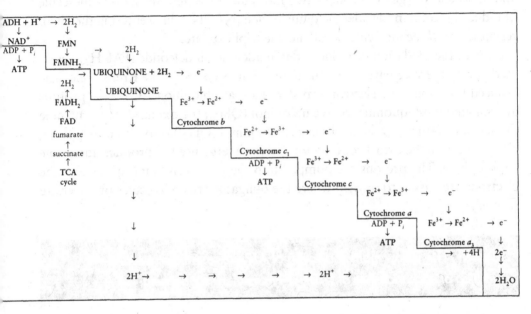

Figure 7.11 Schematic representation of the electron transfer chain, showing the synthesis of three molecules of adenosine triphosphate from nicotinamide adenine dinucleotide and two molecules from flavin adenine dinucleotide

The reactions leading to the reduced form of nicotinamide adenine dinucleotide ($NADH + H^+$) occur in the matrix of the mitochondrion during the Krebs cycle. The reduced form is oxidized by removal of hydrogen protons via *NAD dehydrogenase* providing energy to rephosphorylate adenosine diphosphate to adenosine triphosphate. The oxidized form (NAD^+) is made available to the Krebs cycle again. The electrons and protons pass first to flavin mononucleotide, thereby reducing it ($FMNH_2$), and then to ubiquinone (Q), which in turn is reduced to ubiquinol (QH_2). From here, only electrons are acceptable to the remaining carriers called cytochromes, so ubiquinol is oxidized by the transfer of electrons (e^-) to the cytochrome chain. Physiological pumps move the spare protons (H^+) into the inter-membrane space.

The cytochromes are proteins with a central core of an iron atom (Fe). Electron transfer is facilitated by the presence of the iron atoms, because these atoms can switch between the oxidized ferric (Fe^{3+}) and reduced ferrous (Fe^{2+}) forms. A second molecule of adenosine triphosphate is produced as cytochrome b is oxidized to cytochrome c_1; a third molecule is delivered as the electron passes from cytochrome a to a_3 driven by *cytochrome oxidase*. The final step is reached when two electrons from cytochrome a_3 combine with four protons and molecular oxygen to produce two molecules of water. Thus, every molecule of reduced nicotinamide adenine dinucleotide ($NADH + H^+$) entering the chain resynthesizes *three* molecules of adenosine triphosphate.

Now to the oxidation of reduced flavin adenine dinucleotide ($FADH_2$) generated during the succinate $\rightarrow$ fumarate reaction (Step 16) of the Krebs cycle. The reduced form joins the electron transfer chain at ubiquinone (Q). Two protons are donated to ubiquonine to give ubiquinol (QH_2); the oxidized flavin adenine dinucleotide returns to the Krebs cycle. Ubiquinol (QH_2) is oxidized by passing electrons down the cytochrome chain and the energy used to produce adenosine triphosphate. The protons are pumped into the inter-membrane space, and the electrons are passed to oxygen where the obligatory two molecules of water are formed.

> **Question 7.10**   *How many molecules of ATP are resynthesized from the oxidation of each molecule of $FADH_2$? Figure 7.10 should help.*

Adenosine triphosphate production

Earlier, we learnt that counting the number of adenosine triphosphate molecules produced by oxidative phosphorylation seems to be problematic. In most textbooks, the numbers of adenosine triphosphate molecules quoted are *38* from glucose and *39* from glycogen. However, experimental investigations into aerobic metabolism only produce about *30* molecules. There are two propositions that attempt to bring theory into line with experimental evidence. The first focuses on the reduced nicotinamide adenine dinucleotide ($NADH + H^+$) originating in the sarcoplasm of the muscle during glycolysis. Now, glycolysis takes place outside the mitochondria in the sarcoplasm. The electron transfer chain, however, is located on the inner membrane of the mitochondria. There is an argument, which says that to cross the outer membrane of the mitochondria and gain access to the transfer chain, the reduced nicotinamide adenine dinucleotide must use energy – i.e. adenosine triphosphate. As a result, only *two* rather than *three* molecules of adenosine triphosphate are available from each molecule of reduced nicotinamide adenine dinucleotide originating from Step 6 (glyceraldehyde-3-phosphate $\rightarrow$ 1, 3 diphosphoglycerate) *and* Step 11 (pyruvate $\rightarrow$ acetyl coenzyme A), both of which take place in the sarcoplasm. However, this proposal, if true, says the whole oxidative process still produces *34* molecules from glucose and *35* from glycogen rather than the *30* from direct experimentation.

A second proposition says that the *average* number of molecules of adenosine triphosphate produced during the oxidation of processes of electron transfer is *2.5* molecules from nicotinamide adenine dinucleotide and *1.5* molecules from flavin adenine dinucleotide, not the usual figures of three and two molecules respectively. Combining both propositions leads to *30* molecules of adenosine triphosphate from the aerobic break down of glycogen, a figure that matches experimental data. This argument is a good example of the axiom that scientific knowledge is always provisional, and that the method adopted by scientists is one of speculation followed by attempted refutation.

Fat oxidation

As the time spent in strenuous exercise grows, the glycogen stores are depleted and the fuel used changes to fat or, more correctly, lipids. There are two sources of lipids for muscle contraction; they are stored in the muscle cell as triglycerides, or carried in the blood as free fatty acids. The oxidation of lipids entails the Krebs cycle and electron transfer chain; but before triglycerides can be used as fuel for adenosine triphosphate production, the bond that ties glycerol to the fatty acid chains must be broken. The free fatty acids enter the mitochondria and undergo β-oxidation leading to the production of acetyl CoA. The process is then identical with the oxidation of glycogen.

Question 7.11   *Outline the benefits of lipid versus glycogen oxidation.*

Although each gram of fat stores more than twice the energy of carbohydrate, the oxygen cost of breaking down lipids is greater. The clearest example of this, especially for fun-runners, is the phenomenon of 'hitting the wall' during a marathon. A frequent outcome is a sudden reduction in running speed. Those who have completed about two-thirds of the race in about two hours, often find themselves taking another two to three hours to finish.

If we compare the oxygen cost of glucose and lipid oxidation, described schematically in the following equations, we can see the reason for this phenomenon.

Glucose

$$C_6H_{12}O_6 + 38P_i + 38ADP + \mathbf{6O_2} \rightarrow 6CO_2 + 6H_2O + \mathbf{38ATP}$$

Lipid

$$CH_3(CH_2)_{14}\,COOH + 130P_i + 130ADP + \mathbf{23O_2} \rightarrow 16CO_2 + 16H_2O + \mathbf{130ATP}$$

The increased oxygen demand – 23 versus 6 molecules of oxygen – puts further stress on an already hard-working cardio-respiratory system.

> **Question 7.12**   *Calculate the RER for the aerobic breakdown of carbohydrate compared to lipids. How might this information be used?*

Key points

- Increased oxygen demand from contracting muscle groups is met by vasodilatation of pre-capillary sphincters and increased perfusion of the muscle capillary bed.

- Increases in carbon dioxide and lactate production, and higher muscle temperature, move the oxyhaemoglobin dissociation curve to the right, thereby releasing more oxygen at the same tissue partial pressure.

- Myoglobin is particularly important as an oxygen supplier at very low tissue partial pressures.

- Increased oxygen provided is needed to produce adequate supplies of adenosine triphosphate, the critical energy source for muscle contraction.

- There are two mechanisms for adenosine triphosphate production: substrate-level phosphorylation (without oxygen) and oxidative phosphorylation (with oxygen): and four processes: the phosphagen system, glycolysis, the Krebs (tricarboxylic acid) cycle, and the electron transfer chain.

- The phosphagen system is the first line of defence against low adenosine triphosphate stores and for its resynthesis; but the system is soon exhausted.

- The breakdown of a molecule of glucose, via the Embden–Meyerhof pathway, is called glycolysis.

- It produces two molecules of adenosine triphosphate anaerobically, and eight molecules aerobically.

- The breakdown of glycogen, the preferred fuel for strenuous exercise lasting up to about 2 hours, results in an extra molecule of ATP.

- The end-product of aerobic glycolysis is pyruvate.

- The Krebs cycle and electron transfer chain produce 30 or 31 molecules of ATP from glucose and glycogen respectively.

- The process involves reducing NAD^+ and FAD, and passing hydrogen protons and electrons down an electron transfer mechanism where oxygen is the final electron acceptor.

- The oxygen combines with two protons and two electrons to form two molecules of water.

- Lipid stores are the main source of fuel at rest, during light activity, and when glycogen stores are depleted.

- Lipid provides substantially more ATP per unit than glycogen, but at greater oxygen cost and lower exercise intensity.

Answers to questions in the text

Question 7.1

Arterial blood is 97.5 per cent saturated with oxygen at 10 kPa (760 mmHg).

Question 7.2

At a tissue partial pressure (P_{ti}) of 5.32 kPa (40 mmHg) arterial blood is still 75 per cent saturated with oxygen. This is because of the shape of the oxyhaemoglobin dissociation curve. It is flattest between partial pressures ranging from 13.3 kPa (100 mmHg) to 8 kPa (60 mmHg), so there is a relatively small loss of oxygen for a large change in partial pressure.

Question 7.3

According to the Hagen–Poiseuille equation doubling the radius of a tube increases flow 16-fold. In other words, if the original flow rate is $1\ L \cdot s^{-1}$, doubling the radius of the pre-capillary sphincter leads to a flow rate of $16\ L \cdot s^{-1}$.

Question 7.4

At any particular P_{O_2} more oxygen is released from the haemoglobin when any one or more of the local conditions described above are present. During sustained exercise, all three occur at some point thus encouraging greater oxygen release to the muscle cell.

Question 7.5

Each haemoglobin molecule contains four atoms of iron. This gives it four times the carrying power of myoglobin.

Question 7.6

The breakdown of glucose (glycolysis) results in the production of four molecules of ATP – two molecules at Step 7 and two at Step 10. However, one molecule of ATP is used to phosphorylate glucose to give glucose-6-phosphate at Step 1, and a second molecule is used to phosphorylate fructose-6-phosphate to give fructose-1,6-diphosphate at Step 3, thus giving a net gain of two molecules of ATP.

Question 7.7

The breakdown of glycogen (glycogenolysis) results in the production of four molecules of ATP – two molecules at Step 7 and two at Step 10. However, one molecule of ATP phosphorylates fructose-6-phosphate to give fructose-1,6-diphosphate at Step 3. Thus, the net gain is three molecules of ATP.

Question 7.8

From the anaerobic breakdown of glucose and glycogen.

Question 7.9

From each glucose molecule there is a net gain of 38 (34?) molecules of ATP, and from glycogen there are 39 (35?). This is how those totals are derived. (See Figure 6.8, and take into account of the fact that from Step 5 there are two parallel pathways producing ATP molecules.)

Mechanism	Glucose	Glycogen
Substrate-level phosphorylation		
(a) Glycolysis – without O_2 (Steps 7 and 10 $\times$ 2)	2	3
(b) TCA cycle – GTP $\rightarrow$ ATP (Step 16 $\times$ 2)	2	2
Oxidative phosphorylation		
(via electron transfer chain)		
(a) Glycolysis – with O_2 (Step 6 $\times$ 2)	6 (?4)	6 (?4)
(b) Pyruvate $\rightarrow$ acetyl CoA (Step 11 $\times$ 2)	6 (?4)	6 (?4)
(via TCA cycle and electron transfer chain)		
(c) TCA – NAD^+ (Steps 13, 14, 18 $\times$ 2)	18	18
(d) TCA – FAD (Step 16 $\times$ 2)	4	4
Total	38 (?34)	39 (?35)

Question 7.10

The answer is two molecules of ATP result from the second hydrogen carrier FAD. It enters the electron transfer chain after the first reaction, which has already produce one molecule of ATP from the oxidation of NAD^+.

Question 7.11

There are two main benefits of lipid stores. The first is that there is substantially more fat stored in the average 70 kg man than glycogen or glucose. The second is that significantly more ATP is produced per molecule of fat than glycogen. The costs of these benefits are much slower rates of ATP production via lipid metabolism, and a reduction in sustainable exercise intensity to about 50 per cent of $\dot{V}_{O_2max}$.

Question 7.12

$RER = \dot{V}_{CO_2}/\dot{V}_{O_2}$

Fat breakdown $= 16_{CO_2}/23_{O_2} = 0.7$

Carbohydrate breakdown $= 6_{CO_2}/6_{O_2} = 1.0$

Measuring oxygen consumption and carbon dioxide excretion during steady-state exercise allows the RER at various exercise intensities to be calculated; this gives the relative proportions of lipid and carbohydrate used as fuel for particular intensities.

Answers to exercises in the text

Exercise 7.1

$$\dot{V}_{O_2} \ L \cdot min^{-1} = \dot{Q}_C \ L \cdot min^{-1} \cdot C_{a-\bar{v}O_2} \ mLO_2 \cdot L_{bl}^{-1}$$

$$40 \cdot 200 - 50$$

$$40 \cdot 150$$

$$= 6000 \ mL \cdot min^{-1} \ or \ 6 \ L \cdot min^{-1}$$

Exercise 7.2

Glycolysis, Step 6; breakdown of pyruvate, Step 11; Krebs cycle, Steps 13, 14, 16 and 18.

8

The Interplay between Aerobic and Anaerobic Metabolism

Learning Objectives

By the end of this chapter, you should be able to

- define anaerobic metabolism, and provide examples of the interplay between anaerobic and aerobic metabolism in sports performance

- distinguish between anaerobic capacity and anaerobic power

- explain the importance of nicotinamide adenine dinucleotide in the production of lactic acid

- explain the difference between lactic acid and lactate

- describe how lactate interferes with athletic performance

- list the mechanisms by which lactate is removed from the blood

- outline the importance of the measures such as the anaerobic threshold (An_{Th}), the lactate threshold (La_{Th}), and the onset of blood lactate accumulation (OBLA) for endurance athletes

- describe the principles behind tests to measure An_{Th}/La_{Th} and OBLA

- list the main features of popular tests of anaerobic power

- explain the differences in the Wingate and repeated-sprints test profiles of sprint and endurance athletes

- outline the principles behind and methods used in the maximal accumulated oxygen deficit (MAOD) test of anaerobic capacity

Exercise Physiology: A Thematic Approach   Tudor Hale
© John Wiley & Sons, Ltd   ISBN: 0 470 84682 8 (cloth), ISBN 0 470 84683 6 (pbk)

Objective test

Say whether the following answers are true (T) or false (F). If you do not know, say so (D) – not knowing is not an academic crime, but not finding out is. Try not to look at the answers until you have worked your way through the chapter and completed the test a second time. In this way, you can monitor your progress.

	Pre-test			Post-test		
	T	F	D	T	F	D
1. Lactic acid is a key marker of aerobic metabolism						
2. At rest, there is no detectable lactate in the blood						
3. The 100-m sprint is run fuelled totally by anaerobic glycolysis						
4. Anaerobic glycolysis needs the hydrogen carrier NAD^+ to function						
5. Under anaerobic conditions pyruvate is reduced to lactate						
6. Lactate enters the Krebs cycle and is used to produce ATP						
7. Hydrogen ions block the binding sites on the myosin filament						
8. Hydrogen ions interfere with glycolitic enzyme reactions						
9. Lactic acid is neutralized by buffers in the extracellular fluid						
10. The pyruvate–lactate reaction is not readily reversible						
11. Type IIb muscle fibres readily convert lactate back to pyruvate						
12. Lactate is used in the liver to restore glycogen levels						
13. Myocardial muscle cells use lactate as a substrate for contraction						

	Pre-test			Post-test		
	T	F	D	T	F	D
14. The relationship between exercise and blood lactate is rectilinear						
15. OBLA occurs when lactate levels in the blood exceed <4 mM						
16. A sharp, continuous increase in La_{bl} indicates the lactate threshold						
17. A sharp increase in $\dot{V}_E$ also indicates the lactate threshold						
18. The lactate threshold is positively correlated with 100-m times						
19. Impulse is the change of momentum when two bodies collide						
20. Work is force generated multiplied by the distance travelled						
21. Power is work multiplied by time						
22. The Margaria step test tests anaerobic power						
23. The Wingate test is a reliable measure of aerobic capacity						
24. Wingate profiles of 400-m and marathon runners are very similar						
25. The term 'oxygen debt' was introduced in 1922						
26. Excess post-exercise O_2 consumption reflects anaerobic activity						
27. EPOC is used primarily to refill O_2 stores						
28. Supra-maximal effort is fuelled exclusively by aerobic metabolism						
29. The MAOD test measures anaerobic capacity						
30. MAOD test relies on extrapolation of the $\dot{V}_{O_2}$-power relationship						

Symbols, abbreviations and units of measurement

adenosine triphosphate	ATP	
anaerobic threshold	An_{Th}	
blood lactate	La_{bl}	
blood lactate concentration	$[La_{bl}]$	$mmol \cdot L^{-1}$; mM
excess post-exercise oxygen consumption	EPOC	L
hydrogen ions	H^+	
energy	J	J; kJ; MJ; kcal
lactate dehydrogenase	LDH	
lactate threshold	La_{Th}	
maximum accumulated oxygen deficit	MAOD	L
millisecond	ms	
nicotinamide adenine dinucleotide	NAD^+	
nicotinamide adenine dinucleotide – reduced	$NADH + H^+$	
onset of blood lactate accumulation	OBLA	
oxymyoglobin	$MgbO_2$	
phosphocreatine	PCr	
power	W	$W; J \cdot s^{-1}; kg \cdot m \cdot s^{-1}; N \cdot m \cdot s^{-1}$

Introduction

Some organisms – mainly bacteria – can survive without oxygen; they are obligate anaerobes. As we have seen, athletes do not fall into this category, but they can exercise for limited periods when the oxygen supply is inadequate for the task in hand. The process supplying the energy to undertake that task is anaerobic metabolism, literally the breakdown of substrates 'without air'; the metabolic outcome is lactic acid. Replacing hydrogen ions with metallic elements such as potassium or sodium gives us lactate (La), a salt of lactic acid. We measure the concentration of this salt in capillary blood during and after maximal exercise tests. We can see the outcome in Figure 8.1.

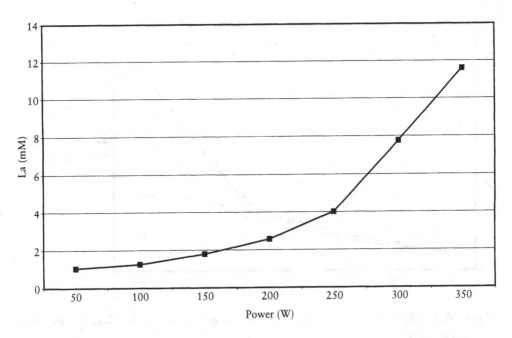

Figure 8.1 Blood lactate concentrations during progressive exercise

Anaerobic metabolism

Strictly speaking, anaerobic metabolism proceeds in the absence of oxygen, but when we consider the exercising athlete there appears to be a paradox. A quick examination of the data from a maximal oxygen uptake test reveals three things. The first is that even at rest, when oxygen is in plentiful supply, blood lactate levels are not zero but typically lie between 0.5 and 0.7 mmol $\cdot L^{-1}$. The second is that increasing oxygen uptake and, eventually, increasing levels of lactate in the blood accompany incremental exercise. Finally, blood lactate levels increase rapidly as exercise approaches maximal intensity. Indeed, one of the second-order criteria for determining whether an individual has reached maximal oxygen uptake is a blood lactate concentration – written $[La_{bl}]$ – of more than 8 mmol $\cdot L^{-1}$. (See Figure 8.2).

Elite endurance athletes routinely perform at 70–80 per cent of their maximal oxygen uptake for long periods with lactate levels of around 4 mmol $\cdot L^{-1}$. Thus, a more reasonable description of the anaerobic metabolism entailed in the exercising human is biochemical activity taking place in individual muscle cells where oxygen is either lacking or transiently unavailable. For example, a sustained contraction of a muscle group – a timed bent-arm pull-up on the beam for example – compresses the capillary walls and interferes

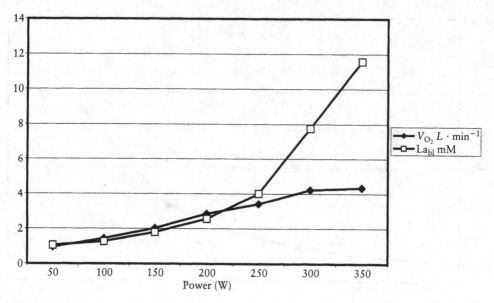

Figure 8.2   Blood lactate concentrations and oxygen uptake values during a maximal oxygen uptake test

with the flow of blood; this prevents access to the oxygen in the blood. The muscle then switches to the oxygen stored in the myoglobin ($MgbO_2$), but it depletes rapidly; the pain that accompanies high lactate concentrations increases, followed by the inability to maintain the isometric contraction.

So when we analyse the physiology of sports performance we must recognize that during activities involving whole body movements – running, cycling, swimming, rowing for example – adenosine triphosphate production is the outcome of an interaction between aerobic and anaerobic metabolism. If we take the two extremes of the athletics running events – the 100-m run in under 9.8 s, and the marathon (42 195 m) run in under 2 hours 6 minutes – the ratio of anaerobic:aerobic metabolism that provides the fuel for adenosine triphosphate resynthesis is roughly 9:1 for the 100-m, and 0.1:9.9 for the marathon. The suggestion that the marathon entails a small measure of anaerobic metabolism may be unsurprising. On the other hand, the fact that aerobic metabolism partly fuels the 100-m sprint, even though the race is over before the oxygen delivery system has had time to respond to the demands of the event, at first sight seems surprising.

Question 8.1   *What explanation can you give for this phenomenon?*

The two anaerobic mechanisms available to skeletal muscle that enable it to continue to contract, and us to engage in severe exercise, when oxygen supplies are inadequate for the task in hand have been outlined briefly in Chapter 7.

> **Question 8.2** *Can you remember what they are?*

However, during that chapter, we dealt mainly with aerobic metabolism, and did not explain in any detail the reactions that led to the production of lactic acid. To rectify that omission we have to return to the glycolitic pathway (see Figure 7.5).

Anaerobic glycolysis

Each molecule of glucose-6-phosphate derived from glucose or glycogen is broken down anaerobically to give two molecules of pyruvate and produce two or three molecules of adenosine triphosphate respectively. A critical reaction occurs at Step 6 when glyceraldehyde-3-phosphate, driven by its *dehydrogenase*, becomes 1,3-diphosphoglyceric acid; this reaction reduces the hydrogen carrier nicotinamide adenine dinucleotide through the addition of hydrogen – i.e. NAD^+ to $NADH + H^+$.

$$\text{glyceraldehyde-3-phosphate} + NAD^+ + P_i$$

$$\downarrow$$

$$\textit{glyceraldehyde-3-phosphate dehydrogenase}$$

$$\downarrow$$

$$\text{1,3-diphosphoglycerate} + NADH + H^+$$

Stores of nicotinamide adenine dinucleotide in the sarcoplasm of the muscle cell are small, but without its involvement in the reaction, glycolysis comes to a halt. To prevent this, the reduced nicotinamide adenine dinucleotide is oxidized by the removal of hydrogen protons and electrons. Under anaerobic conditions, the enzyme *lactate dehydrogenase*, facilitated by pyruvate acting as a hydrogen acceptor in place of the inaccessible molecular oxygen, drives the oxidizing reaction. This means that pyruvate is reduced to lactic acid, but it also leads to the release of the oxidized form of nicotinamide adenine dinucleotide that ensures the continuation of anaerobically produced adenosine triphosphate.

$$\text{pyruvate} + \text{NADH} + \text{H}^+$$

$$\downarrow$$

lactate dehydrogenase

$$\downarrow$$

$$\text{lactate} + \text{NAD}^+$$

The lactate builds up in the muscle cells and eventually diffuses into the blood stream.

> **Question 8.3**　*Can you remember what happens to the reduced form of nicotinamide adenine dinucleotide if sufficient oxygen is present?*

The consequences of anaerobic glycolysis

This physiological mechanism is very important; its main benefit is the rapid production of useful quantities of adenosine triphosphate. The mechanism enables us to run 100-m at speeds of more than $10 \text{ m} \cdot \text{s}^{-1}$, 400-m at about $9 \text{ m} \cdot \text{s}^{-1}$, and 800-m at about $8 \text{ m} \cdot \text{s}^{-1}$, all very useful if our survival is at stake, or we need to sprint to catch the bus, or to win an Olympic medal. However, there is a physiological price to pay for this evolutionary gift. The presence of lactic acid in muscle cells carries two penalties. The first, and the one that we have all experienced, is pain. This particular phenomenon is the first-line safety mechanism designed to prevent us from damaging ourselves; but it can be ignored, and in elite athletes, it usually is. However, we cannot avoid the other penalty, which is the way increased acidity of muscle cells interferes with the mechanics of skeletal muscle contraction. Acids break down (dissociate) into hydrogen ions (H^+) – protons – and bases; lactic acid dissociates into hydrogen ions and lactate ions (La). The hydrogen ions adversely affect the functions of key proteins, particularly the glycolitic enzymes that drive the biochemical reactions; they also interfere with the function of the actin and myosin proteins that make up the myofilaments. In addition, hydrogen ions compete for the binding sites on the actin filament; this reduces the opportunities for myosin head to bind to the actin filament and deliver the power strokes that lead to contraction. As acidity increases, the force generated by muscles diminishes progressively; the athlete is unable to continue at the same early pace and eventually stops. If a cheetah fails to catch its prey in 30 to 40 s it gives up the chase, not because it is not hungry but because of the hydrogen ions derived from lactic acid interfering with muscle contractions. The loss of form and deceleration in and the final 50-m of the 400-m race is another example of the phenomenon.

The fate of lactic acid

Three physiological mechanisms reduce the worst effects of lactic acid. The first is the presence of compounds in the intracellular and extracellular fluids, especially the blood, called 'buffers' – protein, bicarbonate, organic and inorganic phosphate, and haemoglobin for example – that neutralize the acid. We shall deal with this mechanism in more detail when we consider venous blood in Chapter 9.

The second is the ready reversibility of the pyruvate → lactate reaction. In Type I muscle fibres, and particularly those in the non-exercising muscles, the lactate converts back to pyruvate because of the high oxidative capacity of those fibres. The pyruvate then enters the Krebs cycle and electron transfer chain and produces useful amounts of adenosine triphosphate – theoretically 18 molecules per molecule of lactate.

The third is the usefulness of lactate in organs other than skeletal muscle. As the lactate carried by the blood passes through the liver and the heart, it can be converted into useful material. In the liver, glucose resynthesis, and thereby the restoration of glycogen stores, involves the use of lactate. In the heart, lactate is used, along with glucose, as a substrate fuelling the contraction of cardiac muscle; the ability of the myocardium to utilize lactate in this way is very useful, particularly when the metabolic demands of the heart are increased during heavy exercise.

Anaerobic thresholds

At moderate levels of exercise, the moderating mechanisms just described strive to keep a balance between lactate production and removal. Middle- and long-distance runners pay particular attention to the exercise intensity at which the balance between lactate production and removal is disturbed and more lactate is produced than can be removed. This intensity is where the onset of blood lactate accumulation (OBLA), or the anaerobic threshold (An_{Th}), or the lactate threshold occur. The concepts involved illustrate the balance between the two metabolic systems very clearly, and it is worth examining this balance in more detail.

The first step is for the athlete to undertake a progressive exercise test to establish roughly the level of exercise at which there is a sharp rise in the blood lactate concentration. The subject cycles, runs or swims for 5 minutes at a moderate pace, or roughly 50 per cent of their maximum level. This usually allows the subjects to reach the position where oxygen demand and supply are in balance, a position referred to as 'the steady state'. In the fifth minute we note power output for cyclists, or speed for runners and swimmers, record heart rate, and calculate oxygen uptake from expired gas volume and concentrations. Towards the end of that fifth minute, we collect a small sample of blood from a thumb or earlobe, and measure its lactate concentration. The subject continues exercising, and we repeat the procedures at higher intensities. About five of these bouts of incremental exercise is normally sufficient to reveal the pattern of blood lactate concentration plotted against power or speed; a typical plot looks something like that shown in Figure 8.3. The stage at which the slope of the curve becomes steeper indicates the onset of blood lactate accumulation. However, the position of this point may not be precise enough because the relatively large increases in power or speed of each stage may hide the exact power or speed at which lactate to accumulate in the blood.

A second procedure provides a more precise measure. It requires the subject to perform a series of 30-min tests, starting just below the exercise intensity predicted from the original OBLA test but spread over several days. We record power or speed, heart rate, oxygen consumption and blood lactate concentration at 5-min intervals during the 30-min test. After a suitable recovery period, we repeat the whole 30-min test at slightly higher exercise intensities until we reach the point where the subject cannot maintain power or speed for the full 30-min.

In the case of an elite endurance cyclist, shown in Figure 8.4, the incremental increase in power outputs can be as small as 15 w. The sensitivity of the aerobic-anaerobic interface is such that increasing power output from 400 W to 415 W represents the difference between completing a 30-min task and exhaustion in 20 min. Another way of looking at it is that at 400 W lactate removal matches lactate production, but at 415 W, lactate production exceeds removal; it follows that lactate accumulates in the blood and leads quickly to a catastrophic failure of the muscle contraction mechanism.

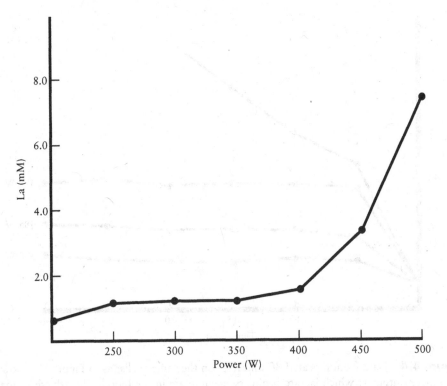

Figure 8.3 Data from an OBLA test on an elite cyclist showing the sharp increase in [La$_{bl}$] at ~400 W. (With permission from Dr P. Keen, British Cycling Federation)

Question 8.4 *What evidence for this catastrophic failure is often seen in some 3000-m – 10 000-m athletic events?*

Monitoring the respiratory responses to progressive exercises provides a non-invasive method of determining the anaerobic/lactate thresholds. Minute ventilation rises with increasing exercise intensity, but there comes a point at which the rise in ventilation increases sharply. This point gives a reasonable estimate of the anaerobic/lactate thresholds. A ramp test accompanied by breath-by-breath monitoring of ventilation is likely to provide a more reliable estimate.

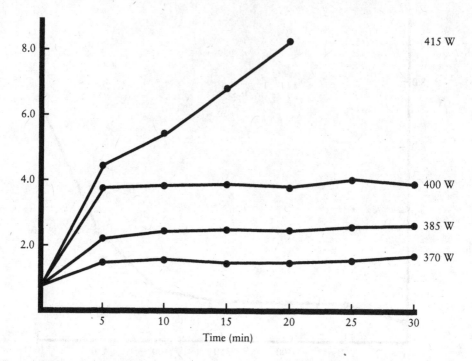

Figure 8.4   Data from repeated 30-min tests on the same cyclist as in Figure 8.3 showing the power output at which lactate begins to accumulate in the blood. The athlete is unable to continue at the required power output of 415 W and the test ends at 20 min. (With permission from Dr P. Keen, British Cycling Federation)

Anaerobic power and capacity

Standing high jump tests

At each end of the scale – the jumps and sprints, and the 400-m and 800-m for example – there is equal interest in the concepts of anaerobic power and anaerobic capacity, together with their measurement. Jumpers are interested in explosive power, based on the mechanical concept 'impulse'. Technically, impulse is the change in the momentum in either body when two bodies collide; in the jumps, it is the change in momentum when an athlete's body collides with the earth at take-off. The imperceptible change of momentum in the earth is set against the much greater change generated in the jumper's body.

We measure impulse most precisely with the aid of force platforms found in the biomechanics laboratories of all good sports science departments. Much cheaper but less accurate measures come when using the Sargent jump and Lewis Nomogram, or its slightly more reliable modern version involving the use of 'jump-mats' that record the time spent in the air following a maximal standing high jump.

Question 8.5 *How much lactate is likely to be generated during these kinds of events: 'hardly any' – 'a small amount' – 'quite a lot'?*

The Margaria test

The 100-m sprinters are interested in slightly longer-term anaerobic effort. An indirect measure that attempts to assess the capacity of the phosphagen system is the long-established Margaria test of anaerobic power; this involves a timed, all-out sprint up a short series of steps. The body mass of the subject and the time to complete the run are recorded; the distance the body mass is lifted from the floor to the top of the steps is known. The work done can be calculated by multiplying the force required to lift the mass by the distance covered; power is work over time.

$$\text{Power} = \frac{\text{Mass (kg)} \cdot \text{Distance (m)}}{\text{Time (s)}}$$

Question 8.6 *How much lactate is likely to be generated during this exercise: 'hardly any' – 'a small amount' – 'quite a lot'?*

The Wingate test

The 400-m and 800-m runners are interested in tests that attempt to assess two things: the *power* of the anaerobic system as a whole, together with its *capacity*. The Wingate test is one attempt to measure anaerobic power that has become a standard test in most laboratories. The test consists of a computer-monitored, 30-s all-out effort on a cycle ergometer. We place a resistive load, related to the subject's body mass, on the weight cradle of a Monark cycle ergometer. From a rolling start, we lower the cradle and require the subject to pedal as fast as possible for the full 30 s; a computer counts the number of revolutions of the flywheel each second. We know the force needed to overcome the resistive load; we calculate the distance the flywheel has travelled from the number of complete revolutions of the flywheel; we standardize the time at 30 s. Theoretically at least, we know all the parts of the equation for calculating power. The computer calculates power output every 25–30 milliseconds (ms) and produces a profile similar to that seen in Figure 8.5. The computer also calculates peak power, time to peak power, total work done, and a fatigue index. Each of these variables may give some insights into the anaerobic capabilities of the subject, although performance on a cycle ergometer may not be transferable to running or swimming events.

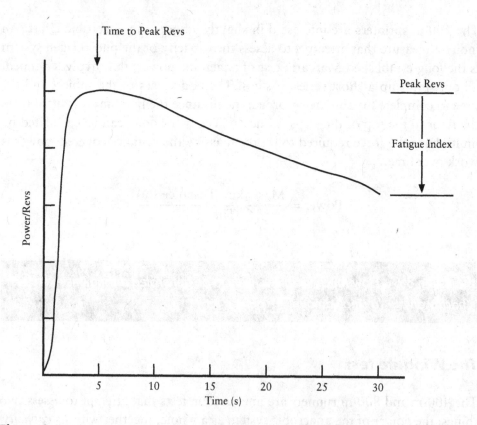

Figure 8.5 A typical power output (flywheel revolutions) profile from a 30-s Wingate test. Note the sharp rise in the first few seconds to peak power, and the gradual decline in power output over the remainder of the time

Question 8.7 *What differences would you expect to see in the profiles of a 400-m and a 10000-m runner?*

However, a problem arises when we express the data in watts (W), the SI unit for power. Two elements create the difficulties. The first is the use of the simple formula for power, i.e. work/time; strictly speaking, we can only use this formula whilst exercising at a relatively constant power output. The profile shows that there is hardly any time when this condition exists – the flywheel is either accelerating or decelerating throughout the 30 s of the test; therefore, we should not apply the formula. The second relates to the characteristics of the individual flywheels, and the weights used to create the resistance. We assume that the mass of these is consistent, but this may not be the case. Therefore, even if applying the formula was justifiable, the results from different ergometers may not be reliable. Unless we check all of the weights, and determine the characteristics of the flywheel by run-down tests, invalid calculations can result. Without these checks, the only reliable piece of evidence we have is the number of flywheel revolutions performed during the test. This is still a useful indicator of anaerobic performance, but it is unwise to equate flywheel revolutions with the Newtonian measure of power.

> **Question 8.8** *How much lactate is likely to be generated during this exercise: 'hardly any' – 'a small amount' – 'quite a lot'?*

The repeated-sprints test

Unlike the traditional track events in athletics, many popular sports require a combination of walking, jogging, and sprinting, interspersed with explosive activities such as jumping, kicking, tackling, and shooting, rather than a sustained, constant effort. The obvious examples are the invasion games that are part of our sporting heritage. The duration of these sports varies between one and two hours, so we need a good aerobic power foundation, with an added ability to produce sustained isometric actions as in a set scrum, explosive actions such as a slam-dunk, or a 50-m sprint ending with a shot on goal. A repeated-sprints test assesses intermittent efforts like these. The Wingate test forms the basis, but instead of a single, 30-s all-out effort, subjects perform a number of short, maximal sprints interspersed with short periods of recovery. The ten profiles indicate the ability of a subject to generate maximum effort repeatedly (Figure 8.6). The increases in time to peak power and the decline in peak power achieved in successive tests are seen, and may be used to monitor the effectiveness of training and rehabilitation programmes. The same reservations expressed about the measurement of power in the Wingate test remain.

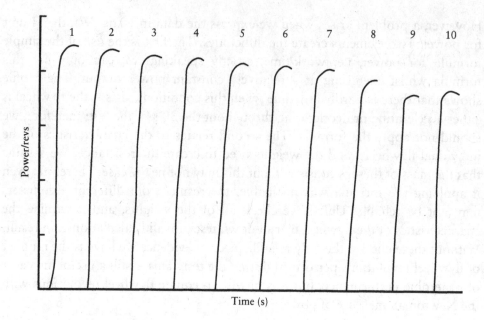

Figure 8.6 Typical power output (flywheel revolution) profiles from a repeated-sprints test

Post-exercise oxygen consumption

We can estimate the energy expenditure of various activities, albeit expensively, via direct calorimetry – 1 W is equivalent to a joule per second ($1J \cdot s^{-1}$), and one litre of oxygen consumed is equivalent to 21.1 kJ – but direct measurement of anaerobic capacity is problematic. Early attempts included the measurement of the 'oxygen debt', a phenomenon first described in 1922 by Archibald Hill and his colleague Hartley Lipton. If we record oxygen consumption at rest, and during and after an all-out effort such as a 400-m run, we find that the amount of oxygen consumed during the actual run is relatively small. During recovery, however, it is higher than the resting level for some time after the end of the run, and it returns to resting levels only slowly. The hypothesis put forward to explain the phenomenon was that the run incurs an 'oxygen debt' during the anaerobic break down of glucose to lactic acid when the supply of oxygen was inadequate. Like all debts, it has to be repaid, with interest. The result is raised oxygen consumption during recovery – repaying the oxygen debt. We describe this now more precisely as excess post-exercise oxygen consumption (EPOC).

Maximum accumulated oxygen deficit

In all-out effort lasting about two minutes, athletes maintain speeds greater than those reached during maximal oxygen uptake tests. We describe such exercise intensities 'supra-maximal' efforts; such intensity clearly calls on anaerobic metabolism. Medbø and his colleagues made an ingenious attempt to assess an athlete's anaerobic capacity through monitoring responses to such supra-maximal exercise; they called it the maximum accumulated oxygen deficit (MAOD) test.

The test uses the linear relationship between steady state oxygen consumption and running speed during sub-maximal exercise to predict the oxygen consumption at supra-maximal exercise through linear extrapolation. Two preliminary tests need to be performed before the MAOD procedure is applied. Firstly, the athlete undertakes a sub-maximal incremental treadmill test to establish the individual oxygen uptake responses to each of the four or five speeds chosen. Secondly, practice establishes the speed designed to exhaust the athlete in about two minutes. From these we calculate the estimated oxygen consumption at the chosen supra-maximal speed. The athlete then performs the 2-min run, during which we measure actual oxygen consumption.

We multiply the oxygen consumption obtained from the extrapolation by the time spent running and derive the *predicted* total oxygen demand for the run. We measure oxygen consumption *during* the run in the usual way. The difference between the demand and the consumption gives the maximum accumulated oxygen deficit that provides a picture of an individual's anaerobic capacity. Figure 8.7 illustrates this procedure.

The major limitation of this test lies in the extrapolation of the well-established sub-maximal rectilinear relationship between exercise intensity and oxygen consumption. We have no real idea of the precise relationship during short-term supra-maximal exercise; it could well remain rectilinear, but equally it may not. We need to undertake more research.

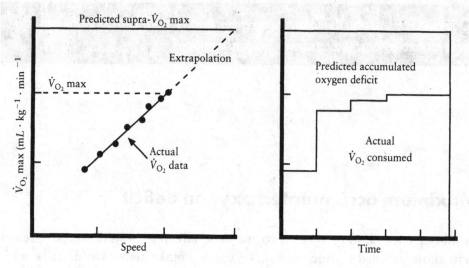

Figure 8.7 A typical maximal accumulated oxygen deficit graph. (Reproduced from Medbø SI *et al* (1988), with permission of the American Physiological Society)

Key points

- The energy for short-term bursts of intense exercise comes from two sources – the phosphagen system, and anaerobic glycolysis.

- The first source relies on the splitting of phosphocreatine to resynthesize adenosine triphosphate, and is exhausted within 10 to 20 s.

- The second source, important for the rapid resynthesis of adenosine triphosphate for about 2 min, comes from the reduction of pyruvic acid to produce lactic acid.

- The hydrogen atom needed for this reduction comes from the oxidation of nicotinamide adenine dinucleotide.

- The equation is pyruvic acid $+ NADH + H^+ \leftrightarrow LDH \leftrightarrow$ lactic acid $+$ NAD^+.

- The enzyme *lactate dehydrogenase* (LDH) drives the reversible reaction.

- The lactic acid, which dissociates into hydrogen ions and lactate ions, stimulates pain receptors in skeletal muscle.

- The hydrogen ions also interfere with key rate-limiting enzyme reactions of the glycolytic pathway, and compete with calcium for binding sites on the actin filaments so that eventually skeletal muscle fails to contract.

- Buffers – haemoglobin, bicarbonate, proteins and phosphates – work to neutralize the acidity produced by the hydrogen ions.

- Type I muscle fibres with their high oxidative capacity can reverse the pyruvate – lactate reaction.

- Lactate is also used as a fuel by cardiac muscle, and is involved in the restoration of glucose stores in the liver.

- The excess post-exercise oxygen consumption (EPOC) is largely due to the continual requirement for adenosine triphosphate to restore blood lactate levels to their resting values.

- Laboratory tests are used to detect the exercise intensity at which lactate begins to accumulate in the blood.

- This exercise intensity is critical for endurance-trained athletes.

- Sports scientists and athletes are also interested in anaerobic power – the rate at which maximal work is done – anaerobic capacity – how much work is achieved before fatigue sets in.

- A range of tests exists to give a picture, albeit a limited one, of power and capacity. These include the Sargent jump, the Margaria test, the Wingate 30-s test, the repeated-sprints test, and the measurement of the maximum accumulated oxygen deficit (MAOD). Each has its limitations.

Answers to questions in the text

Question 8.1
There is oxygen available in the blood perfusing the muscles, and in the myoglobin stores of individual muscle cells, so it is not surprising that some ATP is resynthesized through aerobic metabolism. The fact that so little of that needed – only ~10 per cent – is derived aerobically indicates the slowness of that process, compared to the speed of the phosphagen and anaerobic glycolysis systems.

Question 8.2

The two processes are the phosphagen system, $ADP + PCr = ATP$, and anaerobic glycolysis, the breakdown of glucose and glycogen to lactic acid. The former is exhausted rapidly; the latter can only be sustained at maximal effort for less than a minute.

Question 8.3

Nicotinamide adenine dinucleotide is an essential hydrogen acceptor in the glycolitic process. Without it glycolysis would stop at the point when glyceraldehyde-3-phosphate is transformed into 1,3-diphosphogylcerate. If oxygen is available at this point the reduced $NADH + H^+$ enters the Krebs cycle, and thence the electron transport chain, to be oxidized back to NAD^+, and also provide ATP.

Question 8.4

The best long-distance runners have three advantages over the ordinary runners. The first is the ability to run at a higher percentage of their $\dot{V}_{O_2max}$ over the race distance; the second is the ability to inject a faster lap to break up the rhythm of other runners without accumulating lactate in the blood; the third is the ability to sprint the last 200-m of the race. The first two are important because if runners with relatively low percentage $\dot{V}_{O_2max}$ try to keep up with the better runners they soon experience blood lactate accumulation and soon find themselves dropping further and further behind the front runners. The effect is even more readily seen if a couple of fast laps are injected into the race. Those who are not equipped to match the new pace but try to stay with it are soon dropped by the front-runners and struggle to complete the event.

Question 8.5

'Hardly any' is the answer. Although maximum effort is expended, the time-scale is so short that the effort is completed too quickly for anaerobic glycolysis to be engaged.

Question 8.6

'Hardly any' is again the answer for the same reasons as given in the answer to Question 8.5. It is worth noting that Margaria and his colleagues used the early notion of energy 'debt', and actually divided anaerobic metabolism into either 'lactacid' or 'alactacid' debt. The term 'alactacid' means without lactic acid, and was designed to test the anaerobic power of the phosphagen system as the fuel for short-term, maximal bursts of activity of the kind seen in the test that bears Margaria's name.

Question 8.7

The main differences as shown in Figure 8.8, are (a) a shorter time to reach peak power (peak flywheel revolutions), (b) a greater peak power output (a greater number of flywheel revolutions before deceleration takes over), and (c) a faster decline in power output (flywheel revolutions) for the 400-m runner.

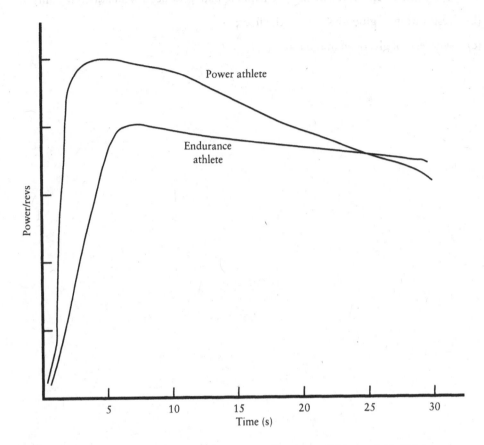

Figure 8.8   A comparison of Wingate test profiles from 400-m and 10 000-m runners

Question 8.8

The best option from those given is probably 'quite a lot', but this problem is difficult to answer simply. It would depend on the lower limb muscle mass, the proportion of fast-twitch (Type IIb) muscle fibres, the training status of the person performing the test, and their ability to pedal quickly. One thing that could be said without too much debate is that more lactate will have been produced during the Wingate test than in the Sargent jump and Margaria tests.

Question 8.9

The homeostasis of the internal environment has been seriously disrupted and needs to be restored. The mechanisms that restore homeostasis require energy in the form of adenosine triphosphate, and include

(a) removal of the accumulated blood lactate via the lactate → pyruvate reaction and entry into the Krebs cycle and the electron transfer chain where oxygen is the final hydrogen acceptor; the adenosine triphosphate produced is an added benefit;

(b) restoration of glucose stores in the liver;

(c) synthesis of glycogen in the muscle.

9 Venous Blood, Carbon Dioxide and Acid–Base Balance

Learning Objectives

By the end of this chapter, you should be able to

♦ explain the ventilatory responses to exercise of increasing intensity

♦ describe the main characteristics of the systemic venous circulation

♦ list the mechanisms that assist in venous return to the right atrium

♦ define normo-, hypo- and hyper-capnia, and say how they occur

♦ describe the mechanisms by which carbon dioxide is carried in venous blood and excreted by the lungs

♦ explain the Bohr effect, the Haldane effect, and the Hamburger (chloride) shift

♦ define an acid and a base, and outline the sources of respiratory and metabolic acids

♦ define pH and neutral pH

♦ give the pHs of intracellular, arterial, and mixed venous blood, and say whether these fluids are acidic or alkaline

♦ list the main components of the buffering system, and explain their function

♦ describe the effects of acids and bases on ventilation

♦ explain how the kidneys respond to metabolic acidosis and metabolic alkalosis

Exercise Physiology: A Thematic Approach   Tudor Hale
© John Wiley & Sons, Ltd   ISBN: 0 470 84682 8 (cloth), ISBN 0 470 84683 6 (pbk)

Objective test

Say whether the following answers are true (T) or false (F). If you do not know, say so (D) – not knowing is not an academic crime, but not finding out is. Try not to look at the answers until you have worked your way through the chapter and completed the test a second time. In this way, you can monitor your progress.

	Pre-test			Post-test		
	T	F	D	T	F	D
1. The walls of veins are much thicker than arteries						
2. In cross-section, veins are circular in shape						
3. At rest ∼ 60% of the total blood volume is stored in the veins						
4. Venoconstriction reduces resistance and increases stored volume						
5. Valves in the veins of the lower limbs assist in venous return						
6. A fall in central venous pressure increases cardiac output						
7. At rest, the P_{CO_2} of mixed venous blood is 6.1 kPa (46 mmHg)						
8. During maximal exercise the P_{aCO_2} rises						
9. Hyperventilation leads to hypocapnia						
10. Cigarette smokers with chronic bronchitis are often hypercapnic						
11. Carbon dioxide is 20 times less soluble than oxygen						
12. ∼ 5% of the CO_2 carried in the blood is in dissolved form						
13. ∼ 5% of the CO_2 carried in the blood combines with haemoglobin						

	Pre-test			Post-test		
	T	F	D	T	F	D
14. The higher the S_{aO_2} the lower the CO_2 carrying capacity of Hb						
15. Carbon dioxide combines with water to form carbonic acid						
16. The enzyme *carbonic anhydrase* is found in the plasma						
17. The erythrocyte membrane is impermeable to anions like HCO_3^-						
18. The Na^+ shift maintains ionic balance between plasma and RBC						
19. More hydrogen carbonate is carried in the plasma than the RBCs						
20. Compounds that accept hydrogen ions are called acids						
21. Compounds that donate hydrogen ions are called bases						
22. The measure of acidity or alkalinity of a solution is its pH						
23. pH = the $\log_{10}$ of the hydrogen ion concentration						
24. The pH scale ranges from 0 to 14. H_2O at 25°C has neutral pH = 7						
25. Increasing acidity raises pH, increasing alkalinity lowers it						
26. At rest arterial blood has a pH = 7.4						
27. Buffers such as Hb, HCO_3^- and proteins remove H^+ from blood						
28. Carbonic acid is excreted by the lungs						
29. Metabolic acids are excreted by the kidneys as ammonia (NH_3)						
30. Altitude acclimatization involves excretion of HCO_3^- in urine						

Symbols, abbreviations and units of measurement

ammonia	NH_3	
ammonium ion	NH_4^+	
arterial carbon dioxide partial pressure	P_{aCO_2}	kPa; mmHg
blood lactate concentration	$[La_{bl}]$	$mmol \cdot L^{-1}$; mM
carbon dioxide	CO_2	
carbamino compounds (free amino acids)	$R \cdot NHCOO^-$	
carbamino-haemoglobin	$Hb \cdot NHCOO^-$	
carbonic acid	H_2CO_3	
chloride ion	Cl^-	
expired volume, minute volume	$\dot{V}_E$	$L \cdot min^{-1}$
hydrogen carbonate, bicarbonate ion	HCO_3^-	
lactic acid	$C_3H_6O_3$	
lactate salt (e.g. sodium lactate)	Na^+La	
maximal oxygen uptake	$\dot{V}_{O_2 max}$	$L \cdot min^{-1}$; $mL \cdot min^{-1}$
measure of acidity/alkalinity	pH	
mixed venous carbon dioxide partial pressure	$P_{\bar{v}CO_2}$	kPa; mmHg
oxygen saturation	S_{aO_2}	%
respiratory frequency	f_R	$br \cdot min^{-1}$
tissue partial pressure of carbon dioxide	$P_{CO_2 ti}$	kPa; mmHg
volume of carbon dioxide excreted	$\dot{V}_{CO_2}$	$L \cdot min^{-1}$; $mL \cdot min^{-1}$

Introduction

The breakdown of dietary carbohydrate, fats and proteins during rest and exercise produces waste materials. The obvious materials are the volatile respiratory acid derived from carbon dioxide, carbonic acid ($H_2CO_3^-$), and the non-volatile metabolic acid, lactic acid ($C_3H_6O_3$). The consequences arising from the production of the two acids during increasing exercise intensity appear in Figure 9.1.

The volume of carbon dioxide excreted ($\dot{V}_{CO_2}$) rises progressively; the blood lactate concentration $[La_{bl}]$ remains fairly low during moderate exercise but rises sharply as intensity increases; expired volume ($\dot{V}_E$) follows a two-phase

Figure 9.1 Schematic representations of minute ventilation ($\dot{V}_E$), carbon dioxide excretion ($\dot{V}_{CO_2}$), blood lactate concentration ($[La_{bl}]$), and pH responses to progressive exercise

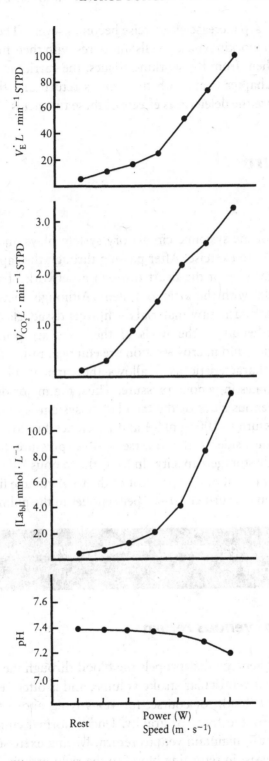

response with a sharp increase as exercise becomes severe. The build-up of these waste materials in working muscle cells interferes with their function, and so we need to remove them from the working tissues; the carrier is the venous blood. The rest of this chapter deals with the venous return and the mechanisms at work that minimize the deleterious effects of these two acids

Venous return

Veins

The venous side of the systemic circulatory system plays an important role in the body's response to exercise. After passing through the capillaries, the blood returns to the right side of the heart through a network of venules and veins that run in parallel with the arterial system. Although veins and arteries are built from the same basic raw materials – fibrous tissue, elastic tissue, smooth muscle and endothelium – the walls of the veins are generally very much thinner than arteries, and in cross-section are elliptical rather than circular. This is an important characteristic as it allows the capacity of veins to increase without large changes in venous pressure. Thus, the major difference between the arterial and venous sides of the circulatory system is that the arterial side presents high pressure ($\sim$100 mmHg) and resistance but low storage capacity, whereas the venous side is the reverse – low pressure ($\sim$15 mmHg) and resistance but high storage capacity. Indeed, the venous side acts as the main blood reservoir. At rest about 60 per cent of the total volume lies in the systemic veins and venules and a further 10–12 per cent lies in the pulmonary vessels.

> **Question 9.1**   *Any suggestions why the walls of veins are thinner than their arterial counterparts?*

Mechanisms of venous return

The main source of energy that propels the blood through the veins is the force generated by the left ventricular stroke volume, and is often referred to as *vis a tergo* (force from behind); of course, for veins lying above the heart venous return is assisted by the force of gravity. Under normal circumstances, these forces are sufficient to maintain venous return. During exercise, however, other mechanisms also assist in returning blood to the right atrium. The first of these is sympathetic innervation of smooth muscle found in the walls of the veins. The resultant venoconstriction increases resistance minimally but substantially reduces the volume of blood stored. The second is the system of valves found in the small to medium-sized veins of the peripheral circulation, particularly in the lower limbs. These valves, consisting of two or three small fibrous flaps, prevent the back-flow of blood towards the feet.

Question 9.2   *Why are valves absent in veins lying above the heart?*

The third mechanism – called the muscle pump – is useful during physical activity. The contraction of skeletal muscles in the limbs squeezes the veins, and in conjunction with the valve flaps, forces the blood towards the heart. Even simple dorsi- and plantar-flexion of the ankles is sufficient to keep lower limb blood moving, and is recommended by airlines to reduce the risk of deep vein thrombosis during long-haul flights. The final mechanism is known as the respiratory pump; it involves an interaction between the abdominal and thoracic cavities during breathing. The heart lies within the thoracic cavity where pressure is below atmospheric pressure. The systemic veins lying outside the thorax are under the influence of atmospheric pressure, and the veins in the abdomen are subject to even greater intra-abdominal pressures as the diaphragm descends during inspiration. The higher pressure outside the thorax, complemented by the lower pressure in the thorax during inspiration, assists in right atrial and ventricular filling.

Central venous pressure

All of these mechanisms affect the pressure in veins near the heart, known as central venous pressure. Changes in central venous pressure produce reflex responses; a fall in pressure leads to reduced cardiac output, and lowered blood pressure. A reflex discharge from sympathetic nerves results in the constriction of smooth muscle in the veins. This, in turn, reduces the storage capacity of the system, raises central venous pressure, and restores cardiac output. During exercise, more blood is required to supply oxygen to the working skeletal muscles. This extra demand results in less blood being stored in the veins, and an accompanying fall in venous pressure. Sympathetic stimulation leads to venoconstriction and the maintenance of pressure and cardiac output.

Venous blood and carbon dioxide

Carbon dioxide (CO_2) was discovered by Jan van Helmont, a Belgian scientist, in the early seventeenth century, and was first isolated by the Scottish scientist, Joseph Black, in 1755. It provides the 'fizz' in drinks ranging from sparkling mineral water to champagne, but its importance here is that it is the major by-product of the metabolism of carbohydrates and fats.

Exercise 9.1

Complete the following equations. Say what they represent.

$$C_6H_{12}O_6 + 6O_2 =$$

$$CH_3(CH_2)_{14}COOH + 23O_2 =$$

At rest, the blood leaves the left ventricle with an arterial carbon dioxide partial pressure (P_{aCO_2}) of 5.3 kPa (40 mmHg). During its passage through the capillaries, the blood picks up the carbon dioxide produced by the working tissues, and returns to the right side of the heart with a venous partial pressure ($P_{\bar{v}CO_2}$) of 6.1 kPa (46 mmHg). It is worth noting here that at rest only ~10 per cent of the total amount of carbon dioxide carried in the blood is excreted at the lungs. This suggests that some level of carbon dioxide in the blood is necessary for normal functions; excessive levels, however, can lead to carbon dioxide poisoning and, if unchecked, death.

Question 9.3 Why is 'some level of carbon dioxide in the blood' necessary?

During exercise, the carbon dioxide partial pressure in the venous blood, particularly in the veins draining large active muscle groups, rises in line with the greater metabolic demands and the increased production of carbon dioxide via the Krebs cycle. Driven by the respiratory centres in the pons and medulla oblongata, ventilation increases to ensure that the respiratory system excretes the excess carbon dioxide produced. The partial pressure of carbon dioxide in the arterial blood leaving the left ventricle provides a measure of the effectiveness of this process. You can see in Figure 9.2 that in spite of increasing

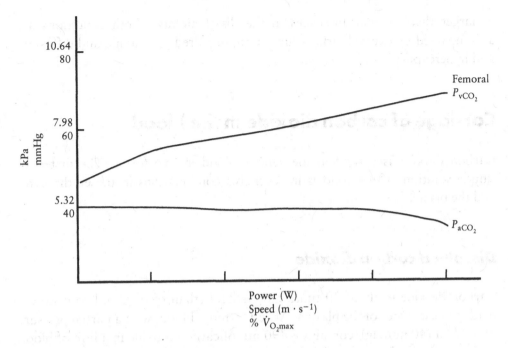

Figure 9.2 Schematic representation of arterial (P_{aCO_2}) and femoral vein (P_{vCO_2}) partial pressures of carbon dioxide response to progressive exercise. (Reproduced with permission of Professor PO Åstrand)

production the arterial partial pressure remains remarkably constant at ~5.3 kPa (40 mmHg). Indeed, during the latter stages of a maximal test it may actually fall below normal values, indicating hyperventilation and transient hypocapnia.

Hypocapnia, defined as carbon dioxide partial pressures of less than 4.7 kPa (35 mmHg), results in respiratory alkalosis; it almost certainly occurs during voluntary hyperventilation prior to an underwater-swimming competition.

Question 9.4   *Why hyperventilate? Why is it dangerous?*

Hypercapnia, defined as partial pressures greater than 6.3 kPa (47 mmHg), results in respiratory acidemia; it occurs in patients with chronic lung disease. Tobacco smoking, the most common source of chronic lung disease, irritates and inflames the airways, reduces the effectiveness of the cilia, and leads to hyper-secretion of mucus in the bronchioles. The end-result is chronic obstructive bronchitis. Emphysema is the destruction of the lung tissue itself resulting in larger than normal air-spaces in the distal airways. Both conditions are accompanied by expired airflow limitation, impaired gas mixing and diffusion, and hypercapnia.

Carriage of carbon dioxide in the blood

Carbon dioxide is carried in the venous blood in two forms. The first is in simple solution. The second is in reversible combinations in the erythrocytes and the plasma.

Dissolved carbon dioxide

Carbon dioxide is about 20 times more soluble than oxygen and so dissolves readily in the water of the plasma. At rest, arterial blood, with a partial pressure of 5.3 kPa (40 mmHg), contains ~490 mL of carbon dioxide in a litre of blood ($mL_{CO_2} \cdot L_{bl}^{-1}$), whereas mixed venous blood with a partial pressure of 6.1 kPa (46 mmHg) contains ~ 530 $mL_{CO_2} \cdot L_{bl}^{-1}$. However, only about 5 per cent of the total amount carried in the blood – ~25 and ~30 $mL_{CO_2} \cdot L_{bl}^{-1}$ respectively – is carried in solution in this unchanged form. However, this amount, though small, is very important because only free carbon dioxide can cross the capillary–alveolar membrane in the lungs easily. The rapid removal of the free gas from the plasma to the alveoli lowers plasma partial pressures, allowing the carbon dioxide carried in the reversible combinations to revert to its free form and complete its removal through expiration.

Reversible combinations

These combinations take two forms: carbamino compounds, of which there are two, and hydrogen carbonate.

Carbamino compounds

Carbamino compounds also take two forms. The first occurs when the carbon dioxide dissolved in the plasma reacts with free amino groups of plasma proteins (R).

$$R \cdot NH_2 + CO_2 \leftrightarrow R \cdot NHCOO^- + H^+$$

The amount of carbon dioxide carried in this way is small enough to be ignored in the general calculations. However, this is not so with the carbon dioxide that diffuses from the plasma into the erythrocyte, where it combines with the amino acids of the globin element of haemoglobin to form carbamino-haemoglobin.

$$Hb \cdot NH_2 + CO_2 \leftrightarrow Hb \cdot NHCOO^- + H^+$$

In resting mixed venous blood ~ 30 $mL_{CO_2} \cdot L_{bl}^{-1}$ is carried in this way. You will notice that both of these reactions result in the production of hydrogen ions (H^+). We shall return to this issue later in the chapter.

Question 9.5 *What is the outcome of increased [H^+] in the blood?*

Hydrogen carbonate

There are also two sources of hydrogen carbonate (HCO_3^-), also known as bicarbonate. The first arises when carbon dioxide dissolves in the water of the *plasma* to form carbonic acid (H_2CO_3), an unstable acid that readily dissociates into hydrogen and hydrogen carbonate (bicarbonate) ions.

$$CO_2 + H_2O \leftrightarrow H_2CO_3 \leftrightarrow H^+ + HCO_3^-$$

However, the process is very slow because the plasma lacks any enzymes that can catalyse the reaction.

The second process, which is very fast, produces hydrogen carbonate from reactions that take place in the *erythrocytes*. Indeed, this is the principal form by which carbon dioxide is carried in the blood. The difference in the rates of reaction is due to the presence in the red blood cell of the enzyme called *carbonic anhydrase*. Under the influence of this enzyme hydrogen carbonate is produced 10 000 times more quickly in the red cell than in the plasma.

$$CO_2 + H_2O \rightarrow carbonic\ anhydrase \leftrightarrow H_2CO_3 \leftrightarrow H^+ + HCO_3^-$$

The partial pressure of carbon dioxide is always higher in the muscle cell than in the plasma and erthyrocytes. Thus, the gas diffuses into the plasma, where some is dissolved; but the majority diffuses into the erythrocyte. Because of the presence of *carbonic anhydrase* the concentration of hydrogen carbonate [HCO_3^-] rises more rapidly in the red blood cell than in the plasma, leading to a concentration gradient from the erythrocyte to the plasma. The erythrocyte membrane is very permeable to anions such as hydrogen carbonate and chloride (Cl^-) ions, and the hydrogen carbonate diffuses into the plasma. This leads to an ionic (electrical) imbalance between the intracellular fluid of the red cell and the extracellular fluid of the plasma. To restore this balance, an equal amount of chloride anions, present in the plasma in large amounts, diffuses into the erythrocyte. This process is known as the Hamburger effect, after its discoverer Viktor Hamburger, and also, more prosaically, as 'the chloride shift'. These reactions lead ultimately to similar hydrogen carbonate concentrations in the red blood cell and the plasma. However, more hydrogen carbonate is carried by the plasma than the erythrocytes.

Question 9.6   *If the concentrations in the red blood cell and plasma are similar, why is more hydrogen carbonate carried in the plasma?*

Figure 9.3 is a schematic representation of the entire process.

The Bohr and Haldane effects

It is very important here to understand the reciprocal nature of the Bohr and Haldane effects. The Bohr or, more precisely, the Bohr–Hasselbalch–Krogh, effect was reported in 1904. These Danish physiologists found that the higher the partial pressure of carbon dioxide in the cell the greater the dissociation of oxygen from the haemoglobin molecule; this is very useful for the hard-working skeletal muscle cell. However, it does not stop there. The level of oxyhaemoglobin saturation affects the carbon dioxide carrying capacity of haemoglobin. The *higher* the oxygen saturation the *lower* the amount of carbon dioxide carried at any given partial pressure of carbon dioxide. Put simply, the greater the amount of oxygen attached to haemoglobin the less room there is for carbon dioxide. As arterial blood passes through the capillary bed of a working skeletal muscle where oxygen partial pressures are low and carbon dioxide partial pressures are high, oxygen is released to fuel the breakdown of glycogen and fat. The higher the carbon dioxide partial pressure the more oxygen is unloaded from the haemoglobin. The result of this enhanced unloading is that there is now room on the haemoglobin

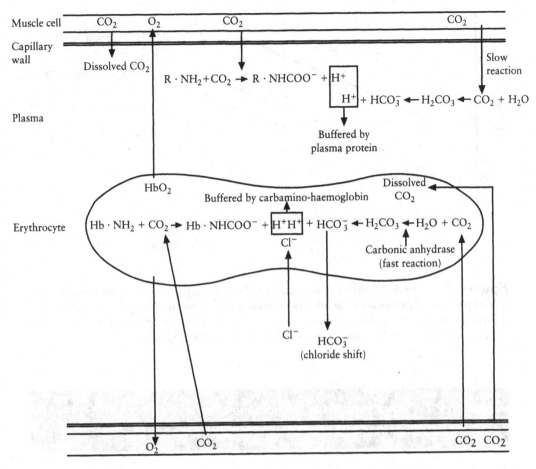

Figure 9.3 Schematic diagram of the carriage of carbon dioxide. The processes are reversed at the lungs where carbon dioxide partial pressure is low and oxygen content high

molecule for the carbon dioxide to combine with the globin element. Equally, it follows that as the mixed venous blood arrives at the alveoli, where the partial pressure of carbon dioxide is low and of oxygen is high, the process is reversed; oxygen binds with the haemoglobin and carbon dioxide is released into the alveoli and exhaled. This reciprocal arrangement is the Haldane effect, after its English discoverer, J. S. Haldane. It is important because it allows the carriage of carbon dioxide from working tissues without a concomitant increase in the partial pressure of the gas (see Figure 9.4).

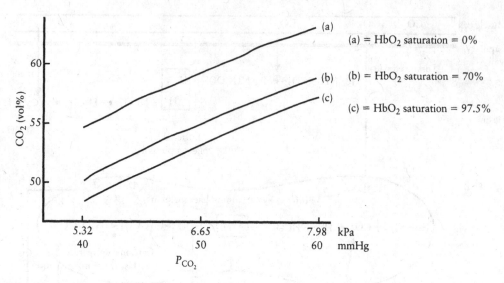

Figure 9.4   The relationship between carbon dioxide partial pressure and content. The partial pressure of carbon dioxide influences oxygen saturation (the Bohr effect), and oxygen saturation influences carbon dioxide content (the Haldane effect). (Reproduced from Comroe (1965) with permission Year Book Medical Publishers, Chicago)

Question 9.7   *What happens to the Haldane effect if you breathe 100 per cent oxygen rather than air? Give reasons for your answer!*

Thus far, we have dealt with carbon dioxide production and carriage. We still have to explain the sharp increase in ventilatory response that occurs as exercise intensity becomes more severe that is responsible for excreting the carbon dioxide. To do this we have to return to the factors that control ventilation. In Chapter 2 we referred to receptors in the lower brain that are sensitive to changes in the acidity of the blood and the cerebrospinal fluid. Severe exercise produces increasing levels of lactic acid in the muscle cell and carbonic acid in the blood. The lactic acid diffuses out of the cell into the blood where it dissociates into hydrogen ions and lactate; the carbonic acid dissociates into hydrogen ions and hydrogen carbonate. The respiratory centre receives stimuli from a variety of sources, but particularly from increased hydrogen ion concentration. Tidal volume and respiratory rate (f_R) increase further, resulting in the sharp increase in minute volume ($\dot{V}_E$). To understand this particular phenomenon we need to look at the general topic of the balance between acids and bases.

Acids and bases

There are several sources of acid in the body. By far the largest source is the production of the respiratory acid carbonic acid (H_2CO_3) from the combination of water with carbon dioxide. Metabolic acids arise from the breakdown of food into amino acids, fatty acids (via digestion), and pyruvic and lactic acids (via glycolysis).

Sport and exercise scientists are particularly interested in the production of large amounts of lactic acid during anaerobic metabolism. At rest, intracellular and extracellular fluids are alkaline, and need to remain so for optimal functioning; this indicates that physiological mechanisms exist to maintain a balance between acid production and its removal. The chemistry of acids and bases is bound up with hydrogen ions or protons (H^+), and compounds known as bases. A substance that *donates* a hydrogen ion is an acid, and a substance that *accepts* hydrogen ions is a base. Thus, adding hydrogen ions increases acidity; on the other hand, bases that accept hydrogen ions reduce it.

All physiological reactions take place in intracellular, extracellular or interstitial fluids; the water in these fluids can dissociate into hydrogen and hydroxyl ions.

$$H_2O \leftrightarrow H^+ + OH^-$$

Pure water at 25°C is neutral, i.e. it is neither acidic nor alkaline; it has the same number of hydrogen and hydroxyl ions. The measure of the acidity or alkalinity of a solution is its pH – defined as the negative logarithm of its hydrogen ion concentration

$$pH = -\log_{10}[H^+]$$

In pure water the concentrations of the hydrogen and hydroxyl ions are 10^{-7} mol $\cdot L^{-1}$; thus

$$\text{Neutral pH} = -\log_{10} 10^{-7} = 7.0$$

The pH scale ranges between 0 and 14.

However, pH is temperature-sensitive; when warmed the ionization of water increases, and the neutral pH is lower than 7; for example, at body temperature neutral pH is 6.8. Acids drive the pH downwards – the stomach contents are very acidic with a pH of ~3–4. Conversely, alkalis drive pH upwards. The typical pHs of arterial blood, mixed venous blood, and intracellular fluid are 7.4, 7.35 and 7.0, respectively.

> **Question 9.8**   *What do these figures tell you about the resting pH of body fluids? Why is intra-cellular pH lower than mixed venous and arterial blood? Why is mixed venous pH lower than arterial blood?*

Any deviation in extracellular pH away from its normal value of 7.4 provokes physiological responses designed to correct the imbalance. During severe exercise, there are two main sources of acid production: the aerobic production of increasing amounts of carbonic acid (the acid from respiration), and the anaerobic production of lactic acid (metabolic acid). To combat the unwanted effects of these acids there are three main regulatory mechanisms: blood buffers (immediate, within milliseconds), the lungs (short-term, within minutes) and the kidneys (long-term, within hours/days).

Blood buffers

Buffers are compounds that do not *remove* hydrogen ions, but carry them in a form that resists a change in pH. Buffers take various forms, and are present in the blood, intracellular and extracellular fluids and urine, as summarized in Table 9.1. Each buffer is important, but some are more effective in resisting the effect of increasing [H$^+$] on pH. Their relative effectiveness is shown in Figure 9.5.

An example of the buffering of the respiratory acid is seen during the carriage of carbon dioxide. As we have seen earlier in this chapter, carbon dioxide combines with water to form carbonic acid; this dissociates into protons and hydrogen carbonate ions. In the erythrocyte, the reaction occurs very rapidly because of the presence of the enzyme *carbonic anhydrase*.

$$CO_2 + H_2O \rightarrow \text{\textit{carbonic anhydrase}} \leftrightarrow H_2CO_3 \leftrightarrow \underline{H^+} + HCO_3^-$$

Table 9.1 The distribution of buffers in body fluids. (Based on data originally published in R. Hainsworth (1986), *Acid–Base Balance*, Manchester University Press)

Buffer	Plasma	RBC	ECF	ICF	Urine
Haemoglobin		×			
Hydrogen carbonate (bicarbonate)	×	×	×	×	×
Proteins	×			×	
Organic phosphate		×		×	×
Inorganic phosphate	×	×	×	×	×
Ammonia					×

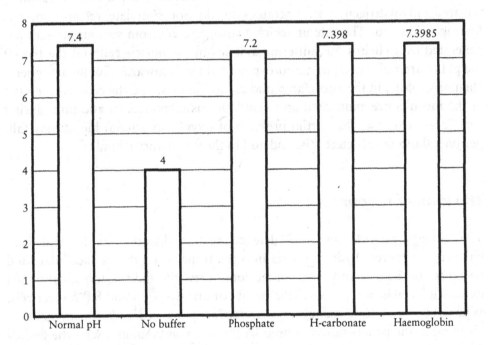

Figure 9.5 The relative effectiveness of particular buffers. (Based on data originally published in R. Hainsworth (1986), Manchester University Press)

The hydrogen carbonate produced diffuses back into the plasma, leaving the hydrogen ion in the red blood cell. Haemoglobin is an important hydrogen ion acceptor; it binds to the hydrogen ions produced by the dissociation of carbonic acid. Importantly, the more desaturated the haemoglobin becomes, the more effective it is as a buffer.

The respiratory response

Although we do not yet fully understand the entire process, we have already seen that the lungs are very effective in dealing with respiratory acid via increased ventilation. In spite of almost doubling the carbon dioxide partial pressure in the femoral vein (from 6 kPa (46 mmHg) to ~11 kPa (80 mmHg)), the partial pressure in the arterial blood is normal (5.3 kPa (40 mmHg)), or even lower near maximal exercise. This suggests that the respiratory sensors in the lower brain are responding to stimulation from a source other than carbon dioxide. The graph showing rising blood lactate concentration, together with the accompanying fall in pH, provides the clue. You know from the chapter dealing with anaerobic metabolism, that the lactic acid produced in the muscle cell quickly diffuses into the blood, where it dissociates into a salt, e.g. sodium lactate, and hydrogen ions. Lactate salts do not stimulate respiration, but hydrogen ions do. The rate at which hydrogen ions from various sources are generated overwhelms the buffering systems in the muscle cell and the blood; the pH of arterial blood and cerebrospinal fluid falls towards 7.0; the peripheral chemoreceptors, in the aortic arch and carotid bodies, and the central receptors in the medulla are stimulated and ventilation is increased. In addition, during very severe exercise, the partial pressure of oxygen in arterial blood may fall; peripheral receptors detect this, and add to the ventilatory stimulus.

The kidney response

The kidneys provide the final defence against disturbances in acid–base balance; we excrete hydrogen ions into the urine when the extracellular fluid becomes too acidic, and bicarbonate ions when the fluid is too alkaline. At extracellular pHs of ~7.0 and 7.8, the pH of urine is ~4.5 and 8.0 respectively. When the pH is low, kidneys use amino acids as fuel rather than glucose, resulting in the production of ammonia (NH_3). This combines with the hydrogen ions to form ammonium ions that are excreted in the urine.

$$NH_3 + H^+ = NH_4{}^+$$

If the pH is high, as the result of hyperventilation or ingestion of bicarbonate for example, the kidneys excrete bicarbonate in the form of sodium bicarbonate in the urine.

$$HCO_3^- + Na^+ = NaHCO_3$$

The clearest example of this process occurs during the initial stages of acclimatization to altitude. The lowered ambient oxygen partial pressure stimulates the respiratory centre and moderate hyperventilation is evident even at rest. This hyperventilation reduces the carbon dioxide stores of the body, raises pH and increases the bicarbonate concentration in the blood. Over the first two or three days of acclimatization, the kidneys restore the balance by excreting the bicarbonate ion attached to sodium.

However, in spite of all of the physiological mechanisms that strive to maintain a stable internal environment, they fail when challenged by highly motivated elite athletes. A blood lactate level of 8 mmol $\cdot$ L_{bl}^{-1} is regarded as an indicator of maximal oxygen uptake, but blood lactate levels of 14 mmol $\cdot$ L_{bl}^{-1} following five minutes of pursuit cycling, and 20 mmol $\cdot$ L_{bl}^{-1} following three minutes of boxing are common. Elite athletes are indeed a race apart.

Key points

- During severe exercise the lungs can excrete the carbonic acid produced; above $\sim$75 per cent of $\dot{V}_{O_2 max}$, arterial partial pressure of carbon dioxide actually falls below the normal value of 5.3 kPa (mmHg) indicating hyperventilation.

- Venous blood carries carbon dioxide blood in solution ($\sim$5 per cent), as carbamino compounds, particularly carbamino-haemoglobin (5–15 per cent), and as hydrogen carbonate (bicarbonate), (80–90 per cent) in the erythrocyte and the plasma.

- The plasma carries more carbon dioxide than erythrocytes.

- The oxygen saturation of the blood (S_{aO_2}) affects the amount of carbon dioxide carried by the protein globin of the haemoglobin molecule. The lower the saturation the more carbon dioxide carried (the Haldane effect).

- Acids are substances that donate protons (H^+); bases are substances that accept protons.

- The pH scale, ranging from 0 to 14, indicates the level of acidity or alkalinity of a solution.

- The pH is the negative log of hydrogen ion concentration. pH of 1 is very acidic, 14 is very alkaline; neutral pH is 7.0, but at body temperature neutral pH = 6.8.

- At rest, the normal value of pH for arterial blood is 7.4; for mixed venous blood it is 7.35.

- During maximal exercise the pH of intra-muscle cells can be as low as 6.8.

- Any disturbance in acid–base balance is corrected by the actions of blood buffers, by the lungs, and ultimately the kidneys.

Answers to questions in the text

Question 9.1

The pressure in the venous system is very low; thus, there is no need for walls of the veins to be any thicker. It is another example of the way the structure of the body reflects the function that needs to be performed. The term given to this process is 'teleology'.

Question 9.2

Valves are absent from the veins lying above the heart because gravity assists venous return.

Question 9.3

Carbon dioxide is the major stimulus to ventilation. Individuals suffering a panic attack hyperventilate, become hypocapnic, feel light-headed, panic ever more etc., etc. The immediate treatment is to rebreathe from a paper bag; the level of carbon dioxide in the bag increases and during rebreathing eventually restores blood carbon dioxide levels.

Question 9.4

Underwater swimming competitors

(a) hyperventilate to load the arterial blood with oxygen in the belief that this will enable them to swim further;

(b) but in so doing they lower their carbon dioxide levels in the blood, diminishing their ventilatory drive;

(c) they then inspire maximally and hold their breath – apneusis.

These three in combination are very dangerous. The muscular actions used in swimming consume the oxygen available, and although carbon dioxide levels in the blood increase, the stimulus to breathe can be resisted voluntarily during breath-holding. The blood oxygen levels become lowered to a critical point at which the individual loses consciousness and may drown.

Question 9.5
Increasing $[H^+]$ leads to higher levels of acid and lowers pH.

Question 9.6
The normal ratio of erythrocytes to plasma is 45:55. Thus, more carbon dioxide is carried in the greater volume of the plasma.

Question 9.7
Breathing 100 per cent oxygen at rest abolishes the Haldane effect. More oxygen is carried in the blood in dissolved form. This raises not only the P_{aO_2} but also the P_{vO_2} leaving the capillary bed. Haemoglobin is more saturated and so carbon dioxide cannot be carried as carbamino-haemoglobin and P_{tiCO_2} rises.

Question 9.8
The blood is slightly alkaline. Intracellular pH is lower than either arterial or venous blood because the rate at which the cells are producing hydrogen ions exceeds the rate at which they diffuse into the blood, so pH falls. The pH of venous blood leaving the capillary bed (pH $\sim$7.35) is lower than arterial blood entering the capillaries (pH $\sim$7.4), even at rest, because the carbon dioxide generated during aerobic metabolism produces carbonic acid. This dissociates into hydrogen ions which lower pH very slightly.

Answer to exercise in the text

Exercise 9.1
(a) $C_6H_{12}O_6 + 6O_2 = 6CO_2 + 6H_2O$
The aerobic breakdown of a carbohydrate.

(b) $CH_3(CH_2)_{14}COOH + 23O_2 = 16CO_2 + 16H_2O$
The aerobic breakdown of a lipid.

10 Epilogue – the Factors Limiting Maximal Oxygen Uptake

Learning Objectives

By the end of this chapter, you should be able to

♦ list the central and peripheral factors that may limit maximal oxygen uptake

♦ describe the physiological mechanisms involved in each factor

♦ evaluate the importance of each mechanism for elite endurance athletes

♦ provide evidence for the hypothesis that there is no single limiting factor applicable to all subjects

Objective test

Say whether the following answers are true (T) or false (F). If you do not know, say so (D) – not knowing is not an academic crime, but not finding out is. Try not to look at the answers until you have worked your way through the chapter and completed the test a second time. In this way you can monitor your progress.

Exercise Physiology: A Thematic Approach   Tudor Hale
© John Wiley & Sons, Ltd   ISBN: 0 470 84682 8 (cloth), ISBN 0 470 84683 6 (pbk)

	Pre-test			Post-test		
	T	F	D	T	F	D
1. Low inspired air oxygen partial pressures limit oxygen uptake						
2. Chronic airflow limitation patients suffer reduced lung volumes						
3. Chronic airflow limitation patients have smaller residual volumes						
4. Chronic bronchitics have high arterial O_2 and low CO_2 values						
5. Emphysema patients suffer from oxygen diffusive limitation						
6. If diffusing distance is halved, diffusing time is doubled						
7. Pulmonary oedema is the appearance of tissue fluid in the lung						
8. O_2 is highly soluble so the tissue fluid aids oxygen transfer						
9. Widening alveolar–arterial oxygen pressures occur in exercise						
10. Increasing alveolar dead space limits gas transfer in the lung						
11. At rest, the average red cell pulmonary transit time is about 1.5 s						
12. At rest, the range of red cell transit times is from 0.5 to 20 s						
13. Large cardiac outputs increase red cell transit times						
14. Large cardiac outputs are linked to high arterial oxygen saturation						
15. High haemoglobin values is known as anaemia						

	Pre-test			Post-test		
	T	F	D	T	F	D
16. Low haemoglobin levels lead to low arterial oxygen content						
17. High maximal oxygen uptake is linked with high cardiac output						
18. Cardiac output is high blood pressure times low stroke volume						
19. Elite endurance athletes have low maximal stroke volumes						
20. Women tend to have smaller heart volumes than men						
21. Smaller heart volumes are linked to smaller cardiac outputs						
22. Increasing age is linked to increasing heart rates						
23. Maximal oxygen uptake falls 10 per cent each decade after the second						
24. Training cannot improve maximal oxygen uptake in the elderly						
25. β_1-blockade increases heart rate and stroke volume						
26. Heart disease patients have low symptom-limited oxygen uptakes						
27. The O_2 content of venous blood leaving skeletal muscle is zero						
28. Some elite athletes have moderate peripheral O_2 extraction rates						
29. Large cardiac outputs are linked to arterial desaturation						
30. Low cardiac outputs are linked to high venous oxygen content						

Symbols, abbreviations and units of measurement

alveolar–arterial oxygen partial pressure difference	$P_{A\text{-}aO_2}$	kPa; mmHg
arterial oxygen content	C_{aO_2}	$mL_{O_2} \cdot L_{bl}^{-1}$
arterial oxygen partial pressure	P_{aO_2}	kPa; mmHg
arterial oxygen saturation	S_{aO_2}	%
blood	bl	$mL; L$
cardiac output, whole body flow	$\dot{Q}_C$	$L \cdot min^{-1}; mL \cdot min^{-1}$
chronic airflow limitation	CAL	
chronic obstructive pulmonary disease	COPD	
dead space – alveolar	V_{DA}	mL
dead space – series	V_{DS}	mL
forced expiratory volume in one second	$FEV_{1.0}$	L
functional residual capacity	FRC	L
heart rate; cardiac frequency	f_C	$bt \cdot min^{-1}$
peak expiratory flow rate	PEFR	$L \cdot min^{-1}; L \cdot s^{-1}$
maximal oxygen uptake	$\dot{V}_{O_2 max}$	$L \cdot min^{-1}; mL \cdot min^{-1}$
maximal oxygen uptake related to body mass	$\dot{V}_{O_2 max}$	$mL \cdot kg_{BM} \cdot min^{-1}$
mixed venous oxygen content	$C_{\bar{v}CO_2}$	$mL_{CO_2} \cdot L_{bl}^{-1}$
residual volume	V_{RES}	L
stroke volume	V_S	$mL \cdot bt^{-1}$
symptom-limited oxygen uptake	$\dot{V}_{O_2 SL}$	$L \cdot min^{-1}; mL \cdot min^{-1}$
total lung capacity	TLC	L
ventilation/perfusion ratio	V_A/Q	
vital capacity	VC	L

Introduction

It is over 230 years since Scheele and Priestley discovered oxygen, over 132 years since Fick and Zuntz measured oxygen consumption, and more than 80 years since Hill and his colleagues introduced the concept of the oxygen plateau as an indicator of maximal oxygen uptake. We think we know a lot more about maximal oxygen uptake than we did 80 years ago. For example, we believe that we are more likely to achieve the oxygen plateau if we use an exercise protocol that

(a) comprises continuous increments (a ramp test);

(b) involves the greatest amount of body mass (ski-ergometer, rowing ergometer, treadmill running, cycling)

(c) is of relatively short duration (7 to 12 minutes) – the longer the duration the less likely a plateau will develop and the lower the actual maximal level achieved;

(d) is applied to highly motivated subjects.

We have also found that in repeated bouts of increasingly vigorous exercise of relatively short duration there appear to be linear relationships between oxygen consumption and power output, heart rate, cardiac output, carbon dioxide in venous blood draining exercising muscles, and perceived exertion. We believe we have unlocked the anatomical, biological, chemical and physical secrets underpinning the physiological mechanisms that transport oxygen from the atmosphere to the electron transfer chain located in the mitochondria of cells that ensure our very existence. We have moved from a position where we proscribed exercise on medical grounds, to aerobic classes, fitness clubs, and medical referral schemes requiring us to exercise for health and fitness. We use maximal tests to establish an individual's current aerobic fitness, and monitor any changes that occur following physical training in groups as divergent as children, students, housewives, elite athletes, the middle-aged, the elderly of both genders, and patients with lung and heart disease. But in spite of these remarkable achievements, we still cannot agree which of the physiological processes is the one that limits maximal oxygen consumption. The rest of the chapter tries to summarize the main arguments that we need to consider when attempting to answer the question: 'Describe the factors that limit maximal oxygen uptake and evaluate the relative importance of each one'.

From the outset, we need to recognize that maximal oxygen uptake is the outcome of a chain of physiological mechanisms linking the delivery of atmospheric oxygen to skeletal muscle contraction. A chain is only as strong as its weakest link, and the issue of which physiological mechanism is the weakest link in the maximal oxygen uptake chain is a matter of continuing, unresolved debate amongst sport and exercise scientists. Most of the debate has centred on two main hypotheses. The first is that the major limitation is a central one, namely, the inability of the heart to deliver oxygen to the working skeletal muscle. The second is that the major limitation is a peripheral one, namely, skeletal muscle cannot take up all of the oxygen delivered to it. Neither of these hypotheses considers the more recent possibility of a limitation arising from less than perfect lung function.

In this chapter, we return to the Fick equation for oxygen

$$\dot{V}_{O_2max} = \dot{Q}_{Cmax} \cdot C_{a-\bar{v}O_2max}$$

to evaluate the strengths and weaknesses of each hypothesis, and examine sequentially the links in the oxygen uptake chain.

Factors affecting arterial oxygen content (C_{aO_2})

Altitude

The most obvious factor affecting arterial oxygen content is the low partial pressure of oxygen seen at altitude. The oxyhaemoglobin dissociation curve gives precise oxygen content values at varying partial pressures and the lower the barometric pressure the lower the oxygen content of arterial blood. Compared to sea level values, maximal oxygen uptake ($\dot{V}_{O_2max}$) falls as altitude increases. In this case, the weakest link is very clear: at maximal cardiac output, the heart is unable to deliver the required amount of oxygen to the working muscle and sustain the maximal power output possible at sea level. The results from endurance events at the Olympic Games held in 1968 at Mexico City reveal the limitations in oxygen delivery imposed by exercise at altitude. In events lasting more than 2 minutes not one world or Olympic track-record was set at these Games. However, the definition of maximal oxygen uptake is 'the maximal amount of oxygen that can be consumed breathing air *at sea-level*', so exercise at altitude is a special case, and sport and exercise scientists treat it as such. We shall not discuss it further here.

Lung disease

There are conditions at sea level that mimic low inspired oxygen concentrations. The commonest condition is lung disease arising from chronic airflow limitation – chronic bronchitis, emphysema and asthma are prime candidates.

Chronic bronchitis is an example of an *obstructive* lung disease; emphysema, on the other hand, is not. Both conditions result in chronic airflow limitation, but the general term 'chronic obstructive pulmonary disease' (COPD) invariably applied to both conditions, is unjustified. In each case, inspired oxygen concentration is normal; but in the case of chronic bronchitis, excessive secretions by mucus glands lining the bronchioles coagulate to form permanent plugs in the small airways that present an obstruction to the diffusion of oxygen into arterial blood. Emphysema, on the other hand, is a condition where lung tissue has been destroyed resulting in relatively large spaces between terminal bronchioles and alveolar ducts (see Figure 10.1).

These large spaces increase the diffusing distance and oxygen diffusion time, thus limiting its presence in the alveoli. Lung function tests reveal two major problems. The first is hyper-inflated lungs – for example, total lung capacity (TLC) of more than 7 litres, residual volumes (V_{res}) greater than 4 litres, and functional residual capacities (FRC) in excess of 5 litres. The second is low flow rates – the ratio of forced expiratory volume to vital capacity ($FEV_{1.0}/VC$) is less than 30 per cent and peak expiratory flow rate (PEFR) is often 25 per cent of normal values (see Figure 10.2). These lead to arterial oxygen partial pressures as low as 4 kPa (30 mmHg), dyspnoea (breathlessness) on minimal exertion, low exercise tolerance and low symptom-limited oxygen uptake ($\dot{V}_{O_2SL}$); this term is preferred to the usual maximal oxygen uptake ($\dot{V}_{O_2max}$). The average maximal value for healthy, 50-year-old sedentary men is approximately $2.5\ L \cdot min^{-1}$; symptom-limited oxygen uptake in 50-year-old men patients with chronic airflow limitation is often less than $1.0\ L \cdot min^{-1}$.

Asthma is a condition characterized by *acute* airflow limitation. It is difficult to diagnose whether the limitation is obstructive or restrictive, since airway narrowing is sometimes accompanied by secretion of mucus, thus offering both characteristics. Restriction rather than obstruction is indicated if rapid relief follows treatment with bronchodilators – for example, intravenous injection of aminophylline, or inhalation of β_2-based drugs. A sustained asthma attack is accompanied by difficulty in breathing and leads to increased residual volume and functional residual capacity. This results in a fall in alveolar oxygen partial pressures and arterial desaturation. In this case, exercise limitation is likely to be the result of psychological and physiological factors. If we insert the term '… in healthy subjects …' into the definition of maximal oxygen uptake, we can treat lung disease patients as a special case also.

Pulmonary oedema

Pulmonary oedema – the appearance of fluid in the tissue spaces of the lung – is a transient condition that affects some athletes. The presence of additional tissue fluid makes oxygen transfer across the alveolar capillary membrane more

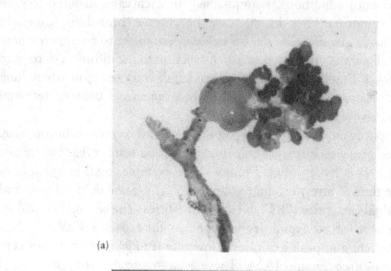

(a)

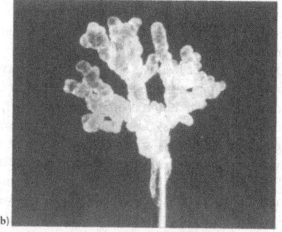

(b)

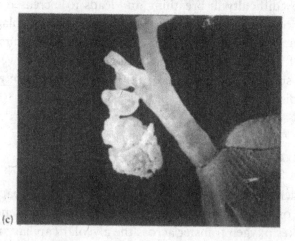

(c)

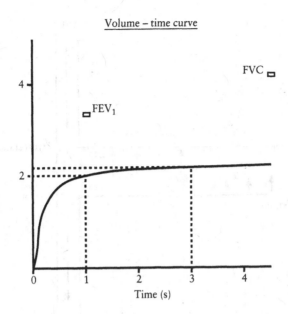

Figure 10.2 Lung function test from an emphysema patient. (With permission of Dr M. Buckman, King Edward VII Hospital, Midhurst)

difficult because the diffusion distance is increased and oxygen is not very soluble. The problem arises because of an imbalance between two physiological mechanisms – hydrostatic pressure and osmosis. The hydrostatic pressure of the capillary blood comes from the force imparted to it during ventricular systole. Osmosis is the movement of water across a membrane to equalize differences in concentrations. In the resting healthy subject, the hydrostatic pressure at the arterial end of the capillary is greater than that of the interstitial fluid. This force squeezes water out of the capillary blood through the porous walls of the capillaries. This water loss increases the osmotic pressure of the blood. As the blood continues towards the venous end of the capillary, its osmotic pressure is than greater that of the interstitial fluid, so water moves back into the blood. This continuous interplay of hydrostatic and osmotic pressures maintains blood volume (see Figure 10.3).

Severe exercise disturbs this resting balance; increased systolic pressure raises hydrostatic pressure and blood velocity through the capillaries. More water

Figure 10.1 Photographs of casts showing destruction of lung tissues resulting from emphysema. From left to right the slides show (a) dilated and destroyed respiratory bronchioles (centrilobular emphysema), (b) dilated alveolar ducts (alveolar emphysema), and (c) the total destruction of the acinus (panacinar emphysema). (With permission of Dr K. Horsfield, Midhurst Medical Research Institute)

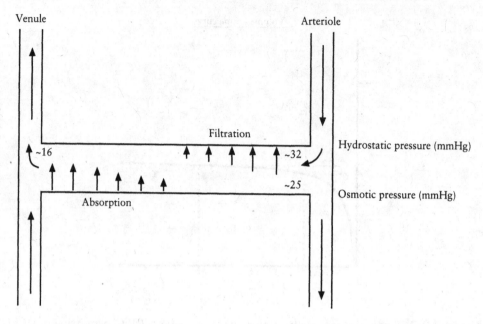

Figure 10.3   Schematic diagram of fluid exchange in the capillary bed

moves into the interstitial space, but the resultant osmotic imbalance has less time to be effective and so water invades the tissue space. In the pulmonary circulation the liquid eventually leaks into the alveoli presenting a barrier to oxygen transfer from alveoli to blood. It is difficult to say whether, or how much this affects oxygen transfer and maximal oxygen uptake; however, it is safe to say that at the very least, it is unlikely to facilitate transfer. In the healthy individual, the excess fluid drains into the lymphatic system during recovery from exercise. In patients suffering with heart failure, diuretic drugs are often needed to remove the excess fluid.

Alveolar ventilation

There has been a widespread consensus amongst sport and exercise scientists that lung ventilation is not a limiting factor in maximal oxygen uptake. However, the progressive widening of the alveolar–arterial oxygen partial pressures ($P_{A\text{-}aO_2}$) that accompanies increasing exercise intensity (see Figure 10.4) suggests a respiratory impairment that is made worse by exercise, a problem that seems to have been largely ignored during this debate.

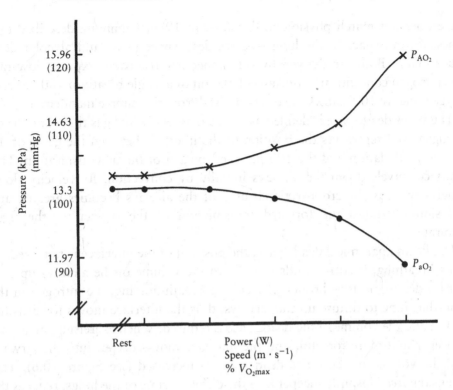

Figure 10.4 Alveolar–arterial oxygen difference ($P_A - P_{aO_2}$) during progressive exercise. Note the increasing divergence as the subject nears maximal oxygen uptake. (Reproduced with permission of Prof. PO Åstrand)

There are various explanations for this widening gap. The first is an inequality in matching ventilation and perfusion (V_A/Q) across the lungs. Research with isotopes shows that exercise actually improves this match, but it is clear that the match between gas and blood is never perfect. This leads to arterio-venous shunts, where blood passes through areas of the lung that are not ventilated and thus not oxygenated. In addition, the lung itself uses oxygen, and the oxygenated depleted bronchial venous blood, draining into the pulmonary veins carrying oxygenated blood to the left side of the heart, adds to the shunt.

Dead spaces

The second is dead space, and therefore wasted, ventilation. The notion of an anatomical dead space was introduced in Chapter 2; but the description given there does not match physiological reality. In 1980, Cumming described two types of dead space in the lung – series dead space (V_{DS}) and alveolar dead space (V_{DA}). Both are derived by simultaneously recording expired flow rate and nitrogen concentration during exhalation of a single breath of 100 per cent oxygen. Figure 10.5 shows the traces derived from this simple manoeuvre.

The series dead space is defined as the volume of expired gas that contains no nitrogen, and represents the position of the interface between the gases of the previous exhalation and the 100 per cent oxygen of the new inspiration. This interface travels down the airways initially by convection. Its velocity slows progressively as the cross-sectional area of the airways becomes greater, and diffusion overtakes the forward transmission of the oxygen in the fresh inspirate.

Unlike an anatomical dead space, the position of the interface is not fixed. In quiet breathing, it corresponds roughly to the volume of the airways up to a third-order respiratory bronchiole. During breath-holding, the nitrogen in the lungs has time to diffuse up the airways, thus the interface moves towards the mouth and the volume of the dead space is reduced. When exercising, breathing is deeper and more forceful, and the interface moves deeper into the airways and the volume of the series dead space is increased (see Figure 10.6). This brings the fresh inspirate deeper into the diffusive zone of the lungs, reduces the length of the diffusion pathway, and has the potential for enhancing gas transfer.

The alveolar dead space is the volume of inspired gas that does not mix with the gases already present in the alveoli. The extent of this mixing is indicated by the typical shape of the expired nitrogen curve; a square-wave would indicate perfect mixing. Inspection of the curve in Figure 10.5 shows that a square-wave does not exist, and suggests that mixing is incomplete. Two explanations have been proffered for this imperfect mixing. The first is that there are differences in regional ventilation of the lung – in other words, some areas are better ventilated than others – and that the sloping nature of the nitrogen plateau is due to asynchronous emptying of different regions of the lung. This explanation relies on an important assumption, namely, that diffusive mixing in the alveoli is complete within the time-span of a single breath. This assumption was the cause of disagreement between physiologists at the start of the twentieth century, and remains the focus of dispute today.

The second explanation argues that diffusive mixing within some acini is not completed within the time-span of a single breath even in resting, healthy individuals. The basis for this argument is that differences in the anatomy of lungs lead inevitably to diffusive pathways of varying lengths. In 1905, Einstein derived a law of diffusion which said that distance covered by a molecule is

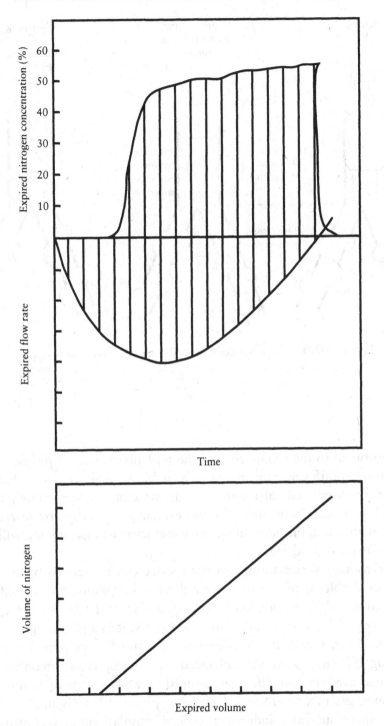

Figure 10.5 Expired flow rate, nitrogen concentration, and volume of nitrogen following a single breath of inhaled oxygen. (Reproduced with permission of Dunod, Paris from the original by Cumming (1980))

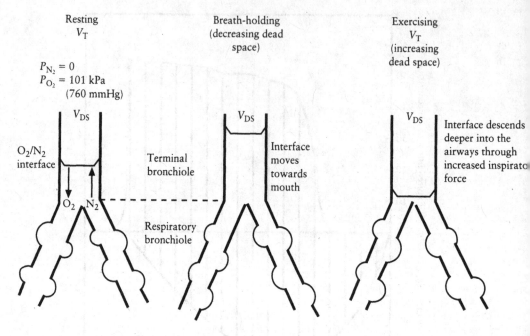

Figure 10.6   The series dead space during rest, breath-holding, and exercise

proportional to the square root of the time taken; thus, if diffusing distance is quadrupled diffusing time increases by a factor of sixteen not a factor of four. Given the asymmetrical nature of lung structure, it seems likely that not all alveoli will contribute equally to gas exchange. As there are upwards of three million alveoli in the adult lung, some inefficiency in gas mixing will contribute to the alveolar dead space.

A reasonable estimate of this dead space can be derived by comparing the measured volume of nitrogen expired with the volume that would have been expired had diffusive mixing been perfect (Figure 10.7). We can calculate the efficiency of gas mixing in the lung and express it as a percentage. In the resting, healthy lung, the efficiency is between 80 and 90 per cent. During exercise, mixing efficiency is initially enhanced; but as respiratory frequency increases, the time available for diffusion diminishes, and in spite of faster, larger tidal volumes, gas mixing efficiency reaches a plateau. The volumes of the alveolar dead space increase, indicating wasted ventilation, and contribute to the growing divergence in the alveolar–arterial oxygen partial pressures and the fall in the partial pressures of oxygen in arterial blood (P_{aO_2}).

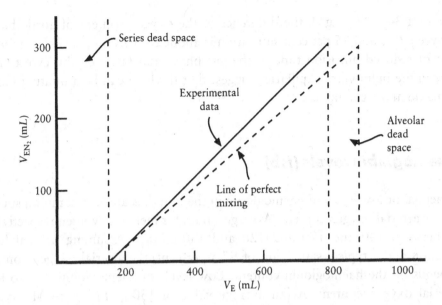

Figure 10.7 Estimation of alveolar dead space, i.e. the inspired volume that does not take part in gas exchange. (Reproduced by permission of Dunod, Paris from the original by Cumming (1980))

Pulmonary capillary transit time

Along with reduced diffusion time in the alveoli, any increases in cardiac output lead to faster erythrocyte transit times through the pulmonary circulation. At a resting cardiac output of $5\ L \cdot min^{-1}$, the average transit time in the healthy lung is about 1.5 s, but depending on which route the red cell takes, the time can vary between a fraction of a second and as many as 20 seconds. Whatever the actual time taken by a single erythrocyte to pass through the pulmonary capillaries, it is sufficient for blood oxygen saturation levels (S_{aO_2}) to reach the typical value of about 97 per cent. During exercise, maximal cardiac output in healthy young adults increases to between 20 and $25\ L \cdot min^{-1}$; but although average erythrocyte transit time is reduced, more capillaries are opened up to give a better match between ventilation and perfusion, and oxygen saturation is maintained at about 97 per cent. However, in 1968 Ekblom and Hermansen reported maximal cardiac outputs in trained endurance athletes ranging from 31.5 to $42.3\ L \cdot min^{-1}$. Cardiac outputs as high as these lead to even faster erythrocyte transit times; the partial pressure of oxygen falls, and oxygen saturation percentage values in the mid-80s have been reported. The effect on the oxygen content of blood of this level of haemoglobin desaturation is marked. Assuming a haemoglobin level of $150\ g \cdot L_{bl}$ and an oxygen-binding rate of $1.34 \ mLO_2 \cdot g^{-1}$, the difference in the oxygen content of aortic blood between 97.5 and 85 per cent saturation is about $26 \ mLO_2 \cdot L_{bl}$. The combination of reduced diffusion time in the gas phase and faster erythrocyte transit time in the pulmonary capillaries suggest that the lung can be a limiting factor in maximal oxygen uptake.

Haemoglobin levels (Hb)

Anaemia, or low levels of haemoglobin in the blood, is another common source of low arterial oxygen content. Average values for men and women respectively, lie between 140 and 170 and 120 and $150 \ g \cdot L_{bl}^{-1}$. Assuming normal lung function and a typical saturation of 97.5 per cent, the arterial oxygen content depends on the haemoglobin content. Low levels of haemoglobin lead to low arterial oxygen content. At an average value of $150 \ g \cdot L_{bl}^{-1}$, arterial oxygen content is about $200 \ mLO_2 \cdot L_{bl}^{-1}$; at a haemoglobin value of $120 \ g \cdot L_{bl}^{-1}$, arterial oxygen content falls to about $157 \ mLO_2 \cdot L_{bl}^{-1}$. Even relative anaemia is a serious weakness in the maximal uptake chain.

Factors affecting cardiac output ($\dot{Q}_C$)

Heart rate and stroke volume

In the view of many sport and exercise scientists, the critical link in the level of maximal oxygen uptake achieved is cardiac output. In the Ekblom and Hermansen study of elite endurance athletes referred to earlier, a strong positive correlation ($+ 0.9$) exists between cardiac output (a mean of $36 \ L \cdot min^{-1}$) and maximal oxygen uptake (a mean of $5.57 \ L \cdot min^{-1}$). However, the relationship between cardiac output and oxygen uptake at maximum exercise was not strictly linear (Figure 10.8), and the rate of increase in cardiac output at maximal effort is declining. There are at least two possible reasons for this decline. The first is the reduced filling time available because of increased heart rate. The second is local vasodilatation at muscle level leads to a fall in peripheral blood pressure; the aortic and carotid sinus stretch receptors respond with a vasoconstrictor response that raises blood pressure but reduces flow.

However, cardiac output is the product of heart rate (f_c) and stroke volume (V_S), so we cannot yet tell which variable is the more important. In the same study, comparative data from trained endurance athletes who had not achieved

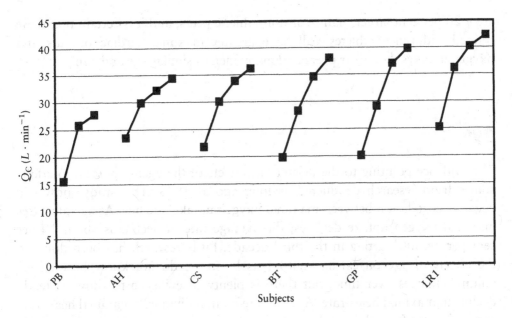

Figure 10.8 The curvilinear nature of cardiac output in elite male endurance athletes. (Based on data originally published by Ekblom, B. and Hermansen, L. (1966).

international recognition revealed that the key variable distinguishing the elite athletes from second division athletes was mean stroke volume. The mean maximal heart rates of the two groups were almost identical -190 bt $\cdot$ min^{-1} for the elite group versus 191 bt $\cdot$ min^{-1} – but the stroke volume of the elite group was 189 mL $\cdot$ bt^{-1} compared to the 149 mL $\cdot$ bt^{-1} of the non-elite group. This difference in stroke volume resulted in an average cardiac output some 20 per cent lower at 28.5 $L \cdot$ min^{-1}, and a mean reduction of 18 per cent in maximal oxygen uptake in the second division group. Two other sources of evidence pointing to the critical nature of cardiac output in oxygen delivery arise from studies into gender differences, and the ageing process.

Gender

Although women's maximal heart rates are similar to men's, their typical heart volumes are ~15–20 per cent smaller. As there is a positive correlation between heart volume and stroke volume, the generally lower stroke volumes will inevitably lead to smaller maximal cardiac outputs and lower absolute maximal oxygen uptakes. Women endurance athletes, however, have heart volumes that are ~20 per cent larger than their non-athletic peers, and it is certain that these trained endurance athletes will have greater maximal cardiac outputs and oxygen uptakes than their peers and many men of similar age and size.

Age

The evidence pointing to the deleterious effects of the ageing process in adults comes from research conducted as long ago as 1938. This study showed a negative correlation between maximal oxygen uptake and age. As age increases maximal oxygen uptake declines; the average rate of decline is about 10 per cent per decade starting in the third decade. Little research has been done on the effects of age on cardiac output itself, so we do not know how stroke volume changes over time, but there is plenty of evidence to show a steady decline in maximal heart rate. An estimate of an individual's maximal heart rate can be derived from the simple equation

$$f_{C_{max}} = 220 - \text{age}$$

This is a very crude rule of thumb, and it conceals a possible error of about ± 20 bt $\cdot$ min^{-1}; thus a 70-year-old may have a maximal heart rate of anywhere between 130 and 170 bt $\cdot$ min^{-1}. In spite of the inadequacies of the equation, what cannot be disputed is the fact that maximal heart rate falls with age. It is unlikely that an increase in stroke volume compensates for the drop in rate, and so maximal cardiac output is reduced. The progressive reduction in cardiac output with age is reflected in progressive decrease in maximal oxygen uptake from ~4 $L \cdot$ min^{-1} for 20-year-old men to ~2.5 $L \cdot$ min^{-1} at 60 years.

These heart rate findings apply equally to both genders, and to active and sedentary groups. However, there are considerable differences in the rate of decline between the active and non-active populations. Those who lead a physically active lifestyle maintain a higher maximal oxygen uptake than those who are essentially sedentary. Furthermore, there is evidence that adults who train can improve their maximal oxygen uptake at any age.

Some of the clearest evidence on the effects of age on aerobic performance comes from published records of running, cycling and swimming times in veterans' competitions. The fall in performance over 1500-m and 10-km running events for men aged between 40 and 70 years lies between 30 and 40 per cent, and reaches 55 per cent in a 1-mile swim; for 80-year-old cyclists, a 25-mile ride performance is reduced by ~45 per cent.

Heart disease

Further evidence highlighting the pre-eminence of cardiac output as the key link in the maximal oxygen uptake chain lies in the performance of patients recovering from a myocardial infarction. This condition is a consequence of coronary heart disease; the coronary arteries that carry oxygenated blood to the myocardium become narrowed by the accumulation of fatty plaques, and less elastic due to calcified deposits in the arterial walls. The Hagen–Poiseuille's equation shows that halving the radius of an artery reduces flow by a factor of 16. When blood flow does not meet the metabolic demands of heart, the muscle is starved of oxygen. This is called ischaemia, and if severe, leads to irreversible structural and functional damage – known as a myocardial infarction – impaired ventricular performance, and reduced cardiac output.

Results from symptom-limited tests on post-infarct patients vary because of a wide range in age and severity of attack, but evidence from studies on patients with an average age of 52 years reveals average symptom-limited heart rates of 163 bt $\cdot$ min^{-1}, lower than the age-predicted maximum heart rate of 170 bt $\cdot$ min^{-1}. Impaired contractile performance also reduces stroke volume. The average symptom-limited oxygen uptake of these patients is 27 mL $\cdot$ kg^{-1} $\cdot$ min^{-1}, some 25 per cent lower than maximal oxygen uptake values of moderately active 50-year-old men.

Beta-blockade

Drugs that control heart rate, such as atenolol, are used to prevent disorders of heart rhythm from developing into full-blown ventricular fibrillation and no cardiac output. In studies investigating cardiac performance in healthy subjects, these β_1-blockers lower maximal oxygen uptake by reducing maximal heart rate and stroke volume.

Training studies

The final source of evidence for the critical nature of cardiac output in maximal oxygen uptake comes from training studies. Previously untrained individuals who undertake a sustained programme of endurance-type exercises show improvements in maximal oxygen uptake sometimes in excess of 20 per cent. The post-training data from a 4-month training programme conducted by Ekblom and his colleagues, show a mean 17 per cent rise in maximal oxygen uptake, from 3.12 to 3.68 $L \cdot min^{-1}$. Increased cardiac output – 22.4 to 24.2 $L \cdot min^{-1}$ – accounts for half of that improvement, due entirely to increased stroke volume; improved peripheral extraction – 138 to 148 $mLO_2 \cdot L_{bl}$ – is responsible for the remaining 50 per cent. It is towards the peripheral oxygen extraction process that we now turn.

Factors affecting venous oxygen content ($C_{\bar{v}O_2}$)

Venous oxygen content is an indicator of the ability of the skeletal muscles to extract and use the oxygen carried there by the blood. If inadequate oxygen delivery via cardiac output is the key factor in high maximal oxygen uptake, we might expect to see the oxygen content of venous blood leaving the capillary bed at, or close to, zero. If we look at data from the Ekblom and Hermansen study, we find mean mixed-venous oxygen content ($C_{\bar{v}O_2}$) of 25 $mLO_2 \cdot L_{bl}^{-1}$, rather than zero. This represents only an 86 per cent extraction rate and introduces the possibility that as the skeletal muscle is not fully able to extract the oxygen made available to it, and peripheral limitation may be the weakest link in the maximal oxygen uptake chain. Difficulties arise when we look at the mixed-venous oxygen content sampled from the right atrium. This sample contains blood returning from all parts of the body, not just the working skeletal muscle, and it is impossible to apportion specific extraction rates to particular body systems. However, if we look at the oxygen content of blood from the femoral vein (C_{vfemO_2}) draining the lower limb during maximal exercise we still see typical values of around 15 $mLO_2 \cdot L_{bl}^{-1}$.

It is worth noting here that in the Ekblom and Hermansen paper, the group of elite endurance athletes with some very high maximal oxygen uptake values still have moderate to poor peripheral extraction rates. On average, about 15 per cent of the oxygen presented to working tissues was unused, but not all of this unused oxygen came from skeletal muscle beds only. Other research, however, has measured the partial pressure of oxygen in femoral venous blood during maximal leg exercise; it reveals venous oxygen partial pressures ranging between 1.3 and 2.7 kPa (10–20 mmHg). As in the pulmonary capillary bed, the erythrocyte transit time in skeletal muscle capillaries may also be shortened. However, unlike the link between pulmonary transit time and arterial oxygen partial pressure, the correlation between cardiac output and the difference in arterial and mixed-venous oxygen content in the Ekblom and Hermansen paper is very low ($r = +0.11$).

Hyperoxia

Attempts to resolve the dispute between central versus peripheral limitations have included the effects of breathing hyperoxic gas mixtures. The hypothesis is that maximal oxygen uptake increases when breathing oxygen-enriched gas. The results tend to show higher maximal oxygen uptakes, but the increase does not match the accompanying increase in arterial oxygen content. This leads to the suspicion that the methods used are open to criticism because of technical problems. One is the difficulty in applying the Geppert–Zuntz–Haldane transformation when breathing oxygen; another concerns the relatively small increases in arterial oxygen content.

Hyperbaric oxygen

A more robust method entails breathing oxygen during exercise in a pressure chamber that significantly enhances arterial oxygen content. In 1970, Kaisjer compared 6 minutes of exhaustive exercise on a cycle ergometer in a pressure chamber breathing air under normal pressure (101 kPa, 760 mmHg), with breathing pure oxygen at three atmospheres (303 kPa, 2280 mmHg). Under high pressure (hyperbaric) conditions, arterial blood was 100 per cent saturated, and its oxygen content, because of the increased oxygen carried in solution, was 30 per cent higher, at $\sim$265 m$LO_2 \cdot L_{bl}^{-1}$, compared to 97 per cent and $\sim$200 m$LO_2 \cdot L_{bl}^{-1}$ during air breathing. The most important findings were that, although maximal heart rate fell about 6 per cent, the difference in oxygen content between arterial and femoral venous blood increased by the same amount, and that maximal oxygen uptake remained constant. In other words, in spite of substantially more oxygen being presented to the maximally working muscle, no more oxygen was consumed. This suggests that, in these young, healthy, averagely fit subjects at least, the limiting factor lies in the muscle's ability to *use* oxygen rather than in the heart's ability to *deliver* it and reinforces the view that the key limitation lies at the periphery of the body rather than in its central pump.

Whether Kaisjer would have discovered similar results in a group of highly trained endurance athletes is open to question. The strenuous, long-term training of the kind undertaken by such athletes also produces changes not only in the heart's performance, but also in skeletal muscle function, particularly of the Type I slow-twitch oxidative fibres. New capillaries appear that enhance perfusion of the muscle bed and increase oxygen availability, and the number and size of the mitochondria increase along with their adenosine triphosphate generating powers. The time-scale for such adaptations is not clear, but it seems that it is in terms of years rather than months and months rather than weeks.

It is also the case that at maximal exercise large amounts of lactate are produced, even though the blood leaving the capillary bed still contains oxygen. This points to an inability of the tricarboxylic acid cycle in the mitochondria of skeletal muscle cells to deal with the large amounts of pyruvate being produced during glycolysis, even though the oxygen capacity of the blood has not been fully deployed. These arguments suggest that the major limitation lies in the use made of the oxygen delivered rather than the delivery itself.

Conclusion

The above data, culled from various sources, deal with average values, because that is how journal articles are accepted for publication. But if we look at individual subjects in both the Ekblom and Hermansen paper, and the Ekblom *et al.* training study, a pattern begins to emerge which points to three groups, albeit rather small ones, of trained individuals. There are those blessed with large cardiac outputs but rather moderate peripheral – that is both pulmonary and skeletal muscle – oxygen extraction rates. The obverse of this is a group who, whilst exhibiting relatively moderate cardiac outputs, have well-developed peripheral extraction capabilities. The final group contain those who are left – they exhibit relatively high capabilities in both characteristics. The data from

Table 10.1 Percentage changes in the Fick equation factors following 4 months of endurance training in eight young male students. (Based on data originally published in Ekblom, B., Åstrand, P. O., Saltin, B. and Wallstrom, B. (1968)

S	$\dot{V}_{O_2 max}$ $(L \cdot min^{-1})$	$\dot{Q}_{max}$ $(L \cdot min^{-1})$	$f_{C\,max}$ $(bt \cdot min^{-1})$	$V_{S\,max}$ $(mL \cdot bt^{-1})$	$C_{a \cdot \bar{v} O_2}$ $(mLO_2 \cdot L_{bl}^{-1})$
1	+16%	+6%	−8%	+15%	+10%
2	+11	+10	−5	+15	+1
3	+18	+27	−2	+30	−8
4	+10	+14	−1	+15	−4
5	+13	+10	−1	+10	+4
6	+1	−8	−11	+3	+9
7	+15	+2	−7	+10	+13
8	+7	+5	−3	+8	+1

Ekblom *et al*'s relatively short-term training study repeat the general picture seen in the elite athlete group. Table 10.1 shows individual responses to the 4-month training programme. Subjects 2, 3, 4 and 8 increase their maximal oxygen uptake largely through increased cardiac output via enhanced stroke volume; subjects 6 and 7 increase their maximal oxygen uptake via greater oxygen extraction; subjects 1 and 5 show improved performance in both central and peripheral responses. These specific characteristics may be due to genetic endowment or the kind of training undertaken. However, this analysis suggests that a single weak link in the oxygen uptake chain that applies to all subjects is unlikely.

Key points

- Factors limiting maximal oxygen uptake can appear at all stages of the oxygen conductance chain.

- In healthy subjects, the lungs seem to offer some barriers to oxygen transfer.

- These include increased series and alveolar dead spaces, pulmonary oedema, and more rapid erythrocyte transits through the pulmonary capillary bed.

- Low haemoglobin content of blood is a serious weakness in the conductance chain.

- Inadequate cardiac output, arising from limitations in rate or stroke volume, is a clear impairment to maximal oxygen uptake.

- Femoral vein oxygen content above zero and significant levels of venous oxygen content in maximally exercising muscles, accompanied by high blood lactate values, suggest that peripheral extraction rate is at least as important as cardiac output in limiting maximal oxygen uptake values.

- A review of two seminal papers reveals individuals with specific central or peripheral limitations, singly or in combination, rather than one overwhelming factor that applies to all subjects.

11 Postscript – Exercise, Fitness and Health

Learning Objectives

By the end of this chapter, you should be able to

♦ distinguish between exercise for fitness, and exercise for health

♦ outline the constituents of cardiovascular disease and distinguish between arteriosclerosis and atherosclerosis

♦ summarize the aetiology of coronary heart disease, outlining the five major attributable risk factors

♦ discuss the evidence linking exercise and reduced risk of heart disease

♦ summarize the outcomes of key epidemiological studies

♦ indicate the risk factors for young children

♦ outline the mechanisms by which protection against heart disease might be conferred

♦ evaluate existing exercise prescription practices

♦ describe briefly the relationships between exercise and other diseases

Exercise Physiology: A Thematic Approach   Tudor Hale
© John Wiley & Sons, Ltd   ISBN: 0 470 84682 8 (cloth), ISBN 0 470 84683 6 (pbk)

Objective test

Say whether the following answers are true (T) or false (F). If you do not know, say so (D) – not knowing is not an academic crime, but not finding out is. Try not to look at the answers until you have worked your way through the chapter and completed the test a second time. In this way, you can monitor your progress.

	Pre-test			Post-test		
	T	F	D	T	F	D
1. Cardiovascular disease accounts for ~4% of all deaths each year						
2. In the UK over 187 000 die a year from heart disease and strokes						
3. Hardening of the arteries is called atherosclerosis						
4. Arteriosclerosis is the build-up of fatty plaques in arterial walls						
5. Atherosclerosis occurs in the large and medium-sized arteries						
6. Arteriosclerosis occurs in the coronary arteries						
7. 1.5 million people suffer angina pectoris						
8. A heart attack results when thrombus blocks a coronary artery						
9. Dead cardiac muscle is called a myocardial infarct						
10. Cholesterol is synthesized in the kidneys from dietary fats						
11. There are three forms of cholesterol: HDL, MDL and LDL						
12. High levels of low-density lipoprotein give protection against CHD						
13. Poor diet is a factor in 80% of cardiovascular disease						

	Pre-test			Post-test		
	T	F	D	T	F	D
14. Increased exercise and low cholesterol reduce the risk of CHD						
15. Average heart volume in healthy men is about 7000 mL						
16. Diseased heart volumes of 3.5 mL have been reported						
17. High levels of physical activity are linked to protection from CHD						
18. Exercise-driven mechanisms leading to reduced risk of CHD are (a) increased cardiac efficiency						
19. (b) higher metabolic cost						
20. (c) shorter diastasis leading to increased coronary perfusion						
21. (d) development of collateral coronary circulation						
22. (e) reduced peripheral resistance due to muscle capillarization						
23. (f) lower levels of HDL-cholesterol						
24. (g) improved control of Type II diabetes						
25. (h) raised post-exercise metabolic rate						
26. One MET is equivalent to oxygen consumption of $3\text{--}4\ \mathrm{m}LO_2 \cdot \mathrm{min}^{-1}$						
27. Walking at $2\ \mathrm{mi} \cdot \mathrm{hr}^{-1}$ is equivalent to 5.5 METs						
28. Moderate exercise in healthy 50-year-old men reduces stroke risk						
29. Moderate exercise can reduce dyspnoea in chronic lung disease						
30. Exercise has no beneficial effect on cancer prevention						

Symbols, abbreviations and units of measurement

basal metabolic rate	BMR	J; kJ; mJ; kcal
body mass index	BMI	$kg \cdot m^{-2}$
cerebral vascular accident – stroke	CVA	
cerebral vascular disease	CeVD	
coronary heart disease	CHD	
high-density lipoprotein (cholesterol)	HDL	$mmol \cdot L^{-1}$
low-density lipoprotein (cholesterol)	LDL	$mmol \cdot L^{-1}$
myocardial infarction	MI	
metabolic equivalent of exercise	MET	$mLO_2 \cdot kg^{-1} \cdot min^{-1}$
respiratory exchange ratio	RER	
symptom-limited oxygen uptake	$\dot{V}_{O_2SL}$	$L \cdot min^{-1}; mL \cdot min^{-1}$
volume of carbon dioxide excreted	$\dot{V}_{CO_2}$	$L \cdot min^{-1}; mL \cdot min^{-1}$
volume of oxygen consumed	$\dot{V}_{O_2}$	$L \cdot min^{-1}; mL \cdot min^{-1}$

Many sport and exercise courses use sporting contexts to illustrate some important physiological point. This is a useful strategy to engage students' interest and attention. However, there are increasing numbers of students interested in exercise physiology as a platform for health-related education rather than improving sports performance. This postscript, in the form of an essay, is an attempt to provide some useful information in a health-related context for such students. The essay title is: 'Discuss the proposition that exercise is good for us'.

Introduction

The belief that exercise is necessary for the fitness and health has its roots in ancient Greece and is a common feature of present health promotion in many rich, industrialized countries of the world. It became manifest in nineteenth-century Britain in the 'muscular Christianity' of the Public Schools, and later with the introduction of physical training, based on the Swedish system, into the state school system. Neither was aimed primarily at health, however. The former was more concerned with moral development, and the notion of 'a sound mind in a sound body'; the latter, regressing to the Platonic view on physical education, was concerned initially with trying to produce soldiers fit enough to fight a war. This specific need became apparent when recruits for the

Boer War were found to be entirely unfit for the physical demands of fighting a guerrilla war in hot conditions and at altitude. The physical *training* provided in the state schools of the first half of the twentieth century was replaced in the second half by the notion of health-related fitness as part of a general programme of physical *education*.

Few sport and exercise scientists would deny that there is strong evidence to support the link between exercise and *fitness*, whether that fitness is general endurance (aerobic fitness), local endurance (anaerobic fitness), strength, or flexibility. There is also evidence of the beneficial effects of exercise for the *restoration* of health. Exercise is a recognized and useful strategy in the rehabilitation of heart, stroke and lung diseases patients, post-operative patients, individuals recovering from injury, and those suffering chronic depression. Exercise also seems to offer *protection* against some diseases, especially those of the cardiovascular system; it also delays the onset of osteoporosis; it can be a factor in the control of obesity; and it may be linked to a reduced incidence of certain cancers.

However, it does not follow that *fitness* leads inevitably to good *health*. As long ago as 380 BC, Plato described the athlete in training as a 'sleepy creature' with health that was 'delicately balanced', and how the smallest deviation from his routine 'leads to serious illness'; the early physicians Hippocrates and Galen were also convinced that athletic activity led to an early death. Even as recently as the early years of the twentieth Century strenuous exercise was not recommended because of a condition called 'athlete's heart'; this was a state of cardiac enlargement similar to that seen in heart disease patients. Today there is much anecdotal evidence that excessive training can lead to depression of the immune system, upper respiratory tract infections, asymmetrical bone and muscular development, the occurrence of acute and chronic over-use injuries, and primary and secondary amenorrhoea in women endurance athletes. It is not only athletes who suffer from the deleterious effects of exercise; recreational exercisers are not immune from some of the above conditions, and can add involvement in traffic accidents, dog bites, and the risk, albeit generally rather slight, of sudden death.

In spite of these caveats, there is a strong consensus that exercise is beneficial for health. The benefits derived from physiotherapy treatment are too obvious to need further discussion, except perhaps in the treatment of chronic depression. In this example of the Hawthorne effect, the beneficial effects of having a pet dog or tropical fish were as great as, and longer-lasting than, those derived from an exercise regime.

Difficulties in other areas also exist. There is a lack of precision regarding the nature of exercise that is needed to provide protection from disease, or to develop the physical, mental and social well-being that lies at the heart of World Health Organization's (WHO) aim of health for all. Whilst it is true that considerable progress has been made in developing training programmes designed to improve fitness and performance of elite performers, the volumes, intensities and durations typical of these programmes are unlikely to be suitable for a health promotion strategy designed to satisfy multi-ethnic groups of both genders ranging from schoolchildren to the elderly. In the rest of this essay, we shall examine critically the complex relationships that exist between exercise and health. We begin with the condition that provided the initial stimulus for the development of the exercise for health movement, namely, diseases of the cardiovascular system.

Cardiovascular disease (CVD)

Cardiovascular disease is the single biggest cause of death in the United Kingdom. It accounts for about 40 per cent of all deaths – over a quarter of a million each year. About 75 per cent of these deaths result from coronary heart disease (CHD) and cerebrovascular disease (CeVD) called strokes, or cerebrovascular accidents (CVA). The two major underlying causes are arteriosclerosis, a stiffening of the arteries, and its near neighbour, atherosclerosis – the development of fatty plaques in the arterial wall.

Arteriosclerosis is found mainly in the arterioles of the viscera, particularly the kidney. The condition is characterized by hyperplasia (increase in number) of endothelial cells in the tunica intima that lines the blood vessel, together with hypertrophy (increase in volume) of the smooth muscles and thickening of the elastic tissue of the tunica media. The loss of elasticity in the blood vessel, together with a reduced diameter, leads inexorably to increased resistance to flow and high blood pressure (hypertension), particularly diastolic pressure. Narrowing of the arterioles of the kidneys leads to secondary hypertension, and can result in an example of the destructive nature of positive feedback mechanisms. In response to the narrowing of the arterioles and a reduction in blood flow, the kidneys secrete large amounts of renin into the bloodstream; the immediate effect is to raise blood pressure further. This exacerbates the existing problem, leading to a downward spiral of function and ultimately to kidney failure.

Atherosclerosis, which often accompanies arteriosclerosis, is found in the aorta and the large and medium-sized arteries of the peripheral circulation –

including the coronary and cerebral arteries. It is characterized by thickening of the tunica intima through accumulation of fatty plaques, which are infiltrated by fibroblasts – the main cell of connective tissue – and undergo calcification. There are two major theories concerning the genesis and subsequent development of atherosclerosis. The first is that it is a natural, irreversible consequence of the ageing process. The second is that it is a problem with lipid, particularly cholesterol, metabolism.

The ageing theory arises from the early appearance of fatty streaks in the first two decades of life, and their progressive development into fully blown atherosclerosis in the seventh decade and beyond. Several phenomena challenge the theory. There are elderly people without significant atherosclerosis; the presence of atherosclerosis may vary in different blood vessels in the same person; the development of the condition varies between countries and ethnic groups; and post-mortem findings reveal significant atherosclerotic development in young adults and even young children.

The metabolic theory is supported by laboratory and epidemiological research. In animal experiments involving ingestion of large quantities of saturated fats, there is evidence of invasion of blood vessel walls by fatty plaques (atheromas). There is a positive relationship between the frequency and severity of atherosclerosis and high levels of cholesterol in humans. Finally there are reports of a lower incidence of atherosclerosis in countries such as Japan where saturated fat and cholesterol intake is low.

Cholesterol is an essential component of the structure of the cell wall. It is synthesized by the liver from dietary fats. It is not absorbed by the blood and therefore has to be transported around the body attached to protein carriers. There are two forms of these carriers – high-density (HDL), and low-density (LDL) lipoproteins. The latter contains mainly cholesterol, and high levels (hypercholesterolaemia) are linked to atherosclerosis. Recent research has focused on the presence of excessive levels of homocysteine in the blood. Homocysteine comes from the protein in our diet, and helps in the building and maintenance of body tissues. In excessive amounts, however, it not only makes blood thicker, and thus more likely to form clots, but it also causes damage to the arterial wall. The damage inflicted provides a site for cholesterol to attach itself to the artery thus beginning the narrowing process.

However, the metabolic theory is not above criticism. For example, the high daily fat intake of the Masai cattle-herders of eastern Africa and Navajo Indians of North America is not always accompanied by coronary heart disease. Heredity, industrialization, and increased intake of simple sugars rather than fats may be confounding factors.

Coronary heart disease (CHD)

The outcome of atherosclerosis is a progressive narrowing and stiffening of the coronary arteries that carry the oxygen needed for the continued contraction of cardiac muscle. Because the lumen of the arteries is reduced, known as stenosis, blood flow also falls in line with the Hagen–Poiseuille equation. An inadequate supply of oxygen, particularly on exercise, leads to the condition known as angina pectoris – literally, 'a pang in the breast'. This is the most common form of coronary heart disease, with about a million and a half sufferers in the United Kingdom.

A heart attack results if a thrombus (from the Greek *thrombos* = a clot) formed from platelets, fibrin and blood cells blocks the narrowed artery and cuts off the blood supply. The area of the myocardium fed by that particular artery becomes ischaemic and, unless given rapid treatment, irretrievably damaged; this is a myocardial infarct (MI). If the thrombosis occurs in a major artery, we see another example of the destructive effects of a positive feedback loop. The myocardium is starved of oxygen; in an attempt to increase the oxygen supply, heart rate increases; the oxygen cost of the contracting cardiac muscle rises, thus requiring even more oxygen, so heart rate increases even further. This vicious spiral continues until ventricular fibrillation occurs – an uncoordinated contraction of individual muscle fibres; this leads to asystole and cessation of cardiac output. About 30 per cent of heart attack patients die before reaching hospital.

The aetiology of coronary heart disease

The study of the causes of coronary heart disease, technically known as its aetiology, reveals a complex picture. The major factors arraigned can be divided into two main groups. The first is our genetic endowment about which we can do nothing but blame our parents. For example, if there has been a familial history of heart disease, particularly related to hyperlipidaemia, the risks of developing the condition are increased. The second group consists of the behavioural characteristics we develop over time. The major attributable risk factors seem to be

(a) hypertension, that is pressures higher than 140 mmHg systolic and 90 mmHg diastolic:

(b) high total blood cholesterol levels of more than 6.5 mmol $\cdot L^{-1}$:

(c) obesity with a body mass index greater than 30 kg/m^2

(d) low levels of fruit and vegetable intake:

(e) smoking:

(f) low levels of physical activity of less than five sessions of 30 min of moderate exercise a week

Positive changes in the above five risk factors would reduce coronary heart disease by almost a third. Other attributable factors include

(g) diabetes:

(h) overweight with waist/hip ratio more than 0.85 for women and 0.95 for men and/or body mass index (BMI) of 25–30 kg/m^2:

(i) acute (binge-drinking) and chronic alcohol abuse (more than 28 units per week):

(j) psycho-social stress, including work stress, lack of social support, depression (including anxiety)

All of these risk factors are, essentially, self-inflicted, and can be avoided, or at least attenuated, by changes in behaviour. Smoking is an expensive, long-drawn-out, ultimately distressful suicide attempt which is frequently successful. Chronic alcoholism adversely affects the metabolic activity of the heart, and leads to myocardiopathy in the form of cardiac enlargement and reduced cardiac output at rest and exercise. On the other hand, it seems that alcohol in moderation – no more than three units a day – has the twin benefits of fleeting pleasure with some protection against heart disease, particularly in the middle-aged rather than the elderly. A sensible diet – low in animal fat, salt and simple sugars intakes, and a high daily intake of fresh fruit and vegetables – combined with regular exercise has been shown to produce beneficial effects on the other risk factors. The benefits of this two-pronged approach include an improved ratio of the high-density lipoprotein fraction of total blood cholesterol values, and a reduction in excess body fat leading, in turn, to a reduced risk of diabetes, lowered blood pressure, and a sense of mental well-being.

The importance of the relationship between diet and cardiovascular health cannot be overstated. It is reinforced by the finding that mortality and morbidity rates were lower during World War II. The decrease was linked to the imposition of rationing, and a reduction in both saturated fat and overall calorific intake. Recent statistics show that diet-related factors are present in more than 80 per cent of cardiovascular disease, and that lowering cholesterol and becoming more physically active could reduce the incidence of coronary heart disease by about 20 per cent. However, the interaction between diet and heart disease is very complex, and is too large a topic to be taken further here. We now focus our attention on the links between physical activity and heart disease.

Exercise and coronary heart disease

As we have already noted, the link between exercise and heart disease was not always regarded as a positive one by the ancient philosophers and physicians, and there is current evidence that *vigorous* exercise is not vital for protection from coronary heart disease, and is proscribed in hypertensive men. In the early 1900s, medical advice was to avoid strenuous exercise because it was thought that the enlarged athlete's heart was a diseased heart. The logic behind this belief arose from X-ray images of the hearts of patients diagnosed with coronary heart disease. The X-rays did not produce direct evidence of the disease, only that heart volume was increased. Post-mortem examination of these patients confirmed cardiac enlargement, and a causal link was made between heart volume and heart disease. In healthy men, average heart volume is about 700 mL and weight is 280–300 g; the average volume of cardiac muscle is about 280 mL. In chronic heart disease, the heart volume increases without any change in muscle volume; this is called cardiac dilatation. On the other hand, high blood pressure results not only in dilatation, but also in increased cardiac muscle mass or hypertrophy. As the disease progresses, any further increases in volume, up to a litre above normal, are the result only of continuing dilatation. Volumes of diseased hearts of 3.5 L do occur, but in coronary heart disease, evidence suggests that enlargement due to hypertrophy seldom exceeds 500–600 mL.

When X-rays of athletes also revealed hearts of above average volumes, it was wrongly concluded that such large hearts were also diseased hearts and that strenuous exercise should be avoided. It was not until post-mortem examination of athletes hearts revealed a highly effective pump that the potential benefits of exercise became apparent.

Epidemiological studies

In the 1950s, the attention of health workers of all kinds was drawn to the link between exercise and coronary heart disease. The prevalence of the disease was rising, and a prime factor in its aetiology was thought to lie in the psycho-emotional stress induced by executive life in an industrialized society. This judgement arose from morbidity data that revealed a high prevalence of coronary heart disease in professional occupations – doctors, clerks, and teachers – but a low prevalence in manual occupations – navvies, labourers and bricklayers. A letter in the *Lancet* remarked that an alternative explanation could be drawn from the data, namely that the prevalence of the disease was highest in those whose occupations required no physical work, and was lowest in those whose did. A spate of epidemiological studies followed. These included death rates from coronary heart disease in London Transport bus drivers and conductors, London Post Office workers, American letter carriers, postal clerks, and railroad workers, farmers in Dakota, Finnish lumberjacks, and members of an Israeli kibbutz.

The studies revealed that morbidity and/or mortality rates from coronary heart disease were lower in those occupations requiring higher levels of chronic habitual physical activity. The bus drivers were likely to die earlier than the conductors. The disease was less prevalent in postal workers who walked or cycled whilst delivering the post compared to those who sat behind the counters. Railroad workers who worked on the track fared better than those who sold the tickets. Farmers, and those members of a kibbutz engaged in physical work, were less like to suffer from coronary heart disease than their sedentary peers. The evidence from these studies pointed to the hypothesis that exercise provided some protection from coronary heart disease.

These early studies were later subjected to severe criticism on the grounds of inadequate control of other risk factors. The study of London Transport workers, for example, reported deaths from coronary heart disease; morbidity was not included, but further scrutiny revealed that the prevalence of angina was higher in conductors. The key issue from which the hypothesis grew – namely differences in habitual physical activity patterns of the two groups – was *assumed* rather than assessed. In a study on the habitual physical activity of Aberdeen policemen, it was found that foot-patrol officers had higher mean heart rates during *work* than car-patrol officers, but with *leisure* time heart rates the reverse was the case, and there was no difference between the groups in physiological responses to a sub-maximal exercise test.

The British Regional Heart Study

A more tightly controlled longitudinal study, involving almost 8000 men aged 40–59 in 24 towns in mainland Britain, was set up in 1978. Follow-up questionnaires were sent in 1983–85, 1992 and 1996, and 4252 (77 per cent) of available survivors were re-examined from 1998 to 2000. Among the findings is significantly stronger evidence for the benefits of increased physical activity as a protective mechanism in coronary heart disease in older men.

Eight years after the initial assessments, the major findings were as follows:

(a) In men without evidence of ischaemic heart disease, moderate or moderately vigorous physical activity patterns were associated with more than a 50 per cent reduction in the risk of a heart attack.

(b) Those with symptomatic ischaemic heart disease undertaking light or moderate levels of physical activity also showed a lower rate of heart attacks.

In a further follow-up 4 to 6 years later these findings were confirmed, and reinforced the view that maintaining or taking up light or moderate physical activity reduces the mortality and heart attacks in older men whether they have diagnosed cardiovascular disease or not. The most recent (2000) report on men with established coronary heart disease showed the highest risk of cardio-vascular mortality in those who remained sedentary.

For sport and exercise scientists engaged in training programmes for fitness and improved sports performance and committed to the mantra of 'no gain without pain', perhaps the most important finding from the study is the kind of physical activity regarded as appropriate for this age group. Data from the study suggest that recreational activity of 4 hours or more a weekend, 40 minutes or more walking daily, or moderate to heavy gardening offers signifi-cantly lower risk of all-cause mortality. Contrary to some expectations, vigor-ous exercise, such as sporting activity, is not essential for this protection and in some cases is even linked to increased risk of heart attack.

The general descriptions of the nature of the physical activity that offers protection against heart attack create problems, however. The data were derived from self-report questionnaires and the subjective nature of descriptors such as light, moderate, moderately vigorous, and vigorous make exercise prescription difficult. The British Heart Foundation seems to offer improved precision in suggesting 30 minutes of moderate exercise five times a week; but when we examine the nature of the 'moderate exercise' prescribed, we find activities ranging from brisk walking and cycling, through dancing and gardening, to stair climbing, and so the difficulties remain. Gardening, for example, encompasses pruning roses, mowing lawns, heavy digging and tree felling; stair climbing, particularly for 30 minutes, presents a serious physiological challenge to healthy, fit young adults. A sensible guideline is that any exercise undertaken should be at an intensity at which conversation is still possible. However, the contrast between this advice and the heart rate driven prescriptions derived from maximal oxygen uptake test data seen in fitness training programmes of healthy young adults and elite athletes is quite obvious, and seems a long way from the minimal activity threshold of 70–75 per cent of maximal work capacity suggested by others.

Cardiovascular disease in children

The discovery of the precursors of atherosclerosis during the first two decades of life has led to concerns over the diminishing levels of physical activity of children of school age. This is particularly so in adolescent girls where puberty is often accompanied by changes to recreational pursuits that exclude sports. The British Heart Foundation's recommendation for school children is 1 hour of moderate exercise a day. To gain a foothold in a prescribed National Curriculum, physical educators have laid claim to a philosophy of health-related fitness as their *raison d'être*. However, research shows that this claim cannot be sustained. Monitoring heart rates during physical education sessions to record the level of exercise intensity reveal two things. First, heart rates seldom exceed a threshold of $120 \ \text{bt} \cdot \text{min}^{-1}$; and second, the total time that the threshold is met seldom reaches 15 min. Indeed, it has been said that children are likely to gain more benefit from cycling or walking to and from school than from the very limited exposure to strenuous exercise provided in current physical education programmes.

What mechanisms might confer protection?

The exercise-driven mechanisms by which the cardiovascular system may be protected against disease are still not clear and are not revealed by epidemiological studies. The most obvious possibilities include changes in cardiac efficiency, the development of collateral circulation, lowered blood pressure, increased high-density lipoprotein cholesterol fraction, modification of insulin-related disease, and weight reduction and prevention of obesity.

Cardiac efficiency

Elite endurance athletes have half the resting heart rate of sedentary groups and double the resting stroke volume. The lowered heart rate (bradycardia) that accompanies chronic exercise is a well-known phenomenon and has two important benefits. The first is the longer diastolic filling time that results in larger end-diastolic volume, greater stretching of the ventricular muscle fibres, and increased stroke volume in line with the Frank–Starling's law. The outcome is a lower metabolic (oxygen) cost for the heart and thus improved efficiency. The second concerns coronary blood supply that occurs during the recovery period (diastasis) of the cardiac cycle. The longer diastasis allows for greater coronary perfusion.

In addition, there is evidence from human autopsies and animal experiments that sustained exercise programmes lead to adaptation of the coronary artery tree. The important finding is that the diameter of the vessels is increased. The result is a reduced resistance and an increased blood flow to the heart in line with the Hagen–Poiseuille equation. For individuals with compromised heart function, these exercise-induced changes confer considerable protective benefits.

Collateral circulation

A seminal study involving experiments on laboratory animals designed to test the exercise hypothesis was reported in 1957. The circumflex coronary artery of each animal was narrowed artificially by mild, moderate or severe ligation to mimic the effects of progressive coronary stenosis. The animals were divided into non-exercising control, and exercising experimental groups. After the conclusion of the exercise treatment, the hearts were examined post-mortem. In the sedentary controls, collateral circulation – in the form of new blood vessels in the myocardium – had developed around the ligatures only if the constriction was moderate or severe. This was seen as a reflex response designed to maintain the oxygen supply to the affected area. The most significant outcome was seen in the exercising group where there was a direct link between the severity of the constriction and the development of collateral vascularization. This was interpreted as strong evidence for the beneficial effects of regular exercise, especially for those with atherosclerosis of the coronary arteries. However, the effectiveness of this reflex response as a protective mechanism is still not clear, and there is always some uncertainty that animal responses are directly transferable to humans.

Reduced blood pressure

As blood pressure is the product of cardiac output and peripheral resistance, any changes in the peripheral blood vessels will affect pressure. There is good evidence that aerobic training results in greater vascularization of skeletal muscle, and that this can lead to lowered systolic and diastolic pressures at rest and, more particularly, during exercise.

Changes in cholesterol and triglycerides

High blood lipid levels (hyperlipidaemia) are associated with increased blood viscosity, platelet stickiness, red cell clumping and blood clotting, all of which have consequences for blood pressure and peripheral oxygen extraction. Reductions in total cholesterol and triglycerides, and a change in the ratio of high- and low-density lipoprotein cholesterol, have occurred following acute and chronic exercise. Increased levels of high-density cholesterol are beneficial because this cholesterol fraction acts as a scavenger, particularly of the low-density variety of cholesterol.

However, it is worth noting that familial hypercholesterolaemia, which is an inherited condition, seems immune to the protective benefits of regular exercise. There is strong evidence of family histories of death from coronary heart disease linking grandparents, parents and siblings. There is also anecdotal evidence that high cholesterol levels remain unaffected by exercise, even in serious joggers, and retired endurance athletes who have maintained a vigorous exercise programme in their retirement. The use of statins – a group of cholesterol-lowering drugs – is likely to offer greater protection, and the key to lowering cholesterol production may lie in reducing the dietary intake of simple carbohydrates such as refined flour and rice, pasta and cakes.

Control of diabetes mellitus – Type II

Type II diabetes, or late-onset diabetes, is related to age and obesity and is a serious risk factor in coronary heart disease. It is the outcome of a limited supply of effective insulin occurring in middle-aged overweight individuals. Insulin is produced by the islets of Langerhans in the pancreas; its function is to provide cells with glucose to fuel metabolism. It does this by changing the permeability of the cell membrane to allow glucose to pass into the intracellular fluid. Insufficient insulin, or resistance to the insulin that is produced, results in hyperglycaemia, high blood sugar levels, and glycosuria, sugar in the urine. It is estimated that if no one was overweight the prevalence of diabetes would be reduced by about two-thirds. Thus, the two major behavioural treatments are dietary control and exercise; the latter is associated with improved insulin sensitivity and reduced insulin resistance.

Prevention of obesity

Exercise is a key component in the prevention of obesity. This is a condition in which energy intake, in the form of food, exceeds the energy expenditure of daily living and the excess energy is stored in the form of adipose tissue made up of fat cells. Two factors facilitate the onset and progressive nature of obesity. The first is the age-related reduction in the energy expended to maintain waking bodily functions – the basal metabolic rate (BMR) – of about 2 per cent every 10 years. The second is the lowered metabolic rate of obese individuals. Combine these two factors with reduced physical activity and the development of obesity is inevitable. Regular aerobic exercise not only increases energy expenditure during the exercise but also for some time afterwards because the non-exercising metabolic rate remains elevated during the post-exercise recovery period. A combination of exercise with reduced dietary intake provides the best strategy for counteracting obesity and the associated cardiovascular diseases.

Exercise prescription

Having established the benefits of regular exercise as a protective mechanism in diseases of the cardiovascular system, we come to the most intractable problem facing the sport and exercise scientist interested in health promotion, namely 'What sort of exercise should we prescribe?' On the one hand, we have those who say that aerobic exercise at 75 per cent of maximum capacity for 30 minutes a day for 5 days a week is needed to enhance aerobic capacity. On the other, we have suggestions that 'regular moderate exercise', whatever those two adjectives mean, is sufficient. There is evidence to suggest that both strategies can be effective; but experience tells us that the likelihood of a mass movement towards adopting the first exercise programme, particularly by the middle-aged and elderly, if not entirely absent, is very low. Exercise adherence to such programmes is traditionally poor; furthermore, a logical case can be made for the moderate approach that depends on replacement of the word 'exercise', with its attendant notions of sweat and pain, by the term 'habitual physical activity'.

If we examine the epidemiological evidence from 50 years ago linking protection from cardiovascular disease with occupation, we find that the key factors appear to be the duration of increased low-intensity physical activity rather than the short, sharp shock approach. Using heart rate as a guide to the level of any exercise intensity, we see that 75 per cent of maximum heart rates lie between 165 bt $\cdot$ min^{-1} for the 20-year-old and 120 bt $\cdot$ min^{-1} for the 60-year-old. Although there is very little in the way of direct evidence, it is difficult to see heart rates of this magnitude being associated with the occupations examined in these epidemiological studies. A more plausible hypothesis suggests that repeated bouts of activity of relatively low intensity – climbing the stairs to the upper deck, the intermittent nature of letter delivery – over an entire 40-hour working week, 48 weeks a year for several years, may be responsible for protection against heart disease.

An alternative approach to estimating exercise intensity is to use the notion of the metabolic equivalent of exercise, known as a MET. Like heart rate, oxygen consumption increases in line with sub-maximal exercise intensity; at rest it is 3–4 mLO$_2$ $\cdot$ kg^{-1} $\cdot$ min^{-1}, which represents 1.0 MET. The metabolic costs of a wide range of activities have been calculated; for example, walking, at 2 mi $\cdot$ hr^{-1} or a brisk 3.5 mi $\cdot$ hr^{-1}, results in energy expenditures of 2.5 and 5.5 METs respectively. If we assume an average energy expenditure of 4 METs, during a 4-hour shift of letter delivery, in a standard 70-kg postman, we get a total expenditure of 67 200 METs. This translates into almost a litre of oxygen a minute for 240 minutes. If we take jogging at 5.0 mi $\cdot$ hr^{-1}, equivalent to about 8 METs, we have to jog for 2 hours to achieve the same energy expenditure. If we wanted to restrict our exercise time to 30 minutes a day, we would need to run at a 4-minute-mile pace (30 METs) for the full 30 minutes to give a total energy expenditure of 63 000 METs, still 4200 short of that expended by the letter deliverer. Although the use of the MET as a measure of energy expenditure is a rather crude instrument, it seems unlikely that many people would accept 30 min of 4-minute mile running as an example of moderate exercise. The major point at issue here is the psychological resistance of ordinary men and women to such a demanding regime.

Another benefit of extended, low-intensity habitual physical activity is its effect on the energy source of that activity. The respiratory exchange ratio (RER) – the ratio of carbon dioxide excreted to oxygen consumed ($\dot{V}_{CO_2}/\dot{V}_{O_2}$) – is related to the intensity of exercise and the main type of fuel used. At rest, the ratio is about 0.75, indicating about 85 per cent of the energy comes from lipids. At 75 per cent of maximal exercise capacity, the ratio is about 0.9 indicating carbohydrates provide about 66 per cent of the energy. Thus, low-intensity exercise relies mainly on lipid metabolism. Comparing high- ($\sim$75 per cent) and low- ($\sim$ 50 per cent) intensity exercise over 30 minutes' duration results, not unexpectedly, in higher energy expenditure for the higher-intensity exercise; the ratio of fat to carbohydrate, however, is 2:1 in favour of carbohydrate and a total energy expenditure of about 80 kJ (332 kcal), of which only 26 kJ (110 kcal) are derived from fats. If we double the duration of the low-intensity exercise to 60 minutes, the energy expenditure is doubled to 160 kJ (664 kcal) but the energy derived from fats increases to 80 kJ (332 kcal). If we combine the MET and RER approaches and look at brisk walking at 3.5 mi · hr^{-1} (5.5 MET) in our standard postman, the estimated oxygen consumption is 1.35 L · min^{-1} and the exchange ratio is 0.8, the energy expended during an hour's walk is 98 kJ (405 kcal), 64 per cent of which comes from fats.

The target of about 3.5 mi · hr^{-1} is the kind of exercise that might be termed 'moderate', and may conform to the British Regional Heart Study's descriptor. This kind of exercise prescription should be couched in everyday language that is understood by all. For example, a suggestion to choose a newsagent located about 1.75 miles away from the house and a target of taking no longer than an hour to collect and return with the daily and Sunday papers, might persuade many more people, especially the middle-aged and elderly, to incorporate this kind of change in their habitual physical activity patterns.

This suggestion should be seen as an attempt to persuade the slothful, probably the majority of the population in the rich, industrialized nations, to take advantage of the beneficial effects of an everyday event. The physiological and psychological benefits are apparent, and there are economic attractions. Assuming the cost of a daily paper is 50p (80$; 30€) and that of a Sunday broadsheet is £1 (1.65$; 60€), the annual cost, including new footwear, would not exceed £300 (495$; 18 000€). This is substantially less than the combined joining fee and annual subscription to the glittering steel and glass of the latest private Health Studios. This strategy is not intended to dismiss the feelings of pleasure brought about by increased endorphin secretion that often accompanies regular exercise of the more strenuous kind. There is also no denying the attractions of the Health Studios and the aerobics class of the local Leisure Centres. These provide an attractive social ambience, and the additional benefit some kind of structure to the exercise regime that many people require. The message is that you can do it more cheaply!

The key question that remains is which protective mechanisms are likely to be induced by this level of habitual activity. It is certain that weight control would be one; although the amount of energy expended during exercise can seem almost trivially small, the cumulative effects over months and years can lead to quite substantial losses in adipose tissue. Lowered triglyceride levels, and total and low-density lipoprotein cholesterol are likely. Improved insulin response is also possible, thereby reducing the risk of developing Type II diabetes. Vascularization of the lower limbs is probable; there is supportive evidence for the beneficial effects of exercise on intermittent claudication, a condition of the lower limbs similar to the angina of the heart muscle. Such a change would also benefit borderline hypertensives by reducing peripheral resistance. The development of adequate vascularization of the myocardium remains uncertain, but there have been reports of beneficial changes in electrocardiograph traces including reduced occurrence of S-T segment depression. It is still not clear if low-intensity exercise can deliver measurable changes in cardiac efficiency.

Exercise and cerebrovascular disease (CeVD)

Data from the British Regional Heart Study indicate that exercise has beneficial effects on cerebrovascular disease in the form of reduced risk from strokes. A stroke results in damage to the brain tissue, through cerebral thrombosis or cerebral haemorrhage. Dependent on its severity, a stroke is accompanied by a range of prognoses from complete or partial recovery, through severe impairment of movement, speech, and sight, to death. In a study involving 7735 men, aged between 40 and 59, physical activity was inversely related to the risk of a stroke. Moderate exercise significantly reduces the risk of strokes in men with and without pre-existing ischaemic heart disease; in addition, vigorous activity did not confer any further benefit.

Exercise and other diseases

Lung disease

The management of patients with chronic airflow limitation accompanying chronic bronchitis and emphysema presents difficult problems for physicians.

The disease produces anxiety, depression and feelings of worthlessness; even minimal exertion often results in dyspnoea, and physical activity is avoided. As a result, the already compromised physical fitness of the patient is made worse, which in turn exacerbates breathlessness on exercise, and sets the patient on the downward spiral of progressive inactivity leading to virtual immobility. However, there is evidence that many respiratory cripples lead needlessly restricted lives, and there are reports of the beneficial effects of exercise with patients with chronic airflow limitation. The clinical benefits include reduced dyspnoea during habitual physical activity, reduced coughing and sputum production in bronchitic patients, and improved sleep. The major practical benefit is the universal finding of increased exercise tolerance. However, subjective assessment of the effects of training by the patients is invariably more positive than that of the changes in objective physiological measures, which are often inconsistent and minimal, and only occasionally statistically significant.

Cardio-respiratory benefits following exercise programmes include: lower resting and sub-maximal exercise heart rates; reduced cardiac output accompanied by increased arterial–mixed venous oxygen difference; and falls in systolic and pulmonary artery pressures. Respiratory function also benefits. Resting spirometric values remain largely unchanged, but breathing exercises often lead to slower respiratory frequency and greater tidal volumes. Maximum voluntary ventilation and minute volume are increased, but ventilation at sub-maximal exercise is lowered; the mechanism at work here appears to be improved respiratory muscle function. Symptom-limited oxygen uptake ($\dot{V}_{O_2SL}$) is increased but consumption at standard work falls. Scintigraphic evidence has revealed changes in the ventilation/perfusion ratio through improved pulmonary perfusion. Even so, it is important to recognize that not all of these benefits are seen in all patients; indeed, there is evidence that subjective assessment of improvement is often accompanied by inconclusive functional data.

The psychotherapeutic benefits of exercise-based rehabilitation programmes cannot be overstated. Some would argue that the initial value of any controlled, supervised programme may be the psychological reassurance that develops, and that an increase in habitual physical activity is indispensable for improvement. This can lead to improved self-image, greater confidence, feelings of well-being, better personal relationships, and reduced fear of exercise and moderately strenuous activity. In some cases, there is return to gainful employment, reducing the financial burden on the family and the National Health Service.

It is also worth noting that the better results are obtained from younger (under 60 years), well-motivated patients in work or seeking employment. Subjects with prominent emphysema, idiopathic lung fibrosis or gravely impaired gas transfer seem less susceptible to exercise training. Despite the positive picture painted here, clear evidence of the effects of training on lifestyle, degree of independence, level of habitual physical activity, recurrence of illness, and eventual cause of death is scarce.

Cancers

The British Regional Heart Study, a 19-year prospective study of nearly 8000 men aged between 40 and 59, showed that moderately vigorous and vigorous physical activity was linked to a significant reduction in total cancers, and in prostate, upper digestive tract, and stomach cancers; but there was an increased risk of bladder cancer linked to vigorous exercise. There was no relationship between activity and colorectal cancer. The mechanisms that provide protection against some cancers are not yet clear.

Conclusion

Since the Industrial Revolution, the physical demands of labour have all but disappeared. The body is a machine designed for action; physiological machines that lie idle suffer the equivalent of poor maintenance, rust and decay. As the energy requirements of everyday living diminish, the human machine needs an injection of voluntary physical effort to maintain its efficiency and effectiveness. Some form of regular, moderate exercise brings with it physical, mental and social benefits. Thus, the answer to the question 'Is exercise good for us?' is almost certainly 'Yes, in moderation, and only if accompanied by good dietary habits and avoidance of nicotine addiction and other equally self-destructive habits.'

Key points

- Exercise for health needs to be distinguished from exercise for sports performance.

- The former is similar to the ongoing maintenance of the family car, whereas the latter is the fine-tuning of a Formula 1 Ferrari.

- There are clear physical and psychological benefits arising out of regular moderate exercise.

- It may minimize the worst effects of cardiovascular diseases, particularly coronary heart disease and strokes, and some cancers.

- It is effective in rehabilitating heart, stroke and lung disease patients, and may provide relief for chronic depression.

- A combination of exercise and a healthy diet lowers the incidence of obesity and the concurrent risk of developing Type II diabetes.

- The social benefits arising from exercise, healthy diet and no smoking in reduced costs for the National Health Service are incalculable.

References and Further Reading

Introduction

In addition to the material that is specific to particular chapters, there is a range of fundamental sources that I have found useful over the years. They include the following:

Encyclopaedia Britannica, Inc. (2002) *Encyclopaedia Britannica, CD Deluxe*

This is a good resource for physiological material, and has access to numerous Internet sites. Copies of the CD-ROM, from about £20, are available for personal computers. The ISBN is 0-7630-3699-4.

Walker PMB (Gen. Ed.) (1995) *The Larousse dictionary of science and technology.* Edinburgh, Larousse plc

This is a useful guide to new scientific terms and definitions. The paperback ISBN is 0-7523-0011-3.

Tortora G and Grabowski SR (2003) *Principles of anatomy and physiology*, 10th edn. New York, John Wiley.

A grasp of the fundamental concepts of anatomy and physiology is vital if we are to make sense of the responses to exercise. I chose this book because of the clarity of the material and the excellent diagrams provided.

Keele CA and Neil E (1971) *Samson Wright's Applied Physiology*, 12th edn. London, Oxford University Press

This book is for the student who discovers an interest and aptitude for exercise physiology, and wishes to understand thoroughly the underlying concepts of applied human physiology.

Åstrand PO and Rodahl K (1986) *Textbook of work physiology*, 3rd edn. Singapore, McGraw-Hill.

This book is still the gold standard against which all other exercise physiology texts are judged. There will be copies in your library.

Exercise Physiology: A Thematic Approach   Tudor Hale
© John Wiley & Sons, Ltd   ISBN: 0 470 84682 8 (cloth), ISBN 0 470 84683 6 (pbk)

Wingate P (1975) *The Penguin medical encyclopedia*. Harmondsworth, Penguin Books.

A great deal of medical terminology occurs during the study of Exercise Physiology, and students can learn a great deal from books such as this.

BLAT Centre for Health and Medical Education. *Audiotapes and booklets on physiology*. British Medical Association, BMA House, Tavistock Square, London WC1H 9JP

This Education Centre produces a wide range of self-instructional audiotapes and supporting booklets dealing with fundamental physiological processes. Demanding, but worth the effort.

Porter R and Ogilvie M (Consultant Editors) (2000) *The Hutchinson dictionary of scientific biography*, Vols I and II, 3rd edn. Oxford, Helicon Publishers Ltd

This is included for those students who like to know the roots of the physical, chemical and biological sciences that contribute to our sub-discipline of exercise physiology. It is interesting and very informative, and gives some notion of the immense history underpinning the progress of science.

www.css.edu/asep *Journal of Exercise Physiology (JEP)* A free on-line journal provided by American Society of Exercise Physiologists.

www.sportsci.org A free on-line source of material.

http://cwis.livjm.ac.uk/psd/DigitalResources/Sport%20Science.htm This is a very good links page.

www.jbriffa.com This is an interesting free site with a substantial list of references for those interested in the impact of diet on health.

Context-based material

Chapter 1   The maximal oxygen uptake test

Astorino TA, Robergs RA, Ghiasvand F, Marks D and Burns S (2000) Incidence of the oxygen plateau at $\dot{V}_{O_2max}$ during exercise testing to volitional fatigue. *JEP* 3(4):1–12 www.css.edu/asep

Consolazio CF, Johnson RE and Pecora LJ (1963) *Physiological measurements of metabolic functions in man*. New York, McGraw-Hill

Douglas CG (1911) A method for determining the total respiratory exchange in man. *J Physiol* London xvi–xvii

Draper SB, Wood DM and Fallowfield J (1999) Effect of test protocol on $\dot{V}_{O_2peak}$ and the incidence of V_{O_2} plateau. *Journ Sports Sci* 17:31

Fox E, Bowers R and Foss M (1993) *The physiological basis for exercise and sport*, 5th edn. Dubuque, Wm C Brown

Geppert J and Zuntz N (1888) Ueber die Regulation der Athmung E *Pflüger Archiv* **XLII**:199

Haldane JS (1912) *Methods of air analysis.* London, Charles Griffin

Luft U, Myhre L and Loeppky J (1973) Validity of the Haldane calculation for estimating respiratory gas exchange. *J Appl Physiol* **35**:864–865

McCardle WD, Katch FI and Katch VL (1994) *Essentials of exercise physiology.* Pennsylvania, Lea & Febiger

Taylor HL, Buskirk E and Henschel A (1955) Maximum oxygen uptake as an objective measure of cardio-respiratory performance. *J Appl Physiol* **8**:73–80

Wyndham CH, Strydom NB, Leary WP and Williams CG (1966) Studies of the maximum capacity of men for physical effort: a comparison of assessing the maximal oxygen uptake. *Int Z agnew Physiol* **22**:285–295

www.btc.Montana.edu/Olympics/physiology/pbo2.html
www.crosslink.net/~cherylW/VO2MAX.htm
www.nismat.org/physcor/maxo2html#op
www.uclan.ac.uk/facs/science/biology/sport/ab214inf.htm
www.udel.edu/HESC/physLab/MaxVO2.htm.

Chapter 2   Oxygen from atmosphere to blood

American College of Sports Medicine (1979) Symposium on ventilatory control during exercise. *Med Sci Sports* **11**:190–226

Comroe JH (1965) *Physiology of respiration.* Chicago, Year Book Medical

Cumming G and Semple SJ (1980) *Disorders of the respiratory system*, Part 1, 2nd edn. Oxford, Blackwell Scientific

Dempsey JA and Reed CE (1977) *Muscular exercise and the lung.* Madison, University of Wisconsin Press

Dempsey JA, Vidruk EH and Mitchell GS (1986) Is the lung built for exercise? *Med Sci Sport Exer* **18**:143–155

Forster HV (2000) Exercise hyperpnoea. *Exerc Sport Sci Rev* **28**:133–137

Horsfield K (1968) Morphology of the bronchial tree. *J Appl Physiol* **24**:373–383

Horsfield K (1968) Functional consequences of airway morphology. *J Appl Physiol* **24**:384–390

Horsfield K (1990) Diameters, generations, and orders of branches in the bronchial tree. *J Appl Physiol* **68**:457–461

Tammeling, GJ and Quanjer, PhH (1980) Contours of breathing. CH Boehringer Sohn, Ingelhein am Rhein

Tortora GJ and Grabowski SR (2003) *Principles of anatomy and physiology*, 10th edn. New York, John Wiley, Chapter 23

Wagner PD, Roca J, Poole DC, Bebout DC and Haab P (1990) Experimental support for the theory of diffusion limitation of maximal oxygen uptake. *Adv Exp Med Biol* **277**:825–833

www.anaesthetist.com/icu/organs/lung/lungfx.htm
www.bartleby.com/107/illus970.html
www.lungusa.org/learn
www.nda.ox.ac.uk/wfsa/html/u12/u1211_01.htm

www.nda.ox.ac.uk/wfsa/html/u02/u02_011.htm
www.mhhe.com/biosci/ap/foxhumphys/student/ok/chap16summary.html
www.umds.ac.uk/physiology/rbm/cvmenu.htm

Chapter 3 Oxygen content of the blood

Bunn HF (1991) Haemoglobin I: Structure and function. In: *Haematology*, 5th edn
Beck WS (Ed). Cambridge, MA, MIT Press
Comroe JH (1974) *Physiology of respiration*, 2nd edn. Chicago, Year Book Medical
Cumming G and Semple SJ (1980) *Disorders of the respiratory system*, Part 1, 2nd edn.
   Oxford, Blackwell Scientific
Cumming G, Crank J, Horsfield K and Parker I (1966) Gaseous diffusion in the airways of
   the human lung. *Respirat Physiol* 1:58–74
Fishman AP and Hecht HH (1969) *The pulmonary circulation and interstitial space*, Part 1.
   Chicago, University of Chicago Press
Tortora GJ and Grabowski SR (2003) *Principles of anatomy and physiology*, 10th edn. New
   York, John Wiley, Chapter 19
www-cryst.bioc.cam.uk/~max/res_hb.html
www.nda.ox.ac.uk/wfsa/html/u10/u1003_01.htm
www.nurseminerva.co.uk.haem.html
www.smd.qmol.ac.uk/biomed/kb/microanatomy/blood/

Chapter 4 Oxygen delivery and the heart

Bakewell S (1995) The autonomic system. *Update in Anaesthesia* 5:3–6
Berne RM and Levy MN (1967) *Cardiovascular physiology*. St Louis, CV Mosby
Cooke WH (1998) Heart rate variability and baroreceptor responsiveness to evaluate
   autonomic cardiovascular adaptation to exercise. *JEP* 1(3) www.css.edu/ asep
Ekblom B and Hermansen L (1966) Cardiac output in athletes. *J Appl Physiol* 25:619–625
Kestin I (1993) Control of heart rate. *Update in Anaesthesia* 3.
Rogers J (1999) Cardiovascular physiology. *Update in Anaesthesia* 10.
Sleight P (Ed) (1978) ICI audio-visual library of cardiology. *Control of the cardiovascular
   system*, Part 3, *The heart as a pump*. ICI Pharmaceuticals Division, London Medi-cine
   Ltd
www.nda.ox.ac.uk/wfsa/html/u01/u01_008.htm
www.nda.ox.ac.uk/wfsa/html/u03/u03_011.htm
www.nda.ac.ox.uk/wfsa/html/u05/u05/010.htm
www. nda.ox.ac.uk/wfsa/html/u10/u1002_01.htm
www.uttyl.edu/mowings/stroke-volume.htm

Chapter 5 Oxygen distribution and the circulation

Berne RM and Levy MN (1967) *Cardiovascular physiology*. St Louis, CV Mosby

Burton AC (1954) Relation of structure to function of the tissues of the wall of blood vessels. *Physiol Rev* 34:619–642

Hester RL and Choi J (2002) Blood flow control during exercise. *Exerc Sport Sci Rev* 30:147–151

Laughlin MH and Armstrong RB (1985) Muscle blood flow during locomotory exercise. *Exerc Sport Sci Rev* 13:95–136

Mellander S and Johansson B (1968) Control of resistance, exchange, and capacitance functions in the peripheral circulation. *Pharmacol Rev* 20:117–196

Raven PB, Potts JT and Xiangrong S (1997) Baroreceptor regulation of blood pressure during dynamic exercise. *Exerc Sport Sci Rev* 25:365–390

Rowell LB (1986) *Human circulation: regulation during physical stress*. Oxford, Oxford University Press

Secher N (1999) Cardiovascular function and oxygen delivery during exercise. In: *Physiological determinants of exercise tolerance in humans*, Whipp BJ and Sargeant AJ (Eds). London, Portland Press, pp. 93–114

Sharma S (1992) Control of arterial blood pressure. *Update in Anaesthesia* 1.

Sleight P (Ed) (1978) ICI audio-visual library of cardiology. *Control of the cardiovascular system*, Part 4, *Cardiac control mechanisms in the intact circulation*. ICI Pharmaceuticals Division, London Medi-cine Ltd

Sleight P (Ed) (1978) ICI audio-visual library of cardiology. *Control of the cardiovascular system*, Part 5, *Structure and function of the vascular system*. ICI Pharmaceuticals Division, London Medi-cine Ltd

Sleight P (Ed) (1978) ICI audio-visual library of cardiology. *Control of the cardiovascular system*, Parts 6 and 7, *The nervous regulation of the cardiovascular system*. ICI Pharmaceuticals Division, London Medi-cine Ltd

Tortora GJ and Grabowski SR (2003) *Principles of anatomy and physiology*, 10th edn. New York, John Wiley, Chapter 21

www.cardiovascular.org/resist.htm

www.cardiovascular.cx/chap1.htm

www.e-cardiovascular.net/heart.html

www.innerbody.com/image/cardov.htm

www.leeds.ac.uk/chb/lectures/anatomy6.html

www.venous.net/

Chapter 6 Oxygen consumption – the structure and contraction of skeletal muscle

Huxley HE (1958) The contraction of muscle. *Sci Am* 19:3

Huxley HE (1965) The mechanism of muscular contraction. *Sci Am* 218:18

Huxley HE (1971) The structural basis of muscular contraction. *Proc R Soc* 178:131

Jones DA and Round JM (1990) *Skeletal muscle in health and disease*. Manchester, Manchester University Press

Komi GV and Karlsson J (1978) Skeletal muscle fibre types, enzyme activities, and physical performance in young males and females. *Acta Physiol Scand* 103:210

Lieber RL (1992) *Skeletal muscle structure and function.* Baltimore, Williams & Wilkins

Lutz GJ and Leiber RL (1999) Skeletal muscle myosin II structure and function. *Exerc Sport Sci Rev* 27:63–78

Otten E (1988) Concepts and models of functional architecture in skeletal muscle. *Exer Sports Sci Rev* 16

Merton P (1972) How we control the contraction of our muscles. *Sci Am* 226:30

Sleight P (Ed) (1978) ICI audio-visual library of cardiology. *Control of the cardiovascular system,* Part 2, *The propagation of the action potential and the contractile cell.* ICI Pharmaceuticals Division, London Medi-cine Ltd

Tortora GJ and Grabowski SR (2003) *Principles of anatomy and physiology,* 10th edn. New York, John Wiley, Chapter 10

www.blackwellscience.com/matthews/myosin.html

www.bms.abdn.ac.uk/microcomputing

www.edb.utexas.edu/syllabus/farrar/lectures/muscle2.html

http://k_2.stanford.edu/~thu/MusclePages/fiber_types.html

www.nau.edu/hp/proj/rah/courses/exs336/lectures/muscle.html

www-rohan.sdsu.edu/course/ens304/public_html/section3/Muscle.htm

www-rohan.sdsu.edu/~ens632/ExcitationContraction.htm

www.shef.ac.uk/~mc/Carey3.html

www.shef.ac.uk/~mc/excont.html

Chapter 7   Oxygen consumption in the muscle cell

Hood DA, Takahashi M, Connor MK and Freyssenet D (2000) Assembly of the cellular powerhouse; current issues in muscle mitochondrial biogenesis. *Exerc Sport Sci Rev* 28:68–73

Maughan R, Gleeson M and Greenhaff PL (1997). *Biochemistry of exercise and training.* Oxford, Oxford University Press

Newsholme EA and Leech A (1983). *Biochemistry for the medical sciences.* Chichester, John Wiley

Ranallo RF and Rhodes EC (1998) Lipid metabolism during exercise. *Sports Med* 26:29–42

Rose S (1991) *The chemistry of life,* 3rd edn. London, Penguin Group

Tonkonogi M and Sahlin K (2002) Physical exercise and mitochondrial function in human skeletal muscle. *Exerc Sport Sci Rev* 30:69–74

Tortora GJ and Grabowski SR (2003) *Principles of anatomy and physiology,* 10th edn. New York, John Wiley, Chapter 3

Wilmore JH and Costill DL (2002) *Physiology of sport and exercise,* 2nd edn. Champaign, Human Kinetics

www.biochem.arizona.edu/classes/bioc460/spring/rlm/lec28.html

www.blc.arizona.edu/courses/181GH/Lectures_WJG.98/metabolism_F.98/ox_pl...

www.omega.dawsoncollege.qc.ca/ray/krebs/redox.htm

www.chem.wsu.edu/Chem102/102-CitrAcCycOxPhos.html

Chapter 8 The interplay between aerobic and anaerobic metabolism

Bar-Or O (1981) The Wingate anaerobic test. *Symbioses* 13:157

Bar-Or O (1987) The Wingate anaerobic test: an update on methodology, reliability, and validity. *Sports Med* 4:381

Coleman SG and Hale T (1998) The effect of different calculation methods of flywheel parameters on the Wingate anaerobic test. *Can J Appl Physiol* 23:409

Gollnick PD and Hermansen L (1973) Biochemical adaptation to exercise: anaerobic metabolism. *Exerc Sport Sci Rev* 1:56

Green S (1995) Measurement of anaerobic capacities in humans. *Sports Med* 19:32–42

Greenhaff PL and Timmons JA (1998) Interaction between aerobic and anaerobic metabolism during exercise. *Exerc Sport Sci Rev* 26:1–30

Hermansen L (1969) Anaerobic energy release. *Med Sci Sport* 1:32

In-bar O, Bar-Or O and Skinner JS (1966) *The Wingate anaerobic test*. Champaign, Human Kinetics

Margaria R, Aghemo I. and Rovelli E (1966) Measurement of muscular power (anaerobic) in man. *J Appl Physiol* 21:1662

Margaria R, Aghemo P and Sassi G (1971) Lactic acid production in supra-maximal exercise. *Pflugers Archiv* 326:152

Medbø JI, Mohn A-C, Tabata RB, Vaage O and Sejersted OM (1988) Anaerobic capacity determined by maximal accumulated O_2 deficit. *J Appl Physiol* 64:50

Russell AP, Le Rossignol PF and Lo SK (2000) The precision of estimating total energy demand: implications for the determination of the accumulated oxygen deficit. *JEP* 3(2) www.css.edu/asep

Russell AP, Le Rossignol PF, Snow RJ and Lo SK (2002) Improving the precision of the accumulated oxygen deficit using $\dot{V}O_2$-power regression points from below and above the lactate threshold. *JEP* 5(1) www.css.edu/asep

Scott CB, Roby FB, Lohman TG and Bunt JC (1991) The maximally accumulated oxygen deficit as an indicator of anaerobic capacity. *Med Sci Sport Exerc* 23:618

Vandewalle GP, Peres G and Monod H (1987) Standard anaerobic exercise tests. *Sports Med* 4:268

www.uclan.ac.uk/facs/science/biology/sport/anaerob.htm
www.pponline.co.uk/encyc/0830.htm
www.shef.ac.uk/~mc/Carey3p2.html

Chapter 9 Venous blood, carbon dioxide and acid–base balance

Åstrand, PO and Rodahl, K (1968) Text book of Work Physiology 3rd edn. McGraw Hill, New York.

Comroe JH (1965) *Physiology of respiration*. Chicago, Year Book Medical

Davenport HW (1958) *The ABC of acid–base chemistry*, 4th edn. Chicago, University of Chicago Press

Hainsworth R (Ed) (1986) *Acid–base balance*. Manchester, Manchester University Press

Drage S and Wilkinson D (2001) Acid base balance. *Update in Anaesthesia* 13

McCardle WD, Katch FI and Katch VL (1994) *Essentials of exercise physiology.* Pennsylvania, Lea and Febiger

Robergs RA (2002) Blood acid base buffering: explanation of the effectiveness of bicarbonate and citrate ingestion. *JEP* 5(3) www.css.edu/asep

Wilmore JH and Costill DL (2002) *Physiology of sport and exercise,* 2nd edn. Champaign, Human Kinetics

Winters W, Engel E and Dell RB (1969) *Acid base physiology in medicine – a self-instruction program.* Cleveland, The London Company

www.anaesthetist.com/icu/organs/lung/lungfx.htm

www.healthsci.utas.edu.au/weller/+docs/respire6.htm

www.leeds.ac.uk/chb/lectures/anatomy6.html

www.nda.ox.ac.uk/wfsa/html/u13/u1312_01.htm

www.qldanaesthesia.com/AcidBaseBook/AB1_2.htm

www.tmc.tulane.edu/anes/acid/physiology.ssi

www.tmc.tulane.edu/anes/acid/production.ssi

www.umds.ac.uk/physiology/rbm/co2carri.htm

www.umds.ac.uk/physiology/rbm/veins.htm

www.venous.net

Chapter 10   Epilogue – the factors limiting maximal oxygen uptake

Astrand, PO and Rodahl, K (1968) Text book of Work Physiology 3rd edn. McGraw Hill, New York.

Amonette WE and Dupler TI (2002) The effects of respiratory muscle training on $\dot{V}_{O_2max}$, the ventilatory threshold and pulmonary function. *JEP* 5(2) www.css.edu/asep

Bassett DR and Howley ET (1997) Maximal oxygen uptake: 'classical' versus 'contemporary' viewpoints. *Med Sci Sport Exerc* 29:591–603

Bassett DR and Howley ET (2000) Limiting factors for maximum oxygen uptake and determinants of endurance performance. *Med Sci Sport Exerc* 32:70–84

Benestad AM (1972) The deteriorative effect of myocardial infarction upon physiological indices of work capacity. *Acta Med Scand* 191:67–75

Bergh U, Ekblom B and Åstrand PO (2000) Maximal oxygen uptake 'classical' versus 'contemporary' viewpoints. *Med Sci Sport Exerc* 32:85–88

Cumming G (1980) The pathophysiology of airways disease. In: *Ventilation-perfusion and gas exchange,* Derenne J-Ph (Ed). Rev fr Mal Resp (Paris), 87–96

Dempsey JA, Vidruk EH and Mitchell GS (1986) Is the lung built for exercise? *Med Sci Sport Exer* 18:143–155

Ekblom B, Åstrand PO, Saltin B and Wallstrom B (1968) Effect of training on circulatory response to exercise. *J Appl Physiol* 24:518–528

Ekblom B and Hermansen L (1968) Cardiac output in athletes. *J Appl Physiol* 25:619–625

Epstein SE, Robinson BF and Kahler RL (1965) Effects of beta-adrenergic blockade on cardiac response to maximal and sub-maximal exercise in man. *J Clin Invest* 44:1745–1753

Hartley LH and Saltin B (1969) Blood gas tensions and pH in brachial artery, femoral vein and brachial vein during maximal exercise. *Med Sci Sport* 3:66–72

Horsfield K (1968) Functional consequences of airway morphology. *J Appl Physiol* 24:384–390

Holloszy JO (1973) Biochemical adaptations to exercise: aerobic metabolism. *Exerc Sports Sci Rev* 1:45–71

Moore DH (1975) A study of age group track and field records to relate age and running speed. *Nature* 253:264–265

Noakes TD (1997) Challenging beliefs: *ex Africa semper aliquid novi. Med Sci Sport Exerc* 29:571–590

Noakes TD (1998) Maximal oxygen uptake: 'classical' versus 'contemporary' viewpoints: a rebuttal. *Med Sci Sport Exerc* 30:1381–1398

Robergs RA (2000) An exercise physiologist's 'contemporary' interpretations of the 'ugly and creaking edifices' of the $\dot{V}_{O_2max}$ concept. *JEP* 4(1)   www.css.edu/asep

Rousseau MF, Brasseur LA and Detry JM-R (1973) Hemodynamic determination of maximal oxygen intake on patients with myocardial infarction: influence of physical training. *Circulation* 48:943–949

Saltin B and Åstrand PO (1967) Maximal oxygen uptake in athletes. *J Appl Physiol* 23:353–358

Whipp BJ and Sargeant AJ (1999) *Physiological determinants of exercise tolerance in humans.* London, Portland Press

Williams J, Powers SK and Stuart MK (1986) Hemoglobin desaturation in highly trained athletes during heavy exercise. *Med Sci Sport Exerc* 18:168–173

www.physiotherapy.Curtin.edu.au/community/educational_resources/ep552_97/limit.background.html#background

www.physiotherapy.Curtin.edu.au/community/educational_resources/ep652_98central.shtml

www.drlenkravitz.com/Articles/limitations.html

Chapter 11 Postscript – exercise, fitness and health

Amsterdam EA, Wilmore JH and DeMaria AN (1977) *Exercise in cardiovascular health and disease.* New York, Yorke Medical Books

Berger M (1984) Exercise in the prevention and management of diabetes mellitus. Symposium Proceedings: *Exercise, health and medicine:37.* The Sports Council

Brody JE (2003) Personal health: statins: miracles for some, menace for a few. http://.nytimes.com/search/article-page.html?res=9906EEDD103BF933A25751C...

Brunner D and Manelis G (1960) Myocardial infarction among members of communal settlements in Israel. *Lancet* 2:1049

de Deuxchaisnes CN (1984) Exercise and the prevention and management of osteoporosis. Symposium Proceedings: *Exercise, health and medicine:39.* The Sports Council

Eckstein RW (1957) Effect of exercise and coronary artery narrowing on coronary collateral circulation. *Circ Res* 5:230–235

Fox SM and Haskell WL (1968) Physical activity and the prevention of coronary heart disease. *Bull New York Acad Med* 44:950–967

Freidberg CK (1966) *Diseases of the heart,* 3rd edn. London, WB Saunders

Glueck CJ, Shaw P, Lang JE, Tracy T, Sieve-Smith L and Wang Y (1995) Evidence that homocysteine is an independent risk factor for atherosclerosis in hyperlipidemic patients. *Am J Cardiol* 75:132–136

Grimby G (1984) Exercise and physical training in the rehabilitation of patients with respiratory impairment. Symposium Proceedings: *Exercise, health and medicine:35*. The Sports Council

Hale T, Hamley EJ and Spriggs J (1976) Effectiveness of an exercise regime on the rehabilitation of COLD patients using heart rate as the parameter. *J Brit Ass Sports Med* 10:71–75

Hale T, Cumming G and Spriggs J (1978) The effects of physical training in chronic obstructive lung disease. *Bulletin Europ Physiopath Resp* 14

Hellerstein HK (1968) Exercise therapy in coronary disease. *Bull New York Acad Med* 44:1028–1047

Kaelin ME, Swank AM, Barnard KL, Adams KJ, Beach P and Newman J (2001) Physical fitness and quality of life outcomes in a pulmonary rehabilitation programme utilizing symptom limited interval training and resistance training. *JEP* 4(3)   www.css.edu/asep

LaPorte RE, Adams LL, Savage DD, Brenes G, Dearwater S and Cook T (1984) The spectrum of physical activity, cardiovascular disease and health: an epidemiological perspective. *Am J Epidemiol* 120:507

Leading article (1951) Cardiac enlargement and hypertrophy *Lancet* 2:671

Morris J, Heady J, Raffle P, Roberts C and Parks J (1953) Coronary heart disease and physical activity of work. *Lancet* 2:1053

Newsholme EA (1984) Exercise and obesity. Symposium Proceedings: *Exercise, health and medicine:41*. The Sports Council

Olsen RE (1968) Diet and coronary heart disease: In: *Revised symposium on coronary heart disease*, 2nd edn, Blumgart HL (Ed). Monograph Number Two. New York American Heart Association

Shaper AG, Wannamethee G, Weatherall R (1991) Physical activity and ischaemic heart disease in middle-aged British men. *British Heart J* 66:384

Solomon H (1975) *The exercise myth*. Melbourne, Angus & Robertson

Wannamethee SG, Shaper AG and Walker M (1998) Changes in physical activity, mortality, and incidence of coronary heart disease in older men. *Lancet* 351(9116):1603

Wannamethee SG, Shaper AG and Walker M (2000) Physical activity and mortality in older men diagnosed with coronary heart disease. *Circulation* 102:1358

Wannamethee SG and Shaper AG (2001) Physical activity in the prevention of cardio-vascular disease. *Sports Med* 31:101

www.bhf.org.uk

www.cheshire-med.com/programs/pulrehab/COPD.htm

www. continuing education.com/nursing/atherosclerosis/descrip_purp/html

www.dphpc.ox.ac.uk/bhfhprg/stats/s000/index.html

www.erjs.org.uk/ERM/Monograph%20 files/6sumaries/whipp3-31.html.htm

www.heartstats.org.uk

www.sghms.ac.uk/ssm/i_raza/Web/pathology.htm

www. ucl.ac.uk/primcare_popsci/brhs/index.htm

Glossary

A-bands areas of the resting sarcomere where actin and myosin filaments overlap.

acceleration the rate of change of velocity measured in metres per second per second $(m \cdot s^2)$.

acetylcholine, ACh an ammonium derivative that is an excitatory neurotransmitter; stored in the vesicles of the synaptic knob it is secreted from nerve endings during an action potential.

acetylcholinesterase an enzyme that removes acetylcholine by converting it to choline, a compound of ammonium hydroxide and acetic acid.

acetyl coenzyme A, acetyl-CoA the key to the Krebs cycle and the oxidation of carbohydrates, fats and proteins; produced from the conversion of pyruvic acid.

acid a substance that donates a proton.

acidity a hydrogen ion concentration below neutral pH = 7.

acidosis an increase in hydrogen ion concentration outside the normal range; also known as acidemia.

acinus the functional unit of the lung, comprising at least two respiratory bronchioles, alveolar ducts and alveoli.

actin globular proteins (G actin) which combine (polymerization) to form the fibres (F actin) that make up the thin filaments of skeletal muscle.

action potential a stimulus that changes the permeability of nerve and muscle cell membranes; this allows sodium to flow into the cell, changing its resting potential of about −70 millivolts (mV) to about +40 millivolts; repeated stimuli lead to tetanus and muscle contraction.

active transport energy requiring movement of material against concentration or electrical gradients – e.g. ionic pumps.

acute (disease) rapid onset and short duration.

adenosine diphosphate, ADP a high-energy compound which combines with phosphate to form adenosine triphosphate.

adenosine triphosphatase, ATPase the enzyme that drives the hydrolysis of adenosine triphosphate to give adenosine diphosphate, inorganic phosphate and energy for cellular activities – e.g. muscular contraction and ionic pumps.

Exercise Physiology: A Thematic Approach Tudor Hale
© John Wiley & Sons, Ltd ISBN: 0 470 84682 8 (cloth), ISBN 0 470 84683 6 (pbk)

adenosine triphosphate, ATP the major high-energy compound essential for cell energetics.

adrenal glands glands lying on the upper surface of the kidneys; consist of an outer portion, the cortex, and an inner portion, the medulla.

adrenaline secreted by the adrenal medulla that acts as a neurotransmitter and hormone for the sympathetic division of the autonomic nervous system; also known as epinephrine.

adrenergic receptors cell receptors that respond to sympathetic stimulation – α and β_2 receptors found in the peripheral blood vessels, β_1 receptors in the myocardium.

aerobes organisms that need oxygen to survive.

aerobic capacity maximum amount of oxygen that can be consumed in unit time.

aerobic metabolism the oxygen-requiring breakdown of food substrates to synthesize adenosine triphosphate.

aetiology study of causes of disease.

afferent nerves nerves carrying information from the periphery of the body towards the central nervous system.

alkaline solution with a pH > 7.

alkalosis a reduction in hydrogen ion concentration below normal range.

all-or-none law a maximal response to an above-threshold stimulus; a below-threshold stimulus results in no response at all.

alveolar–capillary membrane the interface between lung gases and the erythrocyte ~3–5 μm thick; it consists of lung surfactant, alveolar and endothelial membrane, cell membrane and cytoplasm of alveolar cells and endothelial cells, interstitial fluid, capillary walls, plasma, and erythrocyte membranes.

alveolus the small, blind sac within the lung where gas transfer takes place.

ambient pertaining to the immediate surroundings – e.g. ambient temperature.

amino acids basic units of protein molecules.

amenorrhoea absence or suppression of menstrual function.

anabolism metabolic reactions leading to the synthesis of body substances.

anaemia levels of haemoglobin in the blood below defined normal values.

anaerobic literally 'without air', but usually taken to mean without oxygen.

anaerobic respiration energy released in the absence of oxygen.

anaerobic threshold the point when lactate begins to accumulate in the blood.

angina pectoris pain in the chest, and sometimes the throat and arms, resulting from myocardial ischaemia.

angiogram X-ray image of blood vessels, usually of the coronary arteries.

anion negatively charged ion.

anorexia nervosa a chronic eating disorder arising from a psychological distortion of body image and leading to malnutrition and weight loss.

anoxaemia lack of oxygen in the blood (also hypoxaemia).

anoxia lack of oxygen (also hypoxia).

aorta the major artery of the systemic circulation.

apneusis breath-holding after inspiration.

apneustic centre the region of the medulla oblongata controlling inspiration.

apnoea cessation of breathing, usually temporary – e.g. sleep apnoea.

arrhythmia disturbance of the regular rhythm of heart beat.

arterial pertaining to the arteries – e.g. arterial blood.

arteries blood vessels carrying blood from the heart.

arterioles small blood vessels controlling blood flow to the capillaries.

arterio-venous oxygen difference, C_{a-vO_2} the difference in oxygen content between arterial and venous blood.

arteriosclerosis stiffening and thickening of the arteries.

asthma broncho-constriction leading to difficulty in breathing.

asymptote a curve which approaches but never quite reaches the horizontal until infinity.

atheroma invasion of arterial wall by fatty deposits.

atherosclerosis narrowing of arterial blood vessels by fatty deposits.

atom smallest particle taking part in reactions.

atrium entrance chamber of the heart.

atrioventricular valves bicuspid (mitral) and tricuspid valves separating the atria and ventricles.

atrophy wasting of an organ or tissue through disuse.

auricle an extension of each atrium.

autonomic self-regulating – e.g autonomic nervous system.

autonomic nervous system a system of automatic control of the internal environment consisting of two divisions: the largely inhibitory parasympathetic division, and the sympathetic, largely excitatory, division.

axon the long conducting fibre of the neuron (nerve cell).

Bainbridge effect increased heart rate arising from activation of stretch receptors in the right atrium through increased venous return.

baroreceptor stretch receptor located in the aortic arch and carotid sinuses that strive to maintain normal blood pressure.

basal metabolic rate lowest level of resting heat production in an individual following overnight rest and fast; measured by whole body calorimetry, and estimated by measuring oxygen consumption.

beta-blockade drugs that act principally on β-adrenergic receptors in the myocardium and peripheral vessels; they weaken responses to stimulation from the sympathetic division of the autonomic nervous system.

beta-oxidation aerobic breakdown of lipids through removal of carbon atoms from fatty acid chains until two units of 2-carbon acetic acid are produced; these are converted to acetyl coenzyme A which enters the Krebs cycle.

bicarbonate, HCO_3^- a salt derived from the dissociation of carbonic acid, also known as hydrogen carbonate; it is the main extracellular buffer.

bicuspid valve two-flap atrio-ventricular valve in the left side of the heart; also known as the mitral valve.

blood an alkaline suspension consisting of plasma, red cells (erythrocytes), white cells (leukocytes) platelets, proteins, electrolytes, hormones and glucose.

blood pressure   pressure in the arteries generated by contraction of the left ventricle; systolic (central) and diastolic (peripheral) pressures are measured with a mercury or electronic sphygmomanometer.

Bohr effect   greater dissociation of oxygen from haemoglobin in response to increases in the partial pressure of carbon dioxide in the blood.

Borg scale   a numerical system of rating perceived exertion; the RPE scale.

Boyle's law   at constant temperature the volume of a gas is inversely proportional to its pressure – the greater the pressure the smaller the volume.

bradycardia   slow heart rate; seen in the resting heart rate of elite endurance athletes.

bronchi   the main airways of the lung leading from the trachea.

bronchiole   smaller subdivisions of the airways of the lung.

bronchitis   inflammation of the bronchi.

bronchospasm   narrowing of the airway by contraction of smooth muscle, e.g. during an asthma attack.

bronchodilators   drugs that relax the smooth muscle of the airway – e.g. belladonna and salbutamol.

buffers   substances that resist a change in hydrogen ion concentration.

bundle of His   specialized fibres in the myocardium, connecting the atria and the ventricles via the septum, that conduct the electrical impulses generated by the sino-atrial node.

calcium ion, Ca^{2+}   stored in and released from the sarcoplasmic reticulum of muscle cells, it is essential for the contraction of skeletal muscle; it combines with troponin C revealing binding sites on the actin filament onto which the myosin heads can attach.

calorie   heat required to raise one gram of water one degree Celsius; it is a unit of energy now replaced by the joule; a thousand calories = 1 kilocalorie = 4.18 joules.

capillary   thin-walled vessel connecting the arterial and venous sides of the circulatory system from which essential materials and fluid diffuse into the interstitial space between cells.

carbon dioxide, CO_2   a by-product of aerobic metabolism of glucose and lipids; a powerful stimulus of the respiratory system.

carbonic acid, H_2CO_3   a weak acid formed when carbon dioxide dissolves in water $-CO_2 + H_2O = H_2CO_3$; readily dissociates into hydrogen carbonate and a hydrogen ion – $H_2CO_3 + HCO_3^- + H^+$.

carbonic anhydrase   an enzyme in erythrocytes that is essential for the carriage of carbon dioxide in the blood.

cardiac cycle   the sequence of events during a single heart beat.

cardiac muscle   involuntary striated muscle of the heart; however, some voluntary control over heart rate and blood pressure is possible following appropriate training.

cardiac output, Q_C   whole body blood flow; the volume of blood pumped from the ventricle each minute; the product of heart rate and stroke volume.

carotid bodies   tissues situated in the carotid arteries; they are sensitive to changes in the chemistry (chemoreceptors), particularly of oxygen, carbon dioxide and hydrogen ions, of the blood flowing through them; they induce cardio-respiratory reflexes to correct imbalances.

carotid sinus art of the carotid artery sensitive to changes in blood pressure through stretch receptors (baroreceptors) that reflexively try to maintain normal pressure.

catabolism breakdown of complex chemical structures into simpler ones, often accompanied by release of energy.

catecholamines neurotransmitters mainly adrenaline (epinephrine), noradrenaline (norepinephrine) and dopamine.

cation positively charged ion.

cell the basic units capable of independent life; comprising a nucleus and cytoplasm except in erythrocytes and bacteria.

central nervous system the system that consists of the brain and spinal cord which coordinates and controls the body's responses to internal and external stimuli.

cerebral haemorrhage rupture of blood vessel in the brain resulting in a stroke.

cerebral thrombosis blood clot that prevents blood flow to an area of the brain, also resulting in a stroke.

cerebrospinal fluid, CSF fluid bathing the central nervous system.

cerebrovascular accident technical term for a stroke.

Charles–Gay-Lussac's law volume of a gas at constant pressure is directly proportional to its temperature – the higher the temperature the greater the volume.

cholesterol a steroid that is an important component of cell walls, hormones and bile salts; synthesized in all cells and from the diet.

cholesterolaemia excessive production of cholesterol leading to high levels in the blood that are linked with coronary heart disease; can be a genetic problem that runs in families and which is treated by statins – drugs that restore cholesterol homeostasis.

cholinergic receptors responsive to acetylcholine activation such as the sino-atrial node.

chronic (disease): gradual onset, long-term diseased state.

cilia (lung) fine hair-like protrusions covering cell surfaces that undulate constantly; this motion sweeps mucus and inhaled debris upwards towards the upper respiratory tract where they can be expelled.

circulation continuous transport of blood and other fluids by the heart around the arteries, capillaries and veins.

cisternae calcium storage vessels of the sarcoplasmic reticulum.

claudication limping caused by pain in the legs arising from restricted arterial blood flow to the muscles.

collagen protein that forms the major fibrous component of connective tissue.

citric acid cycle alternative name for the Krebs cycle.

collateral circulation development of secondary blood vessels that permit blood to bypass an obstruction (thrombus) in the primary vessel.

concentration the amount of a substance in a given volume.

concentric muscle action shortening of muscle fibres generating force.

conduction   transmission of heat or electrical stimulus through a material.

congenital   present at birth, but not necessarily inherited.

congestion   build-up of material – blood or water – in the body.

congestive heart failure   a condition where venous return exceeds the left ventricular output leading to congestion of the veins. This leads to increased hydrostatic pressure and oedema (the movement of excess water into the interstitial space).

connective tissue   material that separates and supports other tissues – e.g. intramuscular endo-, epi-, and peri-mysium, fibrous tissue, cartilage.

convection   bulk transfer of material – e.g. air through the airways and blood through the arteries and veins.

coronary heart disease   disease of the coronary arteries.

cor pulmonale   failure of the right side of the heart arising from lung disease.

creatine phosphate, CrP high-energy compound that converts adenosine diphosphate to adenosine triphosphate; also known as phosphocreatine (PCr).

cytochromes   compounds found in the electron transfer chain essential for oxidative phosphorylation.

cytoplasm   gel-like substance contained by the cell walls and surrounding the nucleus, consisting mainly of water, proteins and ions and holding the various organelles.

Dalton's law of partial pressures   in a mixture of gases it is the sum of the pressures that each gas would exert if it occupied the same volume at the same temperature on its own, i.e.

$$P_B = P_{N_2} + P_{O_2} + P_{CO_2}$$

dead space, V_D   volume of the lung that does not take part in gas exchange.

dehydrogenase   enzymes driving oxidation by hydrogen atom removal.

dehydrogenation   oxidation by hydrogen atom removal.

density, ρ (rho)   ratio of mass to volume.

depolarization   change in the cell membrane potential from negative (~ -70 mV) to positive ($\sim +30$ mV) resulting from an action potential.

diabetes mellitus   a condition brought about by a lack, or inadequate uptake, of insulin by cells, resulting in high blood sugar levels (hyperglycaemia) and widespread tissue damage if untreated.

diaphragm   dome-shaped sheet of muscle separating thoracic and abdominal cavities that is the major muscle of lung ventilation.

diastole   the relaxation and filling phase of the cardiac cycle.

diastolic blood pressure   representative of the resistance to blood flow in the peripheral vessels.

diffusion   random movement of atoms and molecules, mainly in gases and liquids, via thermal agitation; movement from areas of high to areas of low concentrations.

dilatation   reflex widening of blood vessels to increase flow; also an increased volume of the heart arising from some heart diseases.

dilution   lowered concentration.

dissociation   reversible breakdown of a compound – e.g. oxyhaemoglobin into oxygen and haemoglobin.

dyspnoea   difficulty in breathing.

eccentric muscle action   muscle lengthening whilst generating force.

echocardiography   reflected ultrasound examination of the structure and function of the heart.

ectopic   in the wrong position.

ectopic heart beats   abnormal sino-atrial impulses resulting in arrhythmias.

efferent nerves   nerves carrying impulses away from the central nervous system.

ejection fraction   volume of blood remaining in the ventricles after systole.

electrocardiogram, ECG   recording of the electrical activity of the heart.

electrolytes   compounds that dissociate into ions when dissolved in water – e.g. sodium chloride (NaCl) dissociates into sodium Na^+, and chloride Cl^- ions.

electromyography, EMG   study of the electrical activity of skeletal muscle.

electron   a negatively charged particle that is a constituent of all atoms.

electron transfer chain   the final stage of oxidative phosphorylation; takes place in the mitochondria where electrons are passed through several reactions before combining with molecular oxygen to produce energy, water and carbon dioxide.

emphysema   lung disease involving destruction of lung tissue; it impairs the elastic recoil of the lungs and gas transfer to and from the blood, causing dyspnoea.

end-diastolic volume, EDV   volume of blood in the ventricles at the end of diastole.

endogenous   metabolic process of creation, repair, or renewal of tissue.

endomysium   connective tissue wrapped around individual muscle cells.

enzyme   a protein that facilitates or speeds up chemical reactions but undergoes no permanent change in the process.

epidemiology   study of the incidence and prevalence of disease in populations.

epimysium   connective tissue surrounding a muscle group – e.g. biceps brachii.

epinephrine   the American alternative name for adrenaline.

ergometry   measurement of work done.

erythrocyte   red blood cell.

erythropoiesis   red cell production in bone marrow.

erythropoietin, EPO   hormone produced in the kidney that stimulates erythrocyte production.

etiology   American spelling of aetiology.

eupnoea   normal breathing.

excess post-exercise oxygen consumption, EPOC   above resting levels of oxygen consumption during recovery from exercise; new term for A. V. Hill's concept of an 'oxygen debt'.

excretion   removal of by-products of chemical reactions – e.g. removal of carbon dioxide by the lungs.

exogenous   energy-producing metabolism.

expiration   expulsion of air from the lungs.

expiratory capacity, V_{EC}   maximum volume of gas that can be exhaled from the lungs following normal inspiration

extracellular fluid, ECF fluid that lies outside the cell membrane.

extrapolation estimating further values from previous data – e.g. estimating maximal oxygen uptake from sub-maximal values.

extrasystole arrhythmia arising from a premature heart beat.

farmer's lung lung disease induced by bacterial spores found in mouldy hay that may lead to fibrosing alveolitis.

fasciculus small bundle of muscle cells.

fast-twitch fibres Type II fibres subdivided into two major groups: IIa, fast-twitch oxidative (FOG), and IIb, fast-twitch glycolytic (FG).

fatigue inability to respond fully to a stimulus, or inability to maintain a desired energy output.

fat a lipid, comprising glycerol (glycerine) and fatty acids.

fatty acids chains of carbon and hydrogen atoms that are attached to a glycerol molecule to form mono-, di- and triglycerides; saturated fatty acids have the maximum number of hydrogen atoms, whilst in unsaturated fatty acids there are fewer hydrogen atoms because some carbon atoms bind to each other. The three main dietary fatty acids are oleic, palmitic and stearic acids.

feedback control mechanisms that use information about the consequences of a response to regulate the response; there are negative (inhibiting) and positive (promoting) feedback loops.

fibrillation uncoordinated muscle twitching – e.g. atrial and ventricular fibrillation.

fibrin the basis of a blood clot; formed from the insoluble plasma protein fibrinogen that develops into a network of fibres.

Fick principle method of measuring cardiac output: $\dot{Q} = \dot{V}_{O_2}/C_{a\text{-}\bar{v}O_2}$

filament long protein aggregates, as in the actin and myosin filaments of the sarcomere.

flavine adenine dinucleotide, FAD protein electron carrier of the electron transfer chain.

fluid substance capable of flowing – e.g. gas, liquid or powder.

forced expiratory volume – timed, FEV$_{1.0}$ the volume of air that can be expired in 1 second following maximum inspiration.

Frank–Starling law relationship between end-diastolic volume and stroke volume; increased venous return leads to greater end-diastolic volume and larger stroke volume.

functional residual capacity, FRC residual volume plus vital capacity.

gland an organ that secretes a product which may be used internally, e.g. adrenaline, or externally, e.g. sweat.

glucagon hormone produced by the islets of Langerhans that inhibits glycogenesis and is responsible for breaking down glycogen in the liver and raising blood sugar levels.

glucosuria appearance of sugar in the urine seen in diabetes mellitus.

glucose a monosaccharide providing the major cellular energy source.

glycogen a polysaccharide consisting of chains of glucose molecules, stored mainly in the liver and muscles.

glycogenesis formation of glycogen from glucose.

glycogenolysis breakdown of glycogen to glucose-6-phosphate.

glycolysis breakdown of glucose to pyruvic acid, also known as the Embden–Meyerhof pathway, resulting in the synthesis of adenosine triphosphate. Anaerobic glycolysis results in the conversion of pyruvic acid to lactic acid.

Graham's law of diffusion gas flow is inversely proportional to the square root of its density.

habituation a learning process that leads to a diminution of response – e.g. learning to run on a treadmill so that the validity and reliability of physiological measurements are improved.

haem- a prefix denoting to do with blood; in the USA the prefix becomes 'hem-'.

haem the iron compound that combines with the globin protein to give haemoglobin; the binding site for oxygen.

haematocrit, Hct the ratio of blood cells to plasma.

haemoglobin, Hb a protein with four oxygen binding sites found in the erythrocytes. Carries oxygen and carbon dioxide and also acts as a buffer.

haemolysis the destruction of erythrocytes.

haemorrhage bleeding via a ruptured blood vessel.

Hagen–Poiseuille equation equation that gives the laminar flow rate of a fluid (Q) through a tube given the tube length (L) and radius (R), the driving pressure (P), and the viscosity of the fluid (η) – i.e.

$$Q = \pi PR^4/8L\eta$$

high-density lipoprotein cholesterol, HDL-C one of two forms of cholesterol seen as a protective against coronary heart disease; responsible for removing cholesterol from blood vessel walls to the liver and thus reducing the development of atheroma and atherosclerosis.

heart block damage to heart tissue, e.g. infarct, which interferes with the transmission of nerve impulses from the sino-atrial node to the ventricles.

heart failure inability of the heart to maintain adequate cardiac output to service the body's needs.

heart sounds sounds produced by the closing of the atrio-ventricular and semilunar valves during systole and diastole.

Henry's law the amount of a gas that is dissolved in a liquid at a given temperature is proportional to the pressure of the gas.

high-energy compounds phosphate compounds attached to creatine and adenosine, the hydrolysis of which leads to energy release.

homeostasis tendency of the internal environment of the body to resist change.

hormones substances released by endocrine glands into the blood stream which act on specific tissues.

hydrogen ion positively charged hydrogen atom; a proton.

hydrolysis breakdown of organic compounds by interaction with water – e.g. hydrolysis of adenosine triphosphate to adenosine diphosphate and inorganic phosphate.

hydrophilic   attracted to water.

hydrophobic   repelled by water.

hyperbaric oxygen   oxygen at higher than atmospheric pressure.

hypercapnia   abnormally high level of carbon dioxide in the blood.

hypercholesterolaemia   abnormally high level of blood cholesterol.

hyperglycaemia   abnormally high level of glucose in the blood.

hyperinsulinism   excessive insulin excretion.

hyperlipidaemia   excessive levels of lipids in the blood

hyperoxia   enriched with oxygen.

hyperplasia   tissue growth by increased number of cells.

hyperpnoea   increased lung ventilation.

hypertension   abnormally high blood pressure.

hyperthermia   raised body temperature.

hyperventilation   excessive   lung   ventilation,   leading   to   increased   carbon dioxide excretion and respiratory alkalosis.

hypertonic   increased osmotic pressure of a solution.

hypertrophy   tissue growth by increased size of cells.

hypotension   abnormally low blood pressure.

hypothermia   lowered body temperature.

hypotonic   decreased osmotic pressure of a solution.

hypoventilation   abnormally low lung ventilation leading to hypoxia and respiratory acidosis.

hypoxaemia   lack of oxygen in the blood (also anoxaemia).

hypoxia   oxygen lack.

H-zone   the central area of the resting sarcomere occupied by myosin filaments alone.

I-band   the outer areas of the resting sarcomere occupied by actin filaments alone.

infarct   death of cells arising from blocked blood and oxygen supply.

inhibitor   a substance that diminishes or blocks physiological processes – e.g. hydrogen ions compete for calcium binding sites on actin filaments thereby preventing maximum myosin coupling and reducing muscle contraction.

inspiration   intake of air into the lungs.

inspiratory capacity, IC   maximum volume of air that can be drawn into the lungs following normal expiration.

insulin   hormone produced in the pancreas by the islets of Langerhans.

interstitial fluid   the fluid that bathes all tissues and supplies all nutrients; it is part of the extracellular fluid compartment of the body.

intracellular fluid, ICF   fluid that lies within the cell membrane.

involuntary muscle   smooth and cardiac muscle capable of generating their own intrinsic rhythm, but is under the control of the autonomic nervous system.

ions   electrically charged atoms and molecules.

ischaemia   low tissue oxygen arising from restricted blood flow.

islets of Langerhans   cells in the pancreas that produce insulin and glucagon.

isokinetic contraction muscular contraction at constant speed.

isometric contraction generation of muscular force without muscle fibre shortening.

isotonic having equal osmotic pressures between two fluid compartments.

isotonic contraction contraction that develops constant tension as muscle fibres shorten.

joule, J the SI-derived unit of energy work and quantity of heat; a calorie is 4.18 joules (J) and oxygen consumption of 5.05 litres is the equivalent of 21.1 kilojoules (kJ).

kilogram, kg the SI unit of mass.

Korotkoff sounds sounds heard from the brachial artery during the measurement of blood pressure.

Krebs cycle metabolic pathway in the mitochondria; it converts the pyruvic acid of aerobic glycolysis into carbon dioxide and water via the electron transfer chain with the production of adenosine triphosphate – i.e. oxidative phosphorylation. It is also known as the citric acid cycle and the tricarboxylic acid (TCA) cycle.

lactic acid, $C_3H_6O_3$ the result of the reduction of pyruvic acid during anaerobic glycolysis.

laminar flow flow that has a Reynolds number less than 2000; streamlined flow; flow proportional to the radius of a tube raised to the fourth power – R^4.

larynx part of the upper respiratory tract containing the vocal chords at the entry to the trachea.

latent period time between onset of an impulse and a response to it.

leukocyte white blood cell.

linear relationships rectilinear – a straight line relationship between two variables, e.g. power output and heart rate; curvilinear – a curved relationship, e.g. stroke volume and heart rate.

lipids compounds including fats, oils and waxes found in the body.

lipoproteins compounds that transport fat in the blood, and vital constituents of cell membranes.

litre, L unit for volume in use with the SI.

low-density lipoprotein cholesterol, LDL-C compound consisting mainly of cholesterol thought to be involved in the development of atheroma and atherosclerosis.

lymphatic system network of vessels that carry lymph from tissue interstices to the lymphatic ducts.

mass quantity of a substance, usually measured in kilograms.

mechanoreceptors sense organs that respond to deformation – e.g. stretch receptors, baroreceptors.

medulla oblongata the part of the brain stem which is continuous with the spinal cord; contains the nerve centres controlling respiratory and cardiovascular functions.

metabolic equivalent, MET a method of estimating the metabolic rate of varying activities; resting metabolic rate – 1 MET – is conventionally given as $3.5 \text{ m}L$ $O_2 \cdot kg^{-1} \cdot min^{-1}$

metabolic rate the rate at which energy and heat are produced.

metabolism   the breakdown of substrates to provide energy; it involves anabolism, the construction of large molecules from smaller ones that build and repair body tissues, and catabolism, the conversion of large molecules to smaller ones.

mitochondrion   an organelle of nucleated cells; often referred to as 'the powerhouse of the cells', it is responsible for the production of adenosine triphosphate through oxidative phosphorylation via the Krebs cycle and the electron transfer chain.

mitral valve   the bicuspid atrio-ventricular valve of the left ventricle.

M-line   line of M-filaments that provide structural support for the myosin filaments.

morbidity   the incidence of a disease within a population.

motor end-plate   the connecting point between a motor nerve and a skeletal muscle.

motor unit   a nerve and its associated motor-end plates and skeletal muscle fibres.

multinucleated   containing many nuclei, e.g. in skeletal muscle cells.

muscle   tissue consisting of elongated cells capable of generating force.

muscle cell   a single muscle fibre consisting of several myofibrils made up of myofilaments bound by the sarcolemma.

muscle fibre types   there are three types: Type I, slow oxidative (SO); Type IIa, fast oxidative glycolytic (FOG); Type IIb, fast glycolytic (FG).

myocardial   to do with the myocardium – e.g. myocardial infarction.

myocardium   muscular tissue of the heart.

myofibril   subcellular thread-like structure running the length of the muscle fibre composed of very many sarcomeres arranged end-to-end.

myoglobin, Mgb   an iron containing protein with one oxygen binding site; it is stored in the muscle and releases its bound oxygen only at low partial pressures.

myoneural junction   the connecting site between nerve and muscle fibres.

myopathy   muscle disease.

myosin   the protein fibres making up the thick filaments of the myofibril.

negative feedback   a stabilizing physiological process designed to maintain home-ostasis – e.g. exercise leads to increased core body temperature; sweat glands are stimulated to produce sweat, and subcutaneous blood vessels vasodilate so that blood brought to the outer surface of the body is cooled by evaporation, conduction and convection, thereby lowering core temperature.

negative ion   atom or molecule that has gained an electron; known as an anion.

neurology   study of the nervous system.

neuromuscular junction   the connecting site between nerve and muscle fibres.

neuron   nerve cell and associated conducting fibres.

neurotransmitter   a substance that enables an impulse to progress across the synaptic cleft.

nicotinamide adenine dinucleotide, NAD   the major hydrogen acceptor coenzyme that releases its electrons to the electron transfer chain during oxidative phosphorylation.

Nitrogen, N   an inert gas that in the fasting state does not take part in metabolic reactions.

noradrenaline   hormone of the sympathetic nervous system that induces a constrictor effect in blood vessels; also known as norepinephrine in the USA.

obesity   excessive proportion of body fat – conventionally more than 25 per cent for men and 30% for women.

oedema   accumulation of fluid in tissues – e.g. pulmonary oedema.

onset of blood lactate accumulation, OBLA   a measure of the exercise intensity at which lactate removal is overwhelmed by lactate production, and hydrogen ions begin to impair muscular contraction.

organelle   defined structure within the cytoplasm of the cell – e.g. mitochondria, ribosomes.

osmosis   movement of water from an area of lower concentration across a selectively permeable membrane to an area of higher concentration, thus removing the difference in concentration.

osmotic pressure   the pressure required to prevent water movement across a selectively permeable membrane; solutions with high concentrations of a substance exert a high osmotic pressure and vice versa. A compartment with high osmotic pressure has the capacity to draw water into it.

oxidation   a reaction where oxygen is added or an electron removed; the opposite of reduction.

oxidative phosphorylation   the oxidation of glucose via aerobic catabolism that produces carbon dioxide, water and adenosine triphosphate.

oxygen plateau   the primary indicator of maximal oxygen uptake.

oxyhaemoglobin, $Hb_4(O_2)_4$ the major form of oxygen carriage in the blood.

oxyhaemoglobin dissociation curve   the sigmoid curve indicating the relationship between the oxygen saturation of haemoglobin and partial pressure of oxygen.

palmitic acid, $C_{15}H_{31}COOH$ one of the major dietary fatty acids.

parasympathetic nervous system   generally inhibitory division of the autonomic nervous system consisting of cholinergic nerves.

partial pressure   pressure exerted by one gas in a mixture of gases.

Pascal, Pa   the SI-derived unit of pressure.

passive transport   movement of material by diffusion from an area of high concentration to an area of low concentration.

peak oxygen uptake   maximum amount of oxygen consumed without the appearance of the oxygen plateau.

pericardium   fibrous sac surrounding the heart.

perimysium   connective tissue that supports bundles of fibres.

peripheral nerves   nerves arising from the central nervous system.

pH   the measure of acidity; pH = 7 is neutral, pH < 7 = acid, pH > 7 = alkaline.

phagocyte   white blood cell capable of capturing and digesting bacteria and cell debris.

Phosphocreatine, PCr   the compound that plays a key role in phosphorylating adenosine diphosphate to adenosine triphosphate.

phosphorylation   addition of inorganic phosphate – e.g. adenosine diphosphate plus inorganic phosphate gives adenosine triphosphate.

$$ADP + P_i = ATP$$

pharynx   muscular wall of the mouth and throat extending to the opening of the oesophagus.

plasma   the liquid compartment of the blood.

platelet   a particle suspended in the plasma required for the clotting of blood at the site of an injury; also known as a thrombocyte.

pleura   the double membranes lining the thoracic cavity and surrounding the lungs.

polycythaemia   an excess of erythrocytes – e.g. >6 million per cubic millilitre.

polypeptide   a substance consisting of many amino acids linked by peptide bonds, but shorter than a protein.

positive feedback   excitatory mechanism which, if not controlled, leads to ever-increasing responses – e.g. increasing heart rate in response to myocardial ischaemia which may lead to ventricular fibrillation.

positive ion   atom or molecule that has lost an electron; known as a cation.

power   the product either of force and distance divided by time, $(f \cdot d)/t$, or of force and velocity, $f \cdot v$.

protein   organic compounds essential to living matter, formed from defined sequences of amino acids.

pulmonary   pertaining to the lungs.

pulmonary diffusion   transfer of gases across the alveolar–capillary membrane.

pulmonary ventilation   movement of air into, and expired gases out of, the lungs.

Purkinje fibres   specialized tissue in the heart that conducts the electrical current from the left and right bundle branches to the outer walls via the apex of the heart.

receptors   specialized cells that respond to specific stimuli – e.g. chemoreceptors – adrenergic, cholinergic, and mechanoreceptors – baroreceptors.

red blood cell   erythrocyte; oxygen carrier in the blood.

reduction   a reaction where oxygen is removed or an electron added – the opposite of oxidation.

renal   pertaining to the kidneys.

renin   hormone produced in the kidney that regulates arterial blood pressure.

repolarization   restoration of the ionic balance seen in the resting membrane potential.

residual volume, RV   total lung capacity minus vital capacity; the volume of gas in the lung following maximal expiration.

respiration   gaseous exchange between an organism and its environment.

respiratory bronchiole   the first airways that are involved in gas transfer; the link between the terminal bronchiole and the acinus.

respiratory centre   specialized tissues in the medulla oblongata and pons of the central nervous system that regulate lung ventilation.

respiratory exchange ratio, RER   volume of carbon dioxide excreted by the lung divided by the volume of oxygen consumed: V_{CO_2}/V_{O_2}.

respiratory quotient, RQ   the ratio of the volume of carbon dioxide produced to the volume of oxygen consumed at the cellular level.

resting membrane potential   the ionic imbalance across a cell membrane – negative inside the cell and positive outside it – that is not being stimulated.

Reynolds number, Re   the relationship between the density (ρ), velocity (v) and viscosity (η) and of a fluid flowing in a pipe of a given diameter (d) – Re = $\rho v d/\eta$; a number < 2000 indicates laminar flow, > 2000 indicates turbulent flow.

sarcolemma cell membrane of muscle fibre.

sarcomere the contractile unit of the myofibril.

sarcoplasm the cytoplasm of the muscle cell.

sarcoplasmic reticulum the membranous network of the muscle cell, which synthesizes muscle proteins and passes the action potential from the T-system to the cisternae where calcium that is essential for muscular contraction is stored.

saturated fat fatty acid with the maximum number of hydrogen atoms.

sclerosis hardening of tissue – e.g. arteriosclerosis, hardening of the arteries.

septum a dividing partition of tissue – e.g. the septa dividing the left and right sides of the heart.

sigmoid curve an 'S'-shaped curve – e.g. the oxyhaemoglobin dissociation curve.

sino-atrial node, SA node the site, located in the wall of the right atrium, from which the electrical stimulus for myocardial contraction originates.

sliding filament theory the process by which muscle fibres contract due to the interdigitation of the thick (myosin) and thin (actin) myofilaments.

slow-twitch fibres Type I slow oxidative (SO) fibres that are fatigue-resistant.

smooth muscle involuntary unstriated muscle cell found in blood vessels and bronchioles.

solubility ability of a substance to dissolve in a solvent – e.g. carbon dioxide in water.

solute a substance that has dissolved in a solvent – e.g. carbon dioxide in water.

sphincter a ring of muscle found in hollow organs that can contract and dilate thus changing the diameter of the orifice – e.g. bronchioles, blood vessels.

sphygmomanometer a device for measuring blood pressure

splanchnic contents of the abdominal cavity – the viscera.

standard temperature and pressure 0°C and 101.1 kPa or 760 mmHg.

steady state a dynamic condition of the internal environment where supply matches demand –e.g. oxygen consumption at constant sub-maximal exercise.

stenosis narrowing of an opening or vessel, e.g. mitral stenosis – narrowing of the mitral valve of the heart.

striated muscle characteristic appearance of skeletal and cardiac muscle fibres brought about by the arrangement of myofilaments in the sarcomere.

stroke lack of oxygen to the brain caused by thrombosis or rupture of a blood vessel leading to some form of paralysis.

stroke volume, V_S volume of blood pumped out by one beat of the heart.

substrate substance that reacts with an enzyme.

substrate level phosphorylation reaction involving adenosine diphosphate and inorganic phosphate resulting in the formation of adenosine triphosphate.

summation the effects on a muscle of multiple supra-threshold stimuli leading to increased tension.

suprarenal gland alternative name for the adrenal gland.

surfactant substance secreted by granular pneumocytes that lowers alveolar surface tension and improves lung compliance.

sympathetic nervous system generally excitatory division of the autonomic nervous system consisting of adrenergic nerves.

synapse the junction between nerve cells, and between nerve and muscle cells, where impulses are transmitted by secretion of neurotransmitters such as acetylcholine.

synaptic knob structure at the end of nerve fibres containing vesicles that store the neurotransmitter.

systemic circulation circulatory system for the whole body with the exception of the vessels of the pulmonary circulation.

systole contraction phase of the cardiac cycle when blood is ejected.

tachycardia rapid heart rate.

terminal bronchiole smallest of the conductive airways.

tetanus sustained muscle fibre contraction induced by multiple supra-threshold stimuli.

thick filament the myosin fibre of the sarcomere.

thin filament the actin fibre of the sarcomere.

thoracic pertaining to the thorax.

thorax body compartment enclosed by the ribs and diaphragm.

thrombocyte a blood platelet necessary for clotting.

thrombosis blood clot blocking a blood vessel.

tidal volume, V_T the volume of air inspired in a single breath.

total lung capacity, TLC vital capacity plus residual volume.

trachea cartilaginous tube connecting the upper respiratory tract to the two main bronchi of the lung.

tricarboxylic acid cycle, TCA cycle technically precise name for the Krebs cycle.

tropomyosin protein rods that are attached to the actin filaments of myofibrils.

troponin protein complex that following an action potential facilitates muscle fibre contraction by interacting with calcium and tropomyosin.

T-tubules transverse tubules; extensions of sarcolemma of the skeletal muscle cell taking the form of blind passages that carry the nerve impulses deep into the muscle cell to the sarcoplasmic reticulum.

turbulent flow disturbed flow patterns; non-streamlined; flow with a Reynolds number greater than 2000; flow proportional to the square of the radius (R^2) of a tube.

unsaturated fat fatty acid capable of accepting more hydrogen atoms.

unstriated muscle involuntary, smooth muscle consisting of muscle cells with irregular actin and myosin filament patterns and capable of inherent rhythmicity.

vagus nerve a key nerve of the parasympathetic nervous system affecting the heart and respiratory and digestive systems.

vascular to do with blood vessels.

vasoconstriction narrowing of a blood vessel.

vasodilatation widening of a blood vessel.

vasomotor activity principal means of blood pressure regulation.

vein vessel carrying blood back to the heart.

venae cavae main veins feeding into the right atrium.

venous pertaining to blood circulating in the veins.

ventilatory threshold the point at which the relationship between oxygen consumption, or power, and lung ventilation increases sharply.

ventricles the two larger contractile chambers of the heart.

ventricular fibrillation electrical activity of the ventricles that is rapid and uncoordinated, resulting in no cardiac output.

venule small vein draining the capillary bed.

viscosity resistance to flow of a fluid.

vital capacity, VC maximum amount of air that can be exhaled following maximal inspiratory effort.

volatile substance that readily changes from liquid form into a vapour.

voluntary muscle striated skeletal muscle controlled by the motor centre.

water vapour pressure the pressure generated by the presence of water vapour in the atmosphere.

watt, W SI-derived unit of power; it is equal to 1 joule per second $(J \cdot s^{-1})$.

weight force of gravity acting on a body, measured in newtons.

work, w force generated multiplied by distance covered: $w = f \cdot d$; measured in joules.

Z-line a protein mesh that forms the limit of the sarcomere and to which the actin filaments are attached.

Origins of Some Terms

a-, an	Greek for not, without; e.g. **a**typical – not typical, **an**aerobic – without oxygen.
acinus	Latin for bunch of grapes.
ad	Latin for adjacent to, or at; e.g. **ad**renal gland – adjacent to the kidney.
adeno	Greek *adeno* = gland; e.g. **aden**itis – inflammation of a gland.
aero	Greek *aer* = air; e.g. **aero**bic metabolism.
ambient	Latin *ambire* = to go round.
angio-	Greek *angeion* = vessel.
atom	Greek *atomos* = cannot be cut.
baro-	Greek *baros* = weight.
bio-	Greek *bios* = life; e.g. **bio**logy – the study of living things.
brady-	Greek *bradys* = slow; e.g. **brady**cardia – slow heart beat.
bronch-	Greek *bronkhus* = windpipe.
calorie	Latin *calor* = heat.
capillary	Latin *capillus* = hair.
cardi-	Greek *kardia* = heart.
carotid	Greek *karoun* = stupefied – from loss of consciousness when carotid bodies were stimulated.
chronic	Greek *khronos* = time.
cyto-	Greek *kytos* = cell; e.g. **cyto**logy – the study of cells.
dys-	Greek *dus* = defective, abnormal; e.g. **dys**functional – abnormal function.
endo-	Greek *endos* = within; e.g. **endo**cardium – tissue lining the ventricles of the heart.
epi-	Greek *epi* = upon, over; e.g. **epi**mysium – tissue that encloses muscle.
eu-	Greek *eus* = good, normal; e.g. **eu**pnoea – normal breathing.
extra-	Latin *extra* = outside; e.g. **extra**cellular fluid – fluid outside the cell.
glyc-	Greek *glukus* = sweet; e.g. **glyc**ogen.
haem	Greek *haima* = blood; e.g. **haem**atology – study of blood.
hetero-	Greek *heteros* = other, different; e.g. **hetero**geneous group – a mixed group.

Exercise Physiology: A Thematic Approach Tudor Hale
© John Wiley & Sons, Ltd ISBN: 0 470 84682 8 (cloth), ISBN 0 470 84683 6 (pbk)

homo-　　Greek *homos* = same; e.g. **homo**geneous group – a group exhibiting similar characteristics.

hyper-　　Greek *hyper* = above; e.g. **hyper**aemia – excess of blood.

hypo-　　Greek *hypo* = under; e.g. **hypo**glycaemia – too little sugar.

inter-　　Latin *inter* = between; e.g. **inter**national.

intra-　　Latin *intra* = within; e.g. **intra**cellular fluid – fluid contained within the cell.

iso　　Greek *isos* = equal; e.g. **iso**sceles triangle – triangle with two equal sides.

leuko-　　Greek *leukos* = white; e.g. **leuko**cyte – white blood cell.

myo-　　Greek *myos* = muscle; e.g. **myo**fibril, electro**myo**graphy.

necro-　　Greek *nekros* = dead; e.g. **necro**tic tissue following an infarct.

nephro-　　Greek *nephros* = the kidney; e.g. **nephr**itis – inflammation of the kidney.

neuro-　　Greek *neuron* = nerve; e.g. **neuro**logy – the study of the nervous system.

para-　　Greek *para* = beside; e.g. **para**llel lines.

pent-　　Greek *pente* = five; e.g. **pent**ose – a five carbon sugar.

peri-　　Greek *peri* = around; e.g. **peri**meter, **peri**mysium.

phag-　　Greek *phagein* = eat; e.g. **phag**ocytes.

pneu-　　Greek *pneuma* = breath.

pneumon　　Greek *pneumon* = lung; e.g. **pneumon**ia – inflammation of the lung.

poly-　　Greek *polys* = many: e.g. **poly**gon – many-sided figure.

recti-　　Latin *rectus* = straight; **recti**linear – straight line.

reticul-　　Latin *reticulum* = net; **reticul**ar – a net-like structure.

sarc-　　Greek *sarcos* = flesh.

sclero-　　Greek *sclerosis* = hard.

sept-　　Latin *septum* = partition.

sten-　　Greek *stenos* = narrow.

supra-　　Latin for 'above' or 'over'; e.g. **supra**renal gland – above the kidney.

tachy-　　Greek *tachys* = speed; e.g. **tachy**cardia – fast heart beat.

ultra-　　Latin *ultra* = beyond; e.g. **ultra**filtrate – the interstial fluid.

ur-, uro-　　Greek *uoron* = urine; **uro**logy – study of the urogenital tract.

vaso-　　Latin *vas* = vessel; e.g. **vaso**constriction – narrowing of blood vessels.

Answers to Objective Tests

Chapters

Question	1	2	3	4	5	6	7	8	9	10	11
1	T	T	F	T	F	F	T	F	F	T	F
2	T	T	T	F	F	F	F	F	F	F	T
3	F	F	T	T	T	F	F	F	T	F	F
4	T	F	F	F	T	T	T	T	F	F	F
5	F	F	F	F	T	F	T	T	T	T	T
6	F	T	F	T	F	T	T	F	F	F	F
7	T	T	T	F	T	T	F	F	T	T	T
8	T	T	T	T	T	F	F	T	F	F	T
9	T	F	T	F	F	F	F	T	T	T	T
10	F	F	T	T	T	T	T	F	T	T	F
11	F	F	F	F	F	T	T	F	F	T	F
12	F	T	F	F	F	T	F	T	T	T	F
13	T	F	F	T	T	T	T	T	T	F	T
14	T	T	T	T	F	T	T	F	T	F	T
15	F	T	T	T	T	F	F	F	T	F	F
16	F	T	F	T	T	F	T	T	F	T	F
17	F	F	T	T	T	T	F	T	F	T	F
18	T	F	T	F	F	T	F	F	F	F	T
19	F	T	T	F	F	F	T	T	T	F	F
20	T	F	T	T	F	T	T	T	F	T	F
21	T	F	F	T	T	T	T	F	F	T	T
22	F	T	F	T	T	F	F	T	T	F	T
23	F	T	F	F	F	F	T	F	F	T	F
24	T	T	T	F	F	T	F	F	T	F	T
25	T	T	T	F	T	F	T	T	F	F	T
26	T	F	T	T	T	T	F	T	T	T	T
27	T	T	T	T	F	T	T	F	F	F	F
28	F	F	F	F	T	F	T	F	T	T	T
29	F	F	F	F	F	F	F	T	F	T	T
30	F	F	F	F	F	F	F	T	T	F	F

Exercise Physiology: A Thematic Approach   Tudor Hale
© John Wiley & Sons, Ltd   ISBN: 0 470 84682 8 (cloth), ISBN 0 470 84683 6 (pbk)

Index

Definitions of **technical terms** are in bold type and can be found in the Glossary; those followed by *d* are definitions only. **Page numbers** in bold indicate key information; those followed by *f* or *t* indicate a figure or a table.